Robotic Assistive
Technologies
Principles and Practice

REHABILITATION SCIENCE IN PRACTICE SERIES

Series Editors

Marcia J. Scherer, Ph.D.

President
Institute for Matching Person and Technology
Professor
Physical Medicine & Rehabilitation
University of Rochester Medical Center

Dave Muller, Ph.D.

Visiting Professor
University of Suffolk

Past and Founding Chair of
Chamber of Commerce

Editor-in-Chief
Disability and Rehabilitation

Director
Ipswich Central Ltd.

Published Titles

Ambient Assisted Living, *Nuno M. Garcia and Joel J.P.C. Rodrigues*

Assistive Technology Assessment Handbook, *edited by Stefano Federici and Marcia J. Scherer*

Assistive Technology for Blindness and Low Vision, *Roberto Manduchi and Sri Kurniawan*

Computer Access for People with Disabilities: A Human Factors Approach, *Richard C. Simpson*

Computer Systems Experiences of Users with and Without Disabilities: An Evaluation Guide for Professionals, *Simone Borsci, Maria Laura Mele, Masaaki Kurosu, and Stefano Federici*

Devices for Mobility and Manipulation for People with Reduced Abilities, *Teodiano Bastos-Filho, Dinesh Kumar, and Sridhar Poosapadi Arjunan*

Devices for Mobility and Manipulation for People with Reduced Abilities, *Teodiano Bastos-Filho, Dinesh Kumar, and Sridhar Poosapadi Arjunan*

Geriatric Rehabilitation: From Bedside to Curbside, *edited by K. Rao Poduri, MD, FAAPMR*

Human-Computer Interface Technologies for the Motor Impaired, *edited by Dinesh K. Kumar and Sridhar Poosapadi Arjunan*

Multiple Sclerosis Rehabilitation: From Impairment to Participation, *edited by Marcia Finlayson*

Neuroprosthetics: Principles and Applications, *edited by Justin Sanchez*

Paediatric Rehabilitation Engineering: From Disability to Possibility, *edited by Tom Chau and Jillian Fairley*

Quality of Life Technology Handbook, *Richard Schultz*

Rehabilitation: A Post-critical Approach, *Barbara E. Gibson*

Rehabilitation Goal Setting: Theory, Practice and Evidence, *edited by Richard J. Siegert and William M. M. Levack*

Rethinking Rehabilitation: Theory and Practice, *edited by Kathryn McPherson, Barbara E. Gibson, and Alain Leplège*

Robotic Assistive Technologies: Principles and Practice, *edited by Pedro Encarnção and Albert M. Cook*

Wheelchair Skills Assessment and Training, *R. Lee Kirby*

Robotic Assistive Technologies
Principles and Practice

Edited by
Pedro Encarnação and Albert M. Cook

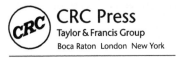

CRC Press
Taylor & Francis Group
Boca Raton London New York

CRC Press is an imprint of the
Taylor & Francis Group, an **informa** business

CRC Press
Taylor & Francis Group
6000 Broken Sound Parkway NW, Suite 300
Boca Raton, FL 33487-2742

First issued in paperback 2019

© 2017 by Taylor & Francis Group, LLC
CRC Press is an imprint of Taylor & Francis Group, an Informa business

No claim to original U.S. Government works

ISBN-13: 978-0-4987-4572-7 (hbk)
ISBN-13: 978-0-367-87513-8 (pbk)

Visit the Taylor & Francis Web site at
http://www.taylorandfrancis.com

and the CRC Press Web site at
http://www.crcpress.com

Contents

Contents

Preface

Robotic assistive technologies are playing an increasingly important role in assisting children and adults who have disabilities and those who need extra help due to aging. These technologies aid in the completion of functional activities, assist with learning, and act as companions, for example. To comprehend the dynamic and rapidly changing field of robotic assistive technologies, it is necessary to understand the characteristics of robots that make them useful to people who have disabilities and the elderly. How can robots be used in a particular context? What are the existing protocols for their use, and what are the known outcomes?

With an evidence-based approach, this book includes a comprehensive overview of current uses of robotic assistive technologies from principles to practice. The underlying principles in each application are followed by a critical review of the technology available, the utilization protocols, user studies, functional outcomes, and existing clinical evidence. The focus is on robots as tools to achieve functional and participation goals. Some of the applications described are in the research and development stage, but many can be acquired off the shelf. Ethical and social implications of robotic assistive technology use are also discussed. At the end of the book a glossary is included. Terms in this glossary are printed in boldface the first time they appear in the book.

The book will be useful for those with a technical background seeking information on how to design robots to meet the needs of individuals who have disabilities and those who are aging. It will also provide an understanding of the expected use and outcomes for practitioners (e.g., physiotherapists, occupational therapists, and teachers) who want to know how to use robotic assistive technologies with persons who have functional limitations. Finally, the book is also aimed at university students in occupational and physical therapy, whose future clients and patients will certainly use robotic assistive technologies.

Acknowledgments

We would like to thank CRC Press for asking us to provide a book on rehabilitation robotics. Their trust in and support of us are appreciated. We are proud of the book and acknowledge the authors of each of the chapters for providing quality content in their areas of expertise. We would like to thank them for their commitment to this project and for their patience and willingness to attend to our comments and suggestions. The book is enriched by the international scope provided by a diverse group of authors from Portugal, Colombia, the Netherlands, Canada, and the United States. Our authors represent industry and academia, adding breadth to the perspectives presented.

We are fortunate to have the expertise of an excellent editorial board: Liliana Alvarez, Kim Adams, Adriana Rios, and Rich Simpson. Thank you for your wise advice and for always being ready to roll up your sleeves and directly contribute to the content of the book when it was necessary. Your efforts are reflected in the quality of the final product.

Pedro Encarnação and Al Cook

When Al Cook, after being contacted by CRC Press, challenged me to coedit a book on robotic assistive technologies, I didn't hesitate to accept. After a sabbatical leave in the Faculty of Rehabilitation Medicine of the University of Alberta working with Al, we have worked together on numerous projects, and I've always admired his intellectual generosity and enjoyed his sense of humor. With little editing experience, I thought that the project would not take too much of my time and that it would be another opportunity for learning from Al. In the end, I have learned a lot and had a lot of fun in the process: Thank you, Al, for that and for your trust in me. But, I did underestimate the time required to put together a multicontributed book such as this. That time was often stolen from my wife, Raquel, and daughter, Joana, and I am indebted to them: I have no words to thank you for your unconditional support.

Pedro Encarnação

Working with Pedro on the project has been a pleasure both intellectually and personally. Certainly, Pedro's expertise in robotic engineering design and application coupled with his clinical research experience in the study of robotic systems for children with disabilities were strong attributes that enhanced the quality of this work. Equally, his drive, attention to detail, and commitment to accurate and readable content have contributed dramatically to this work. I am indebted to Pedro for his willingness to work with me. He talks about his learning from me—I have clearly learned as much from him. Thank you, Pedro.

My wife, Nancy, my three children, Brian, Barbara, and Jen, provide constant support and inspiration. My three grandsons, Ben, Sam, and Arman, continually remind me of the virtues of mixing work with play.

Al Cook

Editorial Board

Liliana Alvarez
Kim Adams
Adriana Rios
Richard Simpson

Contributors

Kim Adams
Faculty of Rehabilitation Medicine
University of Alberta and Glenrose
  Rehabilitation Hospital
Edmonton, Alberta, Canada

Liliana Alvarez
School of Occupational Therapy
University of Western Ontario
London, Ontario, Canada

Sandra Bedaf
Centre of Expertise for Innovative
  Care and Technology
Zuyd University of Applied
  Sciences
Heerlen, the Netherlands

Julianne Bell
University of Waterloo
Waterloo, Ontario, Canada

Arthur Blom
Assistive Innovations Corp.
New York, New York

Cathy Bodine
Department of Bioengineering
University of Colorado
Denver, Colorado

Jaimie Borisoff
Canada Research Chair in
  Rehabilitation Engineering
  Design
British Columbia Institute of
  Technology
Burnaby, British Columbia, Canada

Brian Burne
Department of Bioengineering
University of Colorado
Denver, Colorado

Cecilia Clark
Department of Bioengineering
University of Colorado
Denver, Colorado

Albert M. Cook
Faculty of Rehabilitation Medicine
University of Alberta
Edmonton, Alberta, Canada

Luc de Witte
Centre of Expertise for Innovative
  Care and Technology
Zuyd University of Applied
  Sciences
Heerlen, the Netherlands

Pedro Encarnação
Católica Lisbon School of Business
    and Economics
Universidade Católica Portuguesa
Lisbon, Portugal

Geneviève Foley
Toronto Rehabilitation Institute
AGE-WELL Network of Centres
    of Excellence
University of Toronto
Toronto, Ontario, Canada

Jacqueline S. Hebert
Division of Physical Medicine and
    Rehabilitation
Department of Medicine
University of Alberta
Edmonton, Alberta, Canada

Claire Huijnen
Centre of Expertise for Innovative
    Care and Technology
Zuyd University of Applied
    Sciences
Heerlen, the Netherlands

Mahsa Khalili
Biomedical Engineering Program
University of British Columbia
Vancouver, British Columbia,
    Canada

Wing-Yue Geoffrey Louie
Autonomous Systems and
    Biomechatronics Laboratory
Department of Mechanical and
    Industrial Engineering
University of Toronto
Toronto, Ontario, Canada

Michael Marquez
Department of Bioengineering
University of Colorado
Denver, Colorado

Sharaf Mohamed
Autonomous Systems and
    Biomechatronics Laboratory
Department of Mechanical and
    Industrial Engineering
University of Toronto
Toronto, Ontario, Canada

W. Ben Mortenson
Department of Occupational Science
    and Occupational Therapy
University of British Columbia
Vancouver, British Columbia,
    Canada

Goldie Nejat
Canada Research Chair in Robots
    for Society
Autonomous Systems and
    Biomechatronics Laboratory
Department of Mechanical and
    Industrial Engineering
University of Toronto
Toronto, Ontario, Canada

Patrick M. Pilarski
Division of Physical Medicine
    and Rehabilitation
Department of Medicine
University of Alberta
Edmonton, Alberta, Canada

Adriana Rios
School of Medicine and Health
    Sciences
Universidad del Rosario
Bogotá, Colombia

and

Faculty of Rehabilitation Medicine
University of Alberta
Edmonton, Alberta, Canada

Jim Sandstrum
Department of Bioengineering
University of Colorado
Denver, Colorado

Richard C. Simpson
New York Institute of Technology
New York, New York

Levin Sliker
Department of Bioengineering
University of Colorado
Denver, Colorado

Harry Stuyt
Exact Dynamics BV
Didam, the Netherlands

Andrew Sutcliffe
McGill University
Montreal, Québec, Canada

Renée van den Heuvel
Centre of Expertise for Innovative
    Care and Technology
Zuyd University of Applied
    Sciences
Heerlen, the Netherlands

H. F. Machiel Van der Loos
Department of Mechanical
    Engineering
University of British Columbia
Vancouver, British Columbia,
    Canada

Pooja Viswanathan
University of Toronto
Toronto, Ontario, Canada

1

Fundamentals of Robotic Assistive Technologies

Pedro Encarnação

Contents

Learning Objectives
After completing this chapter, readers will be able to

1. Describe the different conceptualizations of disability.
2. Define **assistive technology**.
3. Describe the **Human Activity Assistive Technology (HAAT) model**.
4. Define and classify a **robot**.
5. Justify the use of robots in **rehabilitation**.
6. Discuss the current international safety standards for **robotic assistive technologies**.
7. List some of the challenges of the rehabilitation robotics market.
8. Explain the goal of a Technology Readiness Levels scale.

Assistive Technology

The term *rehabilitation* in this book refers to the entire process aimed at enabling people with disabilities "to reach and maintain their optimal physical, sensory, intellectual, psychological and social functional levels" (World Health Organization [WHO] 2016a). The concept of disability has evolved through the years. It was first seen as a purely medical problem: a *disease* led to an *impairment* (abnormality of a body structure or

1

appearance or malfunction of an organ or system), which led to a *disability* (limitation to functional performance and activity of the individual), which in turn led to a *handicap* (disadvantage experienced by the individual as a result of the *individual's* disability and impairments) (WHO 1980). Focus was on the impairment that prevented an individual from performing. The social model by Oliver (1990) completely changed the perspective focusing on the barriers erected by society that hinder full participation of people with disabilities. Under this model, it is the society that disables people; disability is not something intrinsic to the individual.

In 2001, WHO adopted the **International Classification of Functioning, Disability, and Health (ICF)** that integrates the medical and the social models of disability into a biopsychosocial model (WHO 2001). In the ICF, disability covers impairments, activity limitations, and participation restrictions. *Impairments* are related to problems in the individual's body function or structure; *activity limitations* refer to the difficulties encountered by an individual in executing a task or action; and *participation restrictions* encompass problems experienced by an individual in involvement in life situations (WHO 2001). *Disability* reflects the negative aspects of the interaction between the individual's health condition and contextual (environmental and personal) factors. Equally relevant in ICF is the concept of functionality covering body functions, body structures, activities, and participation and denoting the positive or neutral aspects of the interaction between the individual's health condition and that individual's contextual factors (WHO 2001). Figure 1.1 illustrates

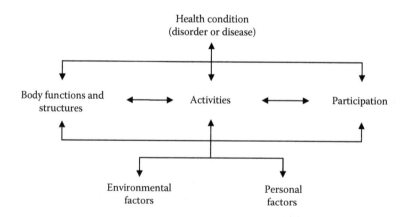

Figure 1.1   Interactions between the components of ICF. (From World Health Organization. *International Classification of Functioning, Disability and Health (ICF)*. Geneva: WHO, 2001.)

the ICF conceptualization of disability as multidimensional and interactive, resulting from the dynamic interaction between body functions and structures, activities, and participation, influenced by the individual's health condition and environmental and personal factors. Despite this paradigm shift, the medical perspective is still omnipresent in statements like "he can't read the newspaper because he's blind."

A major goal in rehabilitation is allowing independence and self-determination for people with disabilities. To bridge the gap between the capabilities of an individual with disabilities and the requirements of an activity the person wants to perform, one or a combination of the following four strategies can be used (EUSTAT 1999): (1) receive training to improve the individual's capabilities; (2) change the environment to reduce the requirements of the activity; (3) use adequate assistive technology to perform the activity; or (4) have a personal helper do or help with the activity.

Assistive Technology means technology designed to be utilized in an assistive technology device or assistive technology service. Note that the term *technology* is used here as "the practical application of knowledge especially in a particular area" ("technology," *Merriam-Webster OnLine*) and not as a machine or piece of equipment that is created by technology. The latter is designated here by the term *technology device*. According to the U.S. Assistive Technology Act of 2004, as amended (Public Law 108-364 2004, 118 STAT. 1709–1710):

> The term "assistive technology device" means any item, piece of equipment, or product system, whether acquired commercially, modified, or customized, that is used to increase, maintain, or improve functional capabilities of individuals with disabilities.
>
> The term "assistive technology service" means any service that directly assists an individual with a disability in the selection, acquisition, or use of an assistive technology device. Such term includes
>
> (A) The evaluation of the assistive technology needs of an individual with a disability, including a functional evaluation of the impact of the provision of appropriate assistive technology and appropriate services to the individual in the customary environment of the individual;
> (B) Services consisting of purchasing, leasing, or otherwise providing for the acquisition of assistive technology devices by individuals with disabilities;
> (C) Services consisting of selecting, designing, fitting, customizing, adapting, applying, maintaining, repairing, or replacing assistive technology devices;
> (D) Coordination and use of necessary therapies, interventions, or services with assistive technology devices, such as therapies, interventions, or services associated with education and rehabilitation plans and programs;

(E) Training or technical assistance for an individual with disabilities, or, where appropriate, the family members, guardians, advocates, or authorized representatives of such an individual; and

(F) Training or technical assistance for professionals (including individuals providing education and rehabilitation services), employers, or other individuals who provide services to, employ, or are otherwise substantially involved in the major life functions of individuals with disabilities.

In other words, *assistive technology* refers to technology that helps an individual carry out a functional activity, taking part in the person's daily life. Technology used in rehabilitative or educational processes, respectively termed rehabilitative or educational technology, is outside the scope of this book.

Several models have been proposed conceptualizing assistive technology. Examples include the HEART (Horizontal European Activities in Rehabilitation Technology) model (Azevedo et al. 1994); the HAAT model (Cook and Polgar 2015); the Enders (1999) model; and the dynamic circles of human activities model by Azevedo (2006). Common to all models is the focus on the activity that the individual with disabilities wants to perform, including the assistive technology necessary to perform the activity and the context in which the activity takes place.

For a comprehensive discussion of the HAAT model, please refer to the work of Cook and Polgar (2015). A short description is provided here. The HAAT model has four components: the human, the activity, the assistive technology, and the context that frames the first three factors. It models an assistive technology system representing a person with a disability doing an activity using an assistive technology within a context.

The activity defines the overall goal of the assistive technology system. Activities can be categorized into **activities of daily living** (e.g., dressing, hygiene, eating, communication); work and productive activities (including home management, educational, vocational, and care-of-others activities); and leisure activities (Canadian Association of Occupational Therapists 2002). The same activity for different persons or in different contexts can be placed in a different category. For example, one person may cook for work while another cooks to relax. Or, the same person may drive a car differently in the role of a professional driver compared to when travelling with the family. The selection of an assistive technology depends on a deep understanding of the activity. Important questions to be addressed include the following: Which skills and abilities does it require from the person? What is the meaning of the activity to the person? In which contexts is the activity performed?

The human component of the HAAT model refers to the person with disabilities with his or her physical and cognitive abilities and emotional states. The human should be the central component in the assistive technology system. It is the person with disabilities who selects the activities he or she would like to perform and within which contexts. It is the gap between the capabilities of the person with disabilities and the requirements of the activity, along with the preferences of the person, that dictates the choice of an assistive technology. The subjective assessment of the person with disabilities plays a leading role when evaluating the effectiveness of an assistive technology system. Even more, persons with disabilities should be involved in the research and development of assistive technologies and not viewed solely as the recipients of the technologies.

The context in which activities are performed includes physical, social, cultural, and institutional facets. Contexts may enable or hinder the use of assistive technology. The physical characteristics of the natural or built environment in which a given activity will be performed have a direct influence on the assistive technology that can be used. For example, they determine the maximum width that a wheelchair can have to be able to cross doorways, or they determine the reflective properties of a display that is supposed to be used under natural light. But, social (referring to those persons who interact with the assistive technology user), cultural, and institutional environments are also of paramount importance when considering assistive technology. Persons with disabilities often report that attitudes of others are frequently more disabling than physical barriers. The use of assistive technology can accentuate disability and contribute to stigmatization (see Chapter 10). Success of assistive technology use depends also on how knowledgeable of assistive technology the persons interacting with the individuals with disabilities are. Examples of cultural factors that affect assistive technology delivery are the degree of importance attributed to physical appearance and to independence, typical coping strategies, and typical roles of a person in society. Finally, funding policies and regulations, accessibility legislation, and standards for product design are examples of factors in the institutional context that affect assistive technology.

The assistive technology component in the HAAT model is what enables the human to perform the activity within a given context. **Assistive technology devices** can be conceptually divided into functional blocks that represent the information flow and the interaction between the device and the other components of the model (Figure 1.2).

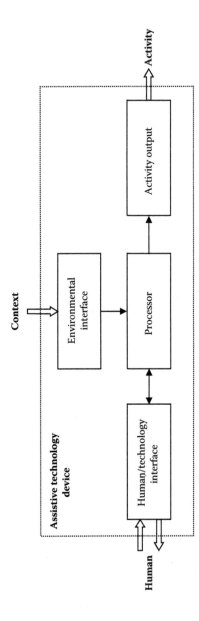

Figure 1.2 Block diagram of an assistive technology device. (Adapted from Cook, A M, and J M Polgar. *Assistive Technologies: Principles and Practice.* 4th ed. St. Louis, MO: Elsevier, 2015.)

The human-technology interface encompasses the interactions from the human to the technology and from the technology to the human. It thus includes positioning devices that enable a person to maintain a functional position to interact with the technology; control interfaces that allow a person to control the technology (e.g., joysticks, keyboards, switches); and displays (visual, auditory, or tactile) that relay information to the user. Chapter 2 discusses the human-technology interface in robotic assistive technologies. The environmental interface is responsible for gathering environmental information necessary for the functioning of the technology. For example, cameras can be used for a **socially assistive robot (SAR)** to perceive the user affect (cf. Chapter 8). The processor block receives and processes the user commands and the environmental inputs, generating the output for the activity and feedback to the user. Activity outputs depend naturally on the activity. They can be synthesized speech for a communication activity, a manipulator movement for a **manipulation** activity, or suggestions of words when writing with the assistance of a word predictor.

All components of the HAAT model need to be considered in assistive technology assessment and intervention. A collaboration should be established between different professionals (e.g., physical and occupational therapists, speech and language pathologists, assistive technology practitioners) and all of those who are involved with the user (e.g., family members, teachers/employers, representatives from the funding source). The role of the different professionals should be advisory to the user, such that he or she can make an informed decision regarding what assistive technology to acquire. In the end, the user choices and preferences should be followed as closely as possible. Failure to meet those preferences will likely result in technology abandonment.

The ICF and HAAT models are closely related. Body functions and structures and the person's health condition in the ICF model are included in the human component of the HAAT model; ICF's activities and participation correspond to the HAAT activity component; and the environmental and personal factors in the ICF model are captured in the context component of the HAAT model. The assistive technology is a separate component in the HAAT model, while in the ICF model the assistive technology is included in the environmental factors. This reflects the fact that the HAAT model is a conceptualization "of the place of assistive technology in the lives of persons with disabilities, guiding both clinical applications and research investigations" (Cook and Polgar 2015, 36), while the ICF is a general classification of health and health-related domains (WHO 2001).

Robots

According to the International Organization for Standardization (ISO), a robot is an "actuated mechanism programmable in two or more axes with a degree of autonomy, moving within its environment, to perform intended tasks" (ISO 2012, 1). In this definition, the robot includes its control system and the interface with the environment and the user.

By stating that a robot should be programmable in two or more axes (i.e., two or more linear or rotary directions of motion), the definition rules out single-axis devices (e.g., ankle-only or knee-only powered orthoses). The number of axes usually coincides with the **degrees of freedom** of a robot, which is the number of variables that need to be specified to locate all parts of the robot.

Robot autonomy is the "ability to perform intended tasks based on current state and sensing, without human intervention" (ISO 2012, 1). Beer, Fisk, and Rogers defined it as "the extent to which a robot can sense its environment, plan based on that environment, and act upon that environment with the intent of reaching some task-specific goal (either given to or created by the robot) without external control" (2014, 77). Robots may exhibit different levels of **autonomy**, ranging from teleoperated (completely controlled by a user) to fully autonomous (robot carries out all actions without human intervention). Several scales of robot autonomy have been proposed (for a review, please refer to the work of Beer, Fisk, and Rogers 2014), the first and most widely cited being the 10-level scale of Sheridan and Verplank (1978) reproduced in Chapter 2.

According to its intended application, a robot can be classified into (a) *industrial robot*, an "automatically controlled, reprogrammable, multipurpose manipulator, programmable in three or more axes, which can be either fixed in place or mobile for use in industrial automation applications," or (b) *service robot*, a "robot that performs useful tasks for humans or equipment excluding industrial automation applications" (ISO 2012). Service robots can be for personal use, used for a noncommercial task, usually by laypersons (*personal service robot*); or for professional use, used for a commercial task, usually operated by a properly trained operator (*professional service robot*) (ISO 2012). Robotic manipulators used in production lines are examples of industrial robots. Robotic manipulators for augmented manipulation (Chapter 3); **robotic prosthesis** (Chapter 4); automated wheelchairs (Chapter 5); **exoskeletons** (Chapter 6); robotic systems to support play, education, and cognitive development (Chapter 7); SARs (Chapters 8 and 9); and domestic servant robots (Chapter 9) are examples of personal service robots. Professional service robots such as delivery robots in hospitals, robots for rehabilitation therapy, or surgery robots are outside the scope of this book.

Within personal service robots, it is useful to refer to three classes that have been defined in the literature: assistive, socially interactive, and SARs (Figure 1.3). Feil-Seifer and Matarić (2005) defined *assistive robots* (ARs) as robots that give aid or support to a human user. Fong, Nourbakhsh, and Dautenhahn (2003) introduced the term *socially interactive robots* (SIRs) to designate robots for which social interaction plays a key role. With this new term, they wanted to distinguish this kind of robot from those for which a "conventional" **human–robot interaction** is involved (e.g., tele-operated robots). SIR characteristics include the ability to "express and/or perceive emotions; communicate with high-level dialogue; learn/recognize models of other agents; establish/maintain social relationships; use natural cues (gaze, gestures, etc.); exhibit distinctive personality and character; and may learn/develop social competencies" (Fong, Nourbakhsh, and Dautenhahn 2003, 145). For a comprehensive survey of SIRs, please refer to Fong, Nourbakhsh, and Dautenhahn's (2002) work. Note that an AR can provide assistance to an individual without any social interaction (e.g., a robotic feeder), and that a SIR can be designed only for entertainment, without providing any assistance to the user. Robots that provide assistance to human users through social interaction are termed *socially assistive robots* (Feil-Seifer and Matarić 2005). These lie at the intersection between ARs and SIRs. The goal of a SAR is to "create close and effective interaction with a human user for the purpose of giving assistance and achieving measurable progress in convalescence, rehabilitation, learning, etc." (Feil-Seifer and Matarić 2005, 465). Similarly, robots that provide assistance to human users through physical interaction can be termed *physically assistive robotics*.

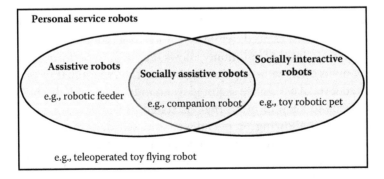

Figure 1.3 Classes of personal service robots.

The term *robotic assistive technologies* in this book refers to robots used to increase, maintain, or improve functional capabilities of individuals with disabilities. These are a subclass of ARs in the sense that they are used by individuals with disabilities, while ARs may be used by individuals in general.

Robotic assistive technologies have been developed since the 1980s. Vlaskamp, Soede, and Gelderblom (2011) provided a brief list of assistive technology milestones, including the following:

- 1980: Utah electronically controlled prosthetic arm (Jacobson et al. 1982)
- 1988: Manus (now *i*Arm) AR manipulator (Römer et al. 2003)
- 2002: Neural interface (Warwick et al. 2003)
- 2003: Paro therapeutic robot (Wada et al. 2005)
- 2003: Bionic arm (Kuiken et al. 2004).

To these we can add

- 2010: eLEGS (now Ekso; http://eksobionics.com/) exoskeleton

This list considers only robotic systems that have been designed as assistive technologies and not the use of mainstream robotic devices as assistive technologies. For example, Cook et al. (1988) reported the use of an industrial manipulator to enable very young children with disabilities to engage in play activities.

There are three characteristics of a robot, as defined previously, that make it a suitable technology device to assist people: It is an *actuated mechanism*, is *programmable*, and has *a degree of autonomy*. As an actuated mechanism, it has a physical presence in the environment and can act on it. Thus, it can assist an individual with physical impairments execute tasks that require physical action. Because a robot is programmable, its use is not restricted to a single task executed in a predefined manner, and it can be adapted to meet a particular user's needs while executing an activity in a given context. Having a certain **level of autonomy** allows the robot to perform part or the total task on its own, without requiring human intervention, thus providing the desired level of assistance required by an individual with disabilities.

One needs to keep in mind that, as stated previously, a major goal in rehabilitation is allowing independence and self-determination of people with disabilities. This is not accomplished with an assistive technology that operates independently when that is not desired by the user. For example, when a child with physical impairments is using a robot to manipulate toys, he or she may prefer to control all the robot degrees of freedom (assuming the child can), instead of specifying only the general goal and expecting the robot to be able to accomplish the task autonomously. That may allow the child to effectively control what to do with the toys, thus enabling free play, instead of choosing an activity from a set of finite choices. Ideally, a robot should be able to dynamically adapt to the user's current needs and preferences and to the context. A robot "capable of performing tasks by sensing its environment and/or interacting with external sources and adapting its behavior" is termed an *intelligent robot* (ISO 2012). Recent advances in machine learning (Wang, Ma, and Zhou 2009) allow a robot to learn from its previous experiences. This is an important feature in robotic assistive technologies because it may maximize the match between the assistive technology and the user, thus preventing technology abandonment. However, intelligent robots raise several ethical concerns (e.g., autonomy of the individual, clinical decision making by a robot without human oversight; see Chapter 10). In Chapter 8, a brief description of current machine learning techniques is given.

Specific design characteristics for different robotic assistive technologies are discussed throughout the book. Because robotic assistive technologies operate side by side with humans, safety is of paramount importance. Current safety guidelines are discussed in the next section.

Safety of Service Robots

The ISO 13482 (ISO 2014) is the currently available international standard defining safety requirements for personal care robots. A personal care robot is a "service robot that performs actions contributing directly towards improvement in the quality of life of humans, excluding medical applications" (ISO 2014, 4). This definition encompasses (a) mobile servant robots (i.e., "personal care robot[s] that [are] capable of travelling to perform serving tasks in interaction with humans, such as handling objects or exchanging information"); (b) physical assistant robots (i.e., "personal care robot[s] that physically assist a user to perform required tasks by providing supplementation or augmentation of personal capabilities"); and (c) person carrier robots (i.e., "personal care robot[s] with the purpose of transporting humans to an intended destination") (ISO 2014, 4). Physical assistant robots may be fastened to a human during use (restraint-type physical assistant robots) or not (restraint-free physical assistant robots). The ISO definition of a personal care robot is thus consistent with our concept of robotic assistive technologies. The ISO 13482 international standard was formulated after acknowledging that personal care robot operation often includes physical human–robot contact; thus, a new set of safety requirements complementing the safety requirements for robots in industrial environments was necessary. ISO 13482 provides guidance for the assurance of safety in the design, construction, integration, installation, and use of personal care robots. Robots manufactured after February 1, 2014, must comply with this standard. ISO 13482 does not apply to robots travelling faster than 20 km/h; robot toys; waterborne robots and flying robots; industrial robots; robots as medical devices; and military or public force application robots.

Different personal care robots present different hazards. ISO 13482 includes a list of typical hazards, but other hazards resulting from a particular design, intended use, or reasonably foreseeable misuse should also be identified. The list in ISO 13482 is considered the minimum set of hazards that a hazard identification methodology should cover. It includes 22 items: (1) battery-charging hazards; (2) energy storage and supply hazards; (3) hazards due to robot startup; (4) hazards due to robot shape; (5) hazards due to noise; (6) hazards due to lack of awareness; (7) hazardous vibration; (8) hazardous substances and fluids; (9) hazardous environmental conditions; (10) extreme temperatures; (11) hazardous nonionizing radiation; (12) hazardous ionizing radiation; (13) electromagnetic interference (EMI)/electromagnetic compatibility (EMC) hazards; (14) stress, posture, and usage hazards; (15) hazards due to robot motion; (16) collision with objects, obstacles, or ground conditions that can cause harm; (17) hazardous physical contact during human–robot interaction; (18) insufficient durability; (19) hazardous autonomous action; (20) hazardous contact with moving parts; (21) hazards due to localization and navigation errors; and (22) other hazard items.

Several hazards are listed under each item and safety requirement clauses are provided for each hazard. Safety requirement clauses include five sections: (1) "General," describing the safety requirement; (2) "inherently safe design," listing requirements for inherently safe design measures; (3) "safeguarding and complementary protective measures," including requirements for protective control functions of the robot to reduce risks arising due to the possible dynamic interactions between objects, obstacles, or ground conditions and the personal care robot; (4) "information for use," providing specific requirements regarding information for use for each hazard; and (5) "verification and validation," recommending methods of verification and validation of various requirements for the significant hazards.

The first and most important step in risk reduction is the use of safe design measures. In fact, safeguarding measures can fail, and information for use may be ignored. Therefore, having an inherently safe robot should be the preferred option for risk reduction.

If protective measures are implemented through a control system, ISO 13482 establishes required performance levels (PLs) or safety integrity levels (SILs) for the control system functions, depending on the type of personal care robot. PLs (ISO 2015) and SILs (International Electrotechnical Commission [IEC] 2005) are discrete levels, each corresponding to a probability of dangerous failure per hour. The PL or SIL shall be defined for each of the following functions when they are used in a personal care robot: (a) emergency stop; (b) protective stop; (c) limits to workspace; (d) safety-related speed control; (e) safety-related force control; (f) hazardous collision avoidance; and (g) stability control (including overload protection). Considerations regarding the design of the user interface are part of the safety-related control system requirements. They include requirements concerning feedback to the user and the operation of the robot control devices. Four operational modes are foreseen in ISO 13482: autonomous, semiautonomous, manual, and maintenance. Table 1.1 summarizes the characteristics of these modes; the first three correspond to different degrees of autonomy of the robot.

Recommended methods of verification and validation of the different requirements include (1) inspection; (2) practical tests; (3) measurement; (4) observation during operation; (5) examination of circuit diagrams; (6) examination of software; (7) review of task-based risk assessment; and

TABLE 1.1   Operational Modes of Personal Care Robots

Characteristic	Operational Mode			
	Autonomous Mode	Semiautonomous Mode	Manual Mode	Maintenance Mode
Initiation of action	By the robot or the user	By the user	By the user	By an authorized person
Frequency of human intervention	Once/rare	Frequently	Constantly	Constantly
Degree of supervision by the human	None/very low	Low to high	High	High

Source: Adapted from the International Organization for Standardization (ISO). *ISO 13482 International Standard: Robots and Robotic Devices—Safety Requirements for Personal Care Robots.* Geneva: ISO, 2014.

(8) examination of layout drawings and relevant documents. Although practical tests and observation during operation are often required, ISO 13482 does not explicitly require or recommend the involvement of end users in these verification and validation methods. There is only a note to the text saying "Consultation with the users is often necessary" (ISO 2014, 55) when possible "user overload" that can result from too many warning signals is under discussion. However, especially when the envisioned end users are people with disabilities, the end user should actively participate in all stages of product development (Cook and Polgar 2015; Newell 2011).

The ISO 13482 standard recognizes that not all users of a personal care robot will be able to read the instruction handbook or notice and understand acoustic or visual warning signs, namely the following: (a) children, elderly persons, mentally impaired persons; (b) animals; (c) guests/visitors in private areas; or (d) third parties near the robot in public areas. However, there are no requirements or recommendations for making information for use accessible to the envisioned end users. The only requirement is that "where it is foreseeable that the information for use will not be available for certain groups of persons, this shall not lead to additional risks" (ISO 2014, 53). Naturally, if personal care robot operation is not understood by the user, it will probably not be used.

Technology Readiness Scale

In this book, currently available robotic assistive technologies, corresponding utilization protocols, and intervention outcomes are reviewed to provide an overview of what can be achieved today by directly acquiring existing technology devices and applying established methodologies. The assistive technology market is challenging. WHO estimates that about 15% of the world's population (over one billion people) experience disability (WHO 2015). However, this population is heterogeneous, not only because people experience different impairments but also because even individuals with the same health condition and body functions and structures may experience different levels of activity limitations and participation restrictions, carry a different personal history and have differing needs and goals, and are within different environments (cf. the ICF model). Of people with disabilities globally, 51% to 53% cannot afford health care (WHO 2015) and thus are dependent on public funding to access assistive technology. This causes fragmentation of the assistive technology market: Industries and services often focus on specific impairments or disabilities, and different countries have different regulations concerning funding for assistive technology (Olive and Le Blanc 2005). The WHO Global Cooperation on Assistive Technology (GATE) initiative (http:// www.who.int/phi/implementation/assistive_technology/phi_gate/en/) published the Priority Assistive Products List (APL), including 50 priority assistive devices, aimed at improving access to high-quality, affordable assistive devices in all countries (WHO 2016b). The European Assistive Technology Information Network (EASTIN) offers a European search engine (http://www.eastin.eu) on assistive technology, working in all languages of the European Union. Initiatives like these broaden the assistive technology market. Other challenges for ARs include (Organization for Economic Co-operation and Development 2012) the following:

1. Their complexity, arising from the need to operate in unstructured environments and in close proximity with humans;
2. Lack of market standardization, component manufacture, and software platforms;
3. High cost of current devices;
4. The need to integrate the assistive robotic industry with the economic ecosystems of health insurance reimbursement providers; and
5. The need to assess and show effectiveness of the robotic devices with end users.

These contribute to not having a single robotic assistive technology in the WHO list of 50 priority assistive devices and to the reasons many of the prototype robotic assistive technologies developed in research projects never reach the market. It is thus important, when describing the currently available robotic assistive technology, to assess its *readiness*, that is, its level of maturity. For that, this book uses a technology readiness level (TRL) scale. Pioneered by NASA in the 1980s, TRL scales were adopted by the U.S. Department of Defense in 1999 (U.S. Department of Defense 2011) and by the U.S. Department of Energy in 2011 (U.S. Department of Energy 2011). TRLs are currently used by many institutions to evaluate the maturity of technology (e.g., the Canadian governmental procurement service [Government of Canada 2015] or the European Union Horizon 2020 Research and Innovation program [European Commission 2016]). Different applications of the concept usually share the number of levels (9), ranging from TRL 1—basic principles observed to TRL 9—actual system proven in operational environment (level designations may differ from application to application). The TRL scale specific for **robotics** proposed by SPARC (http://www.sparc-robotics.net/; SPARC The Partnership for Robotics in Europe 2015) is reproduced in Table 1.2 for reference. Exact interpretation of each TRL depends on the technology under analysis.

TABLE 1.2 Technology Readiness Levels Scale for Robotics

Relative Level of Technology Development	TRL	Designation	Description	Outcomes
Idea development: Basic technology research	1	Basic Principles Observed	Technical feasibility is assessed, basic principles are laboratory tested, technology requirements established, comparative reviews conducted, similar technology in other areas of use assessed.	Technically detailed document which describes a product, application, technical feature, or module and indicates the potential market requirement and likely technical requirements. Typically includes a detailed functional description, customer benefit analysis, ideas for realization, and a detailed technical progression plan.
Concept formation: Basic technology research	2	Technology Concept Formulated	Proof of principle developments including all engineering and systems development (e.g., algorithm development, physical schematics, and simulations). Critical parts of the system are tested in laboratory conditions to show how the technology operates and to provide insights into functional and practical limitations. Assessment of the integration between the proposed components.	Bench demonstration of key technical concepts. Concept formulated with details of potential technical and development risks, including estimated resource requirements and test planning. Understanding of the design and engineering parameters and their inter-relationships with the desired system parameters and key requirements.

(*Continued*)

TABLE 1.2 (CONTINUED) Technology Readiness Levels Scale for Robotics

Relative Level of Technology Development	TRL	Designation	Description	Outcomes
Experimental Development: Technology development	3	Experimental Proof of Concept	Key technical elements developed as subsystems to allow assessment of the core ideas and test practical realization. Realization of parts of the concept to assess the product (e.g., computer simulation models, physical models, assessment of user interaction, consideration of deployment, etc.). Bench development of key technical elements, features, or modules able to validate the viability of the concept within the application parameters. Benchmark testing of system or module performance and comparative assessment with existing systems.	Results and demonstrations that the concept is technically feasible, a first set of modules or components have been developed and tested to show performance compatible with the requirements. Interfaces developed between module and within systems. Detailed future technical scope of work identified.
Experiment: Laboratory demonstration	4	Technology Validated in Laboratory	Technology is demonstrated in a laboratory or development testing environment where testing parameters are designed to demonstrate the limits of the technology with respect to the requirements. Testing of system or major subsystems are validated against established technical benchmarks relevant to the end user. Testing of internal and external inter-connectivity and integration between components in the system. Demonstration and understanding of the impact of the underlying design and engineering parameters on system performance. Initial normative testing with trained users to provide initial usability information.	Demonstration that the technology is expected to scale to achieve end-user relevant technical requirements or shows sufficiently improved performance, over existing systems, using established benchmarks. Usability testing results providing insight into areas for future development and their prioritization. Clear plan for integration and identification of technical risks and their potential impact and severity. Documentation of technical development plan.

(Continued)

TABLE 1.2 (CONTINUED) Technology Readiness Levels Scale for Robotics

Relative Level of Technology Development	TRL	Designation	Description	Outcomes
Laboratory based prototype: Laboratory validation	5	Technology Validated in Relevant Environment	Integrated system developed to perform in an environment that exhibits the main features of the expected operating environment. Performance is sufficient to validate that the technology could scale to achieve useful function in the intended application area. System contains all critical technical elements but not in the desired form factor (shape, size, power consumption, etc.). Core functionality of product, feature, or module can be demonstrated within system and operational context.	Identification and prioritization of the major technical and application risks for the realization of the product, feature or module. Performance characteristics are well understood. Clear evidence is delivered that the different technical components can be integrated into a unified component or system and can perform the intended function.
Functional system: External technology demonstration	6	Technology Demonstrated in Relevant Environment	Main functions perform sufficiently close to requirements such that technology can be validated in an environment that is equivalent to the operational environment. First field trials can be conducted when supported by developers to gain fine grained insight into the issues of product, feature, or module development.	The main functionality of product, feature or module can be demonstrated in a realistic environment under realistic test conditions. The concept is realized to a degree such that there is good usability and impact data, gathered from developer supported customer trials. System design documentation is complete. Expected development plan is complete including a detailed technical progression.

(Continued)

TABLE 1.2 (CONTINUED) Technology Readiness Levels Scale for Robotics

Relative Level of Technology Development	TRL	Designation	Description	Outcomes
Engineering prototype: Product prototype	7	System Prototype Demonstration in Operational Environment	System performance is close to the end product, feature, or module end-user requirement. Development of prototypes with final technology subsystems or close equivalents in a near to complete form factor (size, weight, power consumption, etc.). All functionality required in the end system is capable of being demonstrated. Customer verification trials (independent of developer support) carried out.	Significant reduction in technical risk. Product operation validated in actual end-user environments. Product prototypes realized in close to final form and function. Plan developed for manufacture and deployment including full product testing and certification plan.
Production prototype: Close to market development	8	System Complete and Qualified	Development of production prototypes with final functionality and form factor. System is sufficient for end-user testing in limited launch markets over extended periods of operation. Initial batch production of the product using end manufacturing processes for most parts. Product material and functional quality are at production levels. Product certifiable for use in chosen market.	Product validated for manufacture through extended customer trials, failure mode analysis complete. Certification obtained. All production processes validated and process variations assessed and tested. Full materials and part specifications complete. Product test data validated against end-user requirements. Manufacturability fully assessed.
Product completed: In production	9	Actual System Proven in Operational Environment	Set up of production facilities, production test systems completed, volume components sourced.	Series production and sales.

Source: Adapted from SPARC The Partnership for Robotics in Europe. *Robotics 2020 Multi-Annual Roadmap for Robotics in Europe. Horizon 2020 Call ICT-2016 (ICT25 & ICT 26).* Brussels: SPARC, 2015.

TRLs only apply to whole systems or to modules within a system. When assessing a system, integration issues between different modules should be taken into consideration in addition to the TRLs of each module. Naturally, the TRL of a system cannot be greater than the lowest TRL of its modules. Specific examples of TRLs are provided elsewhere (SPARC The Partnership for Robotics in Europe 2015, 313).

Summary

Robotic assistive technologies are robots used to increase, maintain, or improve functional capabilities of individuals with disabilities. They operate side by side with a person with disabilities, accepting commands from the user to assist in performing a given activity within a particular context and providing feedback to the user.

Chapter 2 discusses the human-technology interface in rehabilitation and assistive robotics (i.e., encompassing robots for rehabilitation therapy and robotic assistive technologies). Chapters 3 to 9 describe different applications of robotic assistive devices. Each of these chapters includes sections that address the following: (a) principles, revealing why and how robots are applied; (b) critical review of the technology available, describing the robotic assistive devices that are now available; (c) critical review of the available utilization protocols, providing currently available information on how to use the robotic assistive technologies; and (d) review of user studies, outcomes, clinical evidence, and reporting results of the assessment of robotic assistive technologies with end users. The actual content of each section depends heavily on the technology readiness level of the devices described. For example, Chapter 3 addresses assistive robotic arms; there are today two commercially available products (TRL 9). It is thus possible to concretely discuss the characteristics and limitations of those devices. On the other hand, most of the SARs discussed in Chapter 8 are investigational robots (TRL 4–5 if considering their application as SARs). Therefore, the section "Critical Review of the Technology Available" mainly summarizes what has been learned from the research projects involving SARs regarding the design of the different robot components. In any case, each chapter aims to answer the following questions for a particular application: What is the rationale for using robots? Which robotic assistive devices are available? How can they be used? With what results? In addition, each chapter discusses directions for future research.

Robotic assistive technologies pose several ethical challenges regarding their design, implementation, and deployment. Autonomy, **beneficence,**

nonmaleficence, justice, and **fidelity** ethical principles in relation to robotic assistive devices are discussed in Chapter 10.

STUDY QUESTIONS

1. What does the ICF biopsychosocial model of disability add to the medical and social models of disability?
2. Does assistive technology designate only items, pieces of equipment, or product systems that are used to increase, maintain, or improve functional capabilities of individuals with disabilities?
3. List the four components of the HAAT model, briefly explaining each component and their relation.
4. Give examples of contextual factors that may affect assistive technology use.
5. Who should be involved in assistive technology assessment and intervention?
6. Define *robot* and describe the differences between industrial and service robots.
7. Describe the assistive robot, socially interactive robot, and socially assistive robot classes of personal service robots.
8. Explain why robots are suitable technologies to use in the rehabilitation of people with disabilities.
9. List five hazard items included in the minimum coverage that should be achieved by any given hazard identification exercise, as set by ISO 13482.
10. Which is the best option regarding safety of personal care robots: Having an inherently safe design or implementing appropriate protective measures? Justify.
11. Comment on the ISO 13482 international standard in light of the HAAT model.
12. List possible causes for many assistive robots never reaching the market.
13. Explain the goal of a technology readiness level scale.

References

Azevedo, L. "A model based approach to provide augmentative mobility to severely disabled children through assistive technology." PhD thesis, Department of Architecture and Computer Technology, Universidad del País Basco, Donostia, San Sebastián, Spain, 2006.

Azevedo, L, H Féria, M Nunes da Ponte, E Wann, and Z Recellado. "HEART Report—Line E E3.2 European Curricula in Rehabilitation Technology Training." Luxembourg: European Comission DG XIII, Telematics Applications Programme, Disabled and Elderly Sector, 1994.

Beer, J, A Fisk, and W Rogers. "Toward a Framework for Levels of Robot Autonomy in Human–Robot Interaction." *Journal of Human–Robot Interaction* 3, no. 2 (2014): 74–99.

Canadian Association of Occupational Therapists. *Enabling Occupation: An Occupational Therapy Perspective.* 2nd ed. Ottawa: CAOT/ACE, 2002.

Cook, A M, P Hoseit, K Liu, R Lee, and C Zenteno-Sanchez. "Using a Robotic Arm System to Facilitate Learning in Very Young Disabled Children." *IEEE Transactions on Biomedical Engineering* 35, no. 2 (1988): 132–137.

Cook, A M, and J M Polgar. *Assistive Technologies: Principles and Practice.* 4th ed. St. Louis, MO: Elsevier, 2015.

Enders, A. "Building a Framework for Collaboration." *Proceedings of the AAATE Conference.* Dusseldorf, November 1999, 1–4.

European Commission. "Horizon 2020 Work Program 2016–2017 General Annexes." 2016. http://ec.europa.eu/research/participants/data/ref/h2020/other /wp/2016-2017/annexes/h2020-wp1617-annex-ga_en.pdf (accessed June 1, 2016).

EUSTAT. *Go for It! A Manual for Users of Assistive Technology.* Deliverable D05.4, Project DE 3402. Milan, Italy: SIVA, 1999.

Feil-Seifer, D, and M Matarić. "Defining Socially Assistive Robotics." *Proceedings of the 2005 IEEE 9th International Conference on Rehabilitation Robotics.* Chicago: IEEE, 2005, 465–468.

Fong, T, I Nourbakhsh, and K Dautenhahn. *A Survey of Socially Interactive Robots: Concepts, Design, and Applications.* Technical Report CMU-RI-TR-02-29. Pittsburgh: CMU, 2002.

Fong, T, I Nourbakhsh, and K Dautenhahn. "A Survey of Socially Interactive Robots." *Robotics and Autonomous Systems* 42, no. 3 (2003): 143–166.

Government of Canada. *Technology Readiness Levels.* February 25, 2015. https:// buyandsell.gc.ca/initiatives-and-programs/build-in-canada-innovation -program-bcip/program-specifics/technology-readiness-levels (accessed June 1, 2016).

International Electrotechnical Commission (IEC). *IEC 62061: Safety of Machinery— Functional Safety of Safety-Related Electrical, Electronic and Programmable Electronic Control Systems.* Geneva: IEC, 2005.

International Organization for Standardization (ISO). *ISO 8373 Robots and Robotic Devices—Vocabulary.* Geneva: ISO, 2012.

International Organization for Standardization (ISO). *ISO 13482 International Standard: Robots and Robotic Devices—Safety Requirements for Personal Care Robots.* Geneva: ISO, 2014.

International Organization for Standardization (ISO). *ISO 13849-1: Safety of Machinery—Safety-Related Parts of Control Systems—Part 1: General Principles for Design.* Geneva: ISO, 2015.

Jacobson, S, D Knutti, R Johnson, and H Sears. "Development of the Utah Artificial Arm." *IEEE Transactions on Biomedical Engineering* BME-29, no. 4 (1982): 249–269.

Kuiken, T A, G A Dumanian, R D Lipschutz, L A Miller, and K A Stubblefield. "The Use of Targeted Muscle Reinnervation for Improved Myoelectric Prosthesis Control in a Bilateral Shoulder Disarticulation Amputee." *Prosthetics and Orthotics International* 28, no. 3 (2004): 245–253.

Merriam-Webster OnLine. s.v. "technology." http://www.merriam-webster.com /dictionary/technology (accessed May 25, 2016).

Newell, A. *Design and the Digital Divide: Insights from 40 Years in Computer Support for Older and Disabled People.* San Rafael, CA: Morgan and Claypool, 2011.

Olive, D, and J Le Blanc. "ICT Accessibility in the U.S.: Developments in Public and Private Sectors." *Fujitsu Scientific and Technical Journal* 41, no. 1 (2005): 10–18.

Oliver, M. *The Politics of Disablement.* Houndmills, U.K.: Macmillan, 1990.

Organization for Economic Co-operation and Development. *The Robotics Innovation Challenge.* DSTI/ICCP/IE(2012)6. Paris: OECD, 2012.

Römer, G, H Stuyt, G Peters, and K van Woerden. "The Current and Future Processes for Obtaining a 'Manus' (ARM) Rehab-Robot within the Netherlands." *Proceedings of the Eighth International Conference on Rehabilitation Robotics,* Daejeon, Korea, 2003, 23–25.

Sheridan, T, and W Verplank. *Human and Computer Control for Undersea Teleoperators.* Cambridge: MIT Man-Machine Systems Laboratory, MIT, 1978.

SPARC The Partnership for Robotics in Europe. *Robotics 2020 Multi-Annual Roadmap for Robotics in Europe. Horizon 2020 Call ICT-2016 (ICT25 & ICT 26).* Brussels: SPARC, 2015.

U.S. Department of Defense. *Technology Readiness Assessment (TRA) Guidance.* Washington, DC: U.S. Department of Defense, 2011.

U.S. Department of Energy. *Technology Readiness Assessment Guide.* Washington, DC: U.S. Department of Energy, 2011.

Vlaskamp, F, M Soede, and G J Gelderblom. *History of Assistive Technology: 500 Years of Technology Development for Human Needs.* Heerlen, the Netherlands: Zuyd University, 2011.

Wada, K, T Shibata, T Saito, K Sakamoto, and K Tanie. "Psychological and Social Effects of One Year Robot Assisted Activity on Elderly People at a Health Service Facility for the Aged." In *Proceedings of the 2005 IEEE International Conference on Robotics and Automation.* Barcelona: IEEE, 2005, 2785–2790.

Wang, H, C Ma, and L Zhou. "A Brief Review of Machine Learning and Its Application." In *2009 International Conference on Information Engineering and Computer Science.* Wuhan, China: IEEE, 2009, 1–4.

Warwick, K, M Gasson, B Hutt, I Goodhew, P Kyberd, B Andrews, P Teddy et al. "The Application of Implant Technology for Cybernetic Systems." *Archives of Neurology* 60, no. 10 (2003): 1369–1373.

World Health Organization (WHO). *International Classification of Impairments, Disabilities, and Handicaps (ICIDH).* Geneva: WHO, 1980.

World Health Organization (WHO). *International Classification of Functioning, Disability and Health (ICF).* Geneva: WHO, 2001.

World Health Organization (WHO). "Disability and Health: Fact Sheet No. 352."
    December 2015. http://www.who.int/mediacentre/factsheets/fs352/en/ (accessed
    June 1, 2016).
World Health Organization (WHO). *Health Topics: Rehabilitation.* 2016a. http://
    www.who.int/topics/rehabilitation/en/ (accessed May 25, 2016).
World Health Organization (WHO). *Priority Assistive Products List: Improving
    Access to Assistive Technology for Everyone, Everywhere.* Geneva: WHO, 2016b.

2

Human–Robot Interaction for Rehabilitation Robots

Wing-Yue Geoffrey Louie, Sharaf Mohamed, and Goldie Nejat

Contents

Learning Objectives

After completing this chapter, readers will be able to

1. Describe the main human–robot interaction (HRI) principles involved in the development of rehabilitation robots.
2. Identify appropriate HRI metrics to evaluate rehabilitation robots.
3. Implement HRI design considerations for rehabilitation robots undertaking either physical or social HRI using the appropriate principles and metrics.
4. Identify the current state-of-the-art HRI systems for rehabilitation robots.
5. Recognize the future directions and open challenges in HRI for rehabilitation robots.

Introduction

Early robotic systems focused on industrial applications that did not involve interactions between human users and robots (Sheridan 1992). In general, these systems were designed for optimal task performance and efficiency. More recently, robots such as personal, service, health care and medical, and space robots are being designed to interact with human users. The relatively new field of human–robot interaction (HRI) focuses on designing, implementing, and evaluating robot systems that interact with humans (Goodrich and Schultz 2007). In particular, HRI research focuses on "human-centered design" with the aim of developing for humans systems that are effective, easy to use, and acceptable (Adams 2002). Human-centered design refers to the process of obtaining the user needs, requirements, and feedback for robot technology throughout the entire robot design process. This human-focused design makes HRI a unique multidisciplinary field requiring expertise in computer science, engineering, psychology, social and behavioral science, anthropology, philosophy, and ethics (Burke et al. 2010).

The first specific applications of HRI to the development of rehabilitation robotics were evident in research conducted in the 1990s, which focused on perceptions of end users of the technology, system reliability, and ease of use (Birch 1993; Chen et al. 1994; Van der Loos 1995). For example, a robot manipulator designed to assist people with physical disabilities in a vocational environment was evaluated for its usefulness through surveys and interviews (Birch 1993). Namely, feedback from individuals with severe physical disabilities as well as able-bodied participants was obtained prior to development of a final product. Chen et al. (1994) investigated an interface design for a robot manipulator for the pick and place of objects using an interface based on command and control; it allowed a user to control the manipulator using speech and gesture inputs, promoting the flexibility of the robot for potential use in different settings and environments by a user with severe physical disabilities. An interface design using spoken commands was also investigated for robot manipulators intended for people with quadriplegia (Van der Loos 1995). Lessons learned from conducting clinical trials with potential users were reported. These works are important to mention here as they provided the motivation needed for the marriage of the HRI and rehabilitation robotics fields and emphasize the importance of designing and obtaining feedback from potential users during the overall design cycle.

As rehabilitation robots interact with users on a physical or social level, there have been two main goals with respect to applying HRI research to the field: (1) to design robots that provide safe physical interaction (e.g., wheelchair robots, and lower and upper limb robotic systems); and (2) to design robots that engage in understandable and acceptable social interactions (e.g., robots that provide prompting and reminders). HRI principles and the corresponding metrics to measure these principles are especially needed for rehabilitation robotics, as rehabilitation robots are being designed for and expected to be used by the general population who are nonexperts. For example, HRI interfaces that are reliable, easy to use, and perceived to be positive will increase the overall effectiveness, success, and acceptance of rehabilitation robotic systems.

This chapter presents a detailed discussion of: (1) the main principles of HRI applied to the development and implementation of rehabilitation robots; (2) the corresponding metrics that measure the effects of the HRI principles; and (3) HRI studies that directly investigate the metrics and principles. We conclude with discussions and future work on these important topics for rehabilitation robots.

Principles

We have identified six main HRI principles that should be considered when designing, implementing, and evaluating rehabilitation robotic systems:

(1) level of robot autonomy; (2) HRI interface; (3) interaction structure; (4) adaptation, training, and learning; (5) aesthetics; and (6) length of exposure. Some of these principles have been adapted from the work of Goodrich and Schultz (2007). We discuss the application of our aforementioned design principles to the field of rehabilitation robotics. The following sections define each design principle and provide examples of their application to rehabilitation robots.

Level of Autonomy

Robot autonomy refers to a robot's ability to accomplish tasks and implement its own actions independent of a human (Goodrich and Schultz 2007). A robot's level of autonomy can be defined according to Sheridan's Levels of Autonomous Decision Making (Sheridan and Verplank 1978). Namely, there are 10 levels of autonomy, ranging from level 1, where a human controls the robot completely through teleoperation and the robot offers no assistance, to level 10, where a robot acts autonomously without requiring any human input or approval (Sheridan and Verplank 1978). A description of each level of autonomy is presented in Table 2.1.

Autonomy is important to the overall HRI design of a rehabilitation robot as it influences the design of the robot, user perceptions toward the robot, and user performance during HRI (Beer, Fisk, and Rogers 2014).

TABLE 2.1 Definitions for Levels of Autonomous Decision Making

Level	Description
1	Human does the whole task up to the point of turning it over to the robot to implement.
2	Robot helps determine action options.
3	Robot helps determine action options and suggests one, which the human need not follow.
4	Robot selects an action, and the human may or may not do it.
5	Robot selects an action and implements it if the human approves.
6	Robot selects an action and gives the human a fixed time to stop it.
7	Robot executes the whole task and tells the human what it did.
8	Robot executes the whole task and only tells the human if explicitly asked.
9	Robot executes task and only tells the human if it feels the need to.
10	Robot executes task independently of the human.

Source: Adapted from Sheridan, T. B., and Verplank, W. L. 1978. *Human and Computer Control of Undersea Teleoperators.* Cambridge, MA: Man-Machine Systems Laboratory, Massachusetts Institute of Technology.

Namely, level of autonomy influences a robot's intelligence, learning capabilities, reliability, and transparency (i.e., the ability of the robot to explain its behavior to a human user). A robot's level of autonomy can also affect human acceptance, situational awareness, trust, and workload during HRI. For example, having a high level of autonomy during robot-assisted movement training (i.e., a robot provides assistance by applying forces to move a patient's limbs) for users with neurological injuries can negatively affect the users' recovery (Marchal-Crespo and Reinkensmeyer 2009). The robot could be assisting too much during the movement training task, encouraging slacking by the user (i.e., decreased motor output, effort, energy consumption, or attention during training).

HRI Interface and Types of Information Exchange

The HRI interfaces are the systems that allow for bidirectional interaction to take place between a human user and a robot. The three common modes of interaction between a human and a robot are auditory, tactile, and visual. These modes of interaction can influence (Goodrich and Schultz 2007): (1) the interaction time required to communicate intent or instructions from the human to the robot or from the robot to the human; (2) the cognitive or mental workload of the human user; (3) the amount of situational awareness the human has of the interaction (i.e., transparency); and (4) the amount of shared understanding between the human and the robot.

Auditory exchanges can include making simple sounds (e.g., beeps) to communicate or more high-level communication through natural language (e.g., speech). Robots use auditory exchanges to provide motivation or feedback to a user during a task (Rosati et al. 2013). Movements of robotic manipulators to assist with activities of daily living by individuals with physical impairments can also be controlled using speech (Volosyak, Ivlev, and Gräser 2005). Tactile exchanges refer to physical contact between a robot and a user. This is common for robots used, for example, in robot-assisted stroke therapy, as a user will perform a rehabilitation task and changing the level of resistance a user feels can motivate the user to use an impaired limb (Johnson et al. 2005). The motion of a robotic wheelchair can also be controlled by a user utilizing a tactile device such as a joystick (Yanco 1998). Visual exchanges refer to communicating information that can be perceived with the eyes, such as pointing gestures and emotional expressions, or pictures, videos, and written words. For example, a combination of facial expressions and gestures can be used to communicate a socially assistive robot's affective intent (Figure 2.1) (McColl, Louie, and Nejat 2013). Users with physical impairments can also use gestures to control a robot manipulator to perform activities of daily living (Gerlich et al. 2007).

In addition to the modes of interaction, HRI interfaces need to be designed such that they take into consideration social norms (e.g., using eye contact when speaking) and user preferences (e.g., comfortable communication distances). For example, studies have shown that increasing the social abilities (e.g., eye contact, nodding while speaking, facial expressions, expressive voice, and apologizing for making mistakes) of a robot can contribute to higher enjoyment and acceptance of the robot (Heerink et al. 2010). A robot providing verbal assistance to a user may also need to understand turn-taking in a conversation to follow human social convention and to make interactions with the user easier and more efficient (Chao and Thomaz 2010). Furthermore, practices in fields such as human-centered design can be used to develop HRI interfaces (Norman 2013). For example, human-centered design concepts such as ensuring that there is spatial correspondence between a device and the configuration of the input control of the device can make the user interface more intuitive and

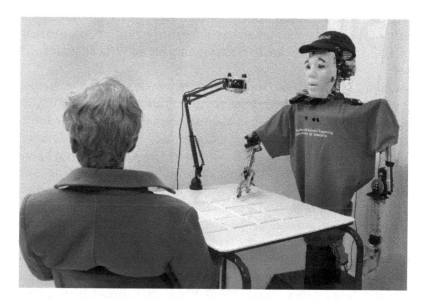

Figure 2.1 The robot Brian 2.1 with a sad facial expression while pointing at a card and requesting a user to flip it over during a memory card game. (© Autonomous Systems and Biomechatronics Lab.)

easy to use (e.g., control for a robot wheelchair going left should be placed on the left side of the user).

Interaction Structure

Interaction structures with rehabilitation robots can include: (1) a single robot interacting with a group of humans; (2) multiple robots interacting with one human; and (3) multiple robots interacting with multiple humans. An example of a *single-robot–multiple-users* scenario would be a socially assistive robot facilitating a cognitively stimulating recreational activity with a group of users (Figure 2.2) (Louie, Vaquero, Nejat, and Beck 2014). An example of a *multiple-robots–single-user* scenario is when multiple robot arms are used to move a user's upper and lower arm simultaneously to practice passive physiotherapy (Toth et al. 2005). With respect to multiple robots interacting with multiple humans, a planning and scheduling problem was introduced that involved multiple social robots interacting with residents in a retirement home environment to provide cognitively and socially stimulating activities, such as bingo

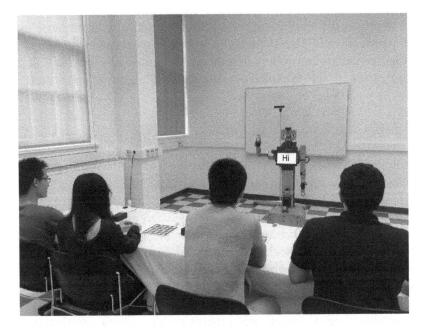

Figure 2.2   The socially assistive robot Tangy facilitating a bingo game with a group of users. (© Autonomous Systems and Biomechatronics Lab.)

and telepresence sessions, throughout the day (Vaquero, Nejat, and Beck 2014).

The interaction structure used directly influences such HRI design decisions as: (1) how many robots should be involved in the overall interaction; (2) what role robots should play during the rehabilitation interaction (i.e., mediator between a therapist and patient or facilitator of the therapy itself); and (3) given conflicts between robot and user, who makes the final decision (i.e., if a robotic wheelchair user wants to drive forward but the robot perceives a dangerous obstacle ahead).

Adaptation, Training, and Learning

Adaptation, training, and learning need to occur on the side of both the robot and the human for rehabilitation robots to be effectively used. For example, a robotic system can adapt and learn the behaviors it needs to interact with a person to improve **engagement** in cognitive training activities (Chan and Nejat 2012). Learning and adaptation have also been used to improve cognitive outcomes in these types of activities by adapting the level of difficulty of the activity to a user's performance (Tapus, Ţăpuş, and Matarić 2009). Similarly, users often need to learn how to use rehabilitation robots as the majority of them, at least initially, will be novice users (Huttenrauch and Eklundh 2002). In some cases, humans will even adapt to their rehabilitation robots despite an unnatural user interface design because they are able to exploit consistent control signals (Jiang et al. 2014).

Aesthetics

Rehabilitation robots are collocated with their users, allowing for proximate interactions (i.e., robot and human interacting in the same location). Due to these proximate interactions and the intended population of interest, physical features of rehabilitation robots often play an important role in the overall acceptance of such systems. For example, healthy adult users prefer a human-like robot for socially assistive tasks, such as exercise instruction (Goetz, Kiesler, and Powers 2003). Alternatively, children with autism are more accepting of interacting with a robot that has no facial features over a human-like robot (Robins, Dautenhahn, and Dubowski 2006). In the case of wearable physical rehabilitation robots such as robotic prosthetics, it is important for such systems to conform to human-like characteristics to be accepted by the intended users (Dellon and Matsuoka 2007).

Length of Exposure

The intended user's length of exposure to a rehabilitation robot has been shown to have varying effects on the HRI. For example, the novelty effect (Kanda and Ishiguro 2013) can be observed: users are excited to interact with the robot at first; however, over time they lose interest, which affect the moods of the users (Wada et al. 2002) and ultimately lead to the user no longer interacting with the robot (Kanda et al. 2004). This, of course, is disconcerting as the user will no longer receive the benefits associated with using these robots. Therefore, it is necessary to consider the interaction time length in the robot design and to investigate the efficacy of rehabilitation robots over long-term studies to ensure that rehabilitation intervention outcomes are not a result of the novelty of the technology.

HRI Metrics

In this section, we define metrics that have been used for HRI in rehabilitation robotics as well as commonly used measures for these metrics. These HRI metrics include: (1) perceptions, attitudes, and acceptance; (2) engagement; (3) compliance; and (4) safety. A summary of these HRI metrics and their associated measures is presented in Table 2.2.

Perceptions, Attitudes, and Acceptance

Overall perceptions and attitudes toward using a robot are a major factors in determining acceptance and use (Davis 1993). To determine if rehabilitation robots will be effective **tools**, we must measure user perceptions and attitudes toward them. Questionnaires are a method of data collection commonly used for measuring user perceptions, attitudes, and acceptance toward robotic rehabilitation technology as they allow researchers to easily gather large amounts of data (Bartneck, Kulic et al. 2009; Heerink et al. 2010). To date, only a handful of questionnaires have been tailored and validated for studying HRI in rehabilitation robotics. These questionnaires include: (1) the Godspeed questionnaire (Bartneck, Kulic et al. 2009); (2) the Almere model (Heerink et al. 2010); (3) the Intrinsic Motivation Inventory (IMI; Ryan 1982); (4) the NASA Task Load Index (NASA-TLX) questionnaire (Hart and Staveland 1988); and (5) the Self-Assessment Manikin (SAM) questionnaire (Bradley and Lang 1994). These questionnaires measure user perceptions toward specific robot characteristics and/or

TABLE 2.2   Summary of HRI Metrics and Measures

Measure	Description
Metric: Perceptions, Attitudes, and Acceptance	
Godspeed questionnaire	Questionnaire to measure a user's overall perceptions of rehabilitation robots
Almere model	Questionnaire to measure an elderly user's acceptance toward socially assistive robots
Intrinsic Motivation Inventory	Questionnaire used to evaluate a user's motivation level when interacting with a robot
NASA-TLX questionnaire	Questionnaire used to assess a user's physical and cognitive workload when operating a robot
Self-Assessment Manikin	Questionnaire used to assess a user's affective reaction when interacting with a robot
Metric: Engagement	
Eye gaze	User's eye gaze toward the robot or the activity itself
Utterances	Number of instances a user verbally communicates with a robot or another person during the interaction
Metric: Compliance	
Cooperative behaviors	Number of cooperative behaviors a user has with respect to a robot's behaviors
Task duration	Total time a user participates in a rehabilitation task
Metric: Safety	
Current measures for safety have not yet been generlized. Presently, they are designed specifically for the activity at hand. Please refer to the Customized Questionnaires category of this section for practical examples of designing for safety.	

functions. Many HRI studies have also used questionnaires designed or customized by the robot designers as they need to study specific user perceptions, demographics, and applications (Kang et al. 2005; Krebs et al. 1998; Tapus, Matarić, and Scassellati 2007).

Godspeed Questionnaire

The Godspeed questionnaire (Bartneck, Kulic et al. 2009) is a Likert scale-based questionnaire used to measure users' overall perceptions of rehabilitation robots. The Godspeed questionnaire categorizes perception using the following: (1) anthropomorphism; (2) animacy; (3) likability; (4) perceived intelligence; and (5) perceived safety. Anthropomorphism refers to attributing human form, human characteristics, and human behaviors to nonhuman agents (Bartneck, Kulic et al. 2009; Duffy 2003; Epley, Waytz, and Cacioppo 2007). The anthropomorphic design aims to allow people to relate to and rationalize with a robot and its behaviors with greater ease (Duffy 2003). Animacy refers to a user attributing lifelike properties to an entity (Bartneck, Kulic et al. 2009). It has been shown that animacy can create deep emotional involvement for the user, and such involvement can be used by the robot to influence users in the desired way (Bartneck, Kulic et al. 2009). Likability is defined as developing positive impressions of a robot (Bartneck, Kulic et al. 2009). For example, visual and vocal behaviors have an impact on likability and lead to evaluations that are more positive (Bartneck, Kulic et al. 2009). Perceived intelligence is defined as the robot's ability to adapt its behaviors to varying situations (Bartneck, Kanda et al. 2009). Perceived safety is a user's perception of the level of danger when interacting with a robot and the user's level of comfort during the interaction (Bartneck, Kulic et al. 2009). If a user feels at risk of being seriously or fatally harmed, the individual will not use the robotic system, regardless of whether the robot is actually harmful (Bartneck, Kulic et al. 2009). Therefore, the robot's appearance, behaviors, and interactions must be designed in a manner that will allow the users to create positive expectations of their safety and comfort. Furthermore, for continual use, these safety expectations must be met by the robot during interaction. User perceptions of robots used for home assistance for the elderly (Cuijpers et al. 2011) to physical rehabilitation for stroke survivors (Shirzad and Van der Loos 2015) have been obtained using the Godspeed questionnaire.

Almere Model

The Almere model (Heerink et al. 2010) is a Likert scale-based questionnaire designed primarily to measure elderly users' acceptance toward socially assistive robots. The questionnaire focuses on the following 12 constructs: (1) anxiety; (2) attitude toward technology; (3) facilitating conditions; (4) intention to use; (5) perceived adaptiveness; (6) perceived enjoyment; (7) perceived ease of use; (8) perceived sociability; (9) perceived usefulness; (10) social influence; (11) social presence; and (12) trust. Anxiety refers to a user's feeling of unease when interacting with a robot. Attitude toward technology refers to a user's positive or negative feelings toward the robot. Facilitating conditions refer to factors in the environment that facilitate the use of the system (e.g., being trained to use a robot). A user's intent to use the robot over a period of time is defined as intention to use. Perceived adaptability is the perceived ability of the robot to adapt to the needs of the user. Perceived enjoyment refers to a user's feelings of pleasure associated with the use of the robot. The degree to which a user believes that he or she can use a robot without effort is defined as ease of use. Perceived sociability refers to the perceived ability of the robot to perform appropriate social behaviors. Perceived usefulness refers to the degree that a user believes a robot would be assistive. A user's perception that their social network would want or not want them to use the system is defined as social influence. Social presence refers to the user's experience of sensing a social entity when interacting with the robot. Last, trust refers to the user's belief that the robot behaves with integrity and reliability. The Almere model has been used for measuring attitudes and acceptance toward: (1) animal-like robots for companionship (Heerink et al. 2010); (2) human-like socially assistive robots to assist with activities of daily living (McColl, Louie, and Nejat 2013; Louie, McColl, and Nejat 2014); and (3) telepresence robots to provide a medium for communication with family and caregivers (Bevilacqua et al. 2014).

Intrinsic Motivation Inventory

The IMI (Ryan 1982) is a questionnaire used to evaluate a user's motivation level when interacting with a robot. This questionnaire determines motivation based on: (1) interest/enjoyment; (2) perceived competence; (3) effort/importance; (4) pressure/tensions; (5) perceived choice; (6) value/usefulness; and (7) relatedness. Answers are provided on a scale of 1 (not at all true) to 7 (very true). Interest and enjoyment are used to determine if the activity kept the user's attention and whether it was fun or boring. Perceived competence is how skilled the user believes he or she is at the activity, as well as how satisfied the user was with his or her performance. Effort and importance define how hard the user tried to accomplish the task, as well as how important the user considered the task. Pressure/tension is how nervous and anxious the user felt while performing the task. Perceived choice is the level of self-determination the user felt when choosing to do the activity. Value/usefulness is how beneficial the user thought the activity was to them, as well as to others. Relatedness is a combination of: (1) how much the user trusted the robot; (2) how much the user desired to interact with the robot; and (3) how friendly the person thought the robot was. The IMI has been used primarily in studies that involve the use of physical rehabilitation robotic systems in which the users play video games (Burke et al. 2010; Colombo et al. 2007; Novak et al. 2014). The main goal in the inclusion of video games is usually to increase the user's motivation for the therapy.

NASA Task Load Index

The NASA-TLX tool (Hart and Staveland 1988) is designed to assess physical and cognitive workload. The NASA-TLX consists of users performing a pairwise comparison of workload factors, as well as giving a rating to each factor individually. The results from the pairwise comparison in conjunction with the individual ratings are used to produce an overall score for the workload. Workload is defined as a hypothetical construct that represents the cost incurred by a human operator to achieve a particular level of performance. The questionnaire divides workload into six factors: (1) mental demand; (2) physical demand; (3) temporal demand; (4) performance; (5) effort; and (6) frustration level. Mental demand is defined as the amount of mental and perceptual activity required (e.g., easy/demanding, simple/complex, and exacting/forgiving). Physical demand is the amount of physical activity required (e.g., easy/demanding, slow/brisk, slack/strenuous, and restful/laborious). How much time pressure was felt due to the pace of the task is defined as temporal demand (e.g., slow and leisurely/rapid and frantic). Performance is how successful the user believed he or she was in accomplishing the task goals (e.g., self-satisfaction). Effort is how hard the user had to work to accomplish the level of performance, and frustration level is how frustrated the user felt during the task (e.g., insecure/secure, irritated/relaxed, and stressed/content). The NASA-TLX tool is most commonly used for rehabilitation applications involving exoskeletons, as these tasks tend to be extremely stressful and demanding on users (Schiele 2009; Zimmerli et al. 2012); furthermore, the questionnaire has also been used with other, nonwearable, robotic systems (Chen and Kemp 2010; Shirzad and Van der Loos 2015).

Self-Assessment Manikin Questionnaire
The SAM questionnaire (Bradley and Lang 1994) is a pictorial assessment technique for measuring a person's affective reaction when interacting with a robot. The questionnaire models affect as three categories: (1) pleasure; (2) arousal; and (3) dominance. Each category consists of pictures of a character figure drawing expressing different levels of the corresponding affect. The user rates each category by circling the picture that best depicts the way the user feels, or the user may choose to circle in between two pictures. This gives the user an option to rate all three categories on a scale from 1 to 5. The SAM questionnaire has been used in assessing user affect with respect to a **lower limb exoskeleton** used to assist a user in walking (Koenig et al. 2011) and a robotic manipulandum used for reaching exercises (Shirzad and Van der Loos 2015).

Customized Questionnaires
Customized questionnaires using Likert scales are often designed by HRI researchers to measure a user's perceptions toward a specific HRI topic

that has not been covered by the aforementioned questionnaires or to combine constructs from these questionnaires with new constructs they have defined. For example, perceptions of users toward the Pioneer 2-DX mobile robot were measured for monitoring, assisting, and encouraging users during poststroke rehabilitation exercises (Tapus, Matarić, and Scassellati 2007). A Likert scale questionnaire was developed to determine if users thought the robot's character was unsociable and whether they thought the robot's personality was a lot like their own. User perceptions were measured for the mobile robot Clara performing cardiac physical therapy exercises (Kang et al. 2005). Namely, users were asked to fill out a Likert scale questionnaire that investigated if the robot was helpful, enjoyable, likable, and useful for spirometry exercises.

User tolerance was measured for the MIT-MANUS robot arm physically assisting stroke patients in completing goals within a video game (Krebs et al. 1998). The robot was able to move, guide, or perturb the movement of a stroke patient's upper limb. In this study, a questionnaire was developed that asked users to answer questions on a scale from 0 (strongly disagree) to 7 (strongly agree). The questionnaire was used to measure users' comfort levels, enjoyment of the therapy, perceived usefulness of the session, perceived value of the robot, and future intent to use the robot.

Engagement

Engagement in the context of robots can be defined as the process by which a human user establishes, maintains, and ends his or her perceived connection with the robot itself or the task (Castellano et al. 2012). User engagement is important to the success of robot rehabilitation therapy as users who are not engaged will not directly benefit from the therapy programs. User engagement during HRI can be measured by eye gaze direction and/or the number of utterances toward the robot. The duration of eye gaze toward the robot or the assistive activity itself is often used as a measure of a user's engagement (McColl, Louie, and Nejat 2013). For socially assistive robots, the number of utterances, defined as the number of instances that a user verbally communicates with the robot or another person during the interaction, is another metric often used to determine engagement of users (Feil-Seifer and Matarić 2008; McColl and Nejat 2013). For physical rehabilitation robots, engagement has been measured using a 5-point Likert scale where the user responded to multiple questions about his or her enjoyment, perceived productivity, perceived engagement, and perceived boredom (English and Howard 2014).

Compliance

Compliance has been defined as the extent to which a person's behavior coincides with medical advice (Melnikow and Kiefe 1994). Compliance is important as it will positively affect the health efficacy of the rehabilitation interventions (Rosenstock 1975). As such, compliance is a common metric utilized to measure the effectiveness of HRI (Steinfeld et al. 2006). Compliance can be measured by observing the number of cooperative behaviors a user performs with respect to a robot's behaviors (McColl, Louie, and Nejat 2013) and the total time a user participates in a rehabilitation task (Colombo et al. 2007; Matarić et al. 2007).

Safety

When designing rehabilitation robots, the user's safety is a high priority. For robots that engage in physical HRI, where the robot is constantly in contact with an impaired user, safety is an important metric incorporated in the design of the robot. To address this, safety protocols and standards have been applied from other fields, such as industrial robotics (Furusho et al. 2005). In many HRI studies with physical rehabilitation robots, safety considerations are taken by limiting robots' physical capabilities, for example, limiting range of motion, velocity, acceleration, and torque of the motors (Fleischer et al. 2009; Gopura and Kiguchi 2009; Klein et al. 2010; Morales et al. 2011). Another commonly used safety feature is to have emergency stop switches/buttons on the robot (Culmer et al. 2010; Dovat et al. 2008; Gassert et al. 2006). It is desired that the user is capable of activating one of these switches/buttons for psychological comfort as well as to prevent harm in case of great physical discomfort. In addition, it is considered advantageous in terms of user comfort to have a lightweight system when developing wearable robots (Junius et al. 2013; Van der Linde and Lammertse 2003).

With the use of wheelchairs, safety features are considered specifically to prevent collisions and increase user comfort by providing full control to the wheelchair in potentially dangerous situations (Jain and Argall 2014; Lopes, Pires, and Nunes 2013; Taha, Miro, and Dissanayake 2008). These safety features include: (1) if the user moves toward a wall or an obstacle, automatically slowing or stopping (Alonso-Mora et al. 2014; Mandel, Huebner, and Vierhuff 2005; Urdiales et al. 2013) or planning a safe trajectory to follow (Carlson and Demiris 2012); and (2) providing navigation assistance in difficult-to-navigate situations, such as driving through doorways (Derry and Argall 2013; Wang and Liu 2014), narrow corridors (Wang and Liu 2014), and crowded rooms (Lin and Song 2014; Pires et al. 1998; Wang and Liu 2014).

Safety considerations for robotic manipulators placed on wheelchairs are mainly used to protect the user from being hit by the manipulator (Schrock et al. 2009; Shiomi et al. 2015). These safety features include: (1) scaling down the motions of the user when controlling the manipulator (Alqasemi and Dubey 2007); (2) automatically stopping the manipulator if an impending collision is detected (Palankar et al. 2009); and (3) providing the user control to modify the course of ongoing movements and stop the system if there is uncertainty (Buhler et al. 1995; Song, Lee, and Bien 1999; Van der Loos et al. 1999).

With respect to robotic prosthetic limbs, safety considerations are taken to primarily prevent injury to a user (Dedic and Dindo 2011; Hargrove et al. 2013). Such safety features include: (1) using compliant actuators as they can absorb large forces due to shocks (Hitt et al. 2009; Junius et al. 2013); (2) providing smooth, slow, and safe corrective movements from large positional errors to return the user to the correct trajectory during trajectory tracking (Junius et al. 2013); and (3) limiting the range of motion of prosthetic joints (Bellman, Holgate, and Sugar 2008).

In 2014, the International Organization for Standardization (ISO) released international standards defining safety requirements for personal care robots. These are briefly reviewed in Chapter 1.

Discussion

The most commonly utilized metric for both social and physical HRIs are the perceptions, attitudes, and acceptance of the users toward the rehabilitation robotic technology. This is the most important metric because for robots to be effectively used in rehabilitation interventions, they must be accepted and adopted by the intended population. The most popular method to measure this metric has been to use either standard or customized questionnaires for the specific rehabilitation scenario. This is often because questionnaires are a fast way to gather large samples of user perceptions and perspectives toward new technology. In addition, user engagement and compliance during robot-assisted rehabilitation tasks have been used as metrics. The majority of user engagement measures for social HRI focus on observing eye gaze direction toward a robot and task, as well as verbal utterances toward the robot. **User compliance** measures include the number of cooperative behaviors a user performs with respect to a robot's behaviors and the total time a user participates in a rehabilitation task.

Review of User Studies, Outcomes, and Clinical Evidence

Human–robot interaction in rehabilitation robotics can be divided into two main categories based on the modes of interaction between the human and robot (Feil-Seifer and Matarić 2005; Fong, Nourbakhsh, and Dautenhahn 2003): social HRI and physical HRI. Rehabilitation robots engaged in social HRI focus on providing assistance through social interactions (e.g., conversation, gestures, and establishing social relationships), whereas rehabilitation robots engaged in physical HRI assist using physical contact (e.g., moving a person or object from location to location, moving a limb, or exerting forces on impaired limbs). Social HRI robots are discussed in detail in Chapters 8 and 9. Physical HRI robots are discussed in Chapters 3 to 7. In the subsequent sections, we discuss the literature with respect to these two HRI categories. We discuss and evaluate HRI principles and metrics for different rehabilitation robotic applications to highlight which characteristics have been effective in designing for HRI.

Social HRI

Level of Autonomy

One main motivation for social HRI is often to assist in minimizing the overload of health care staff by using robots to assist in facilitating, prompting, instructing, monitoring, motivating, and engaging individuals in various rehabilitation activities (Tapus, Matarić, and Scassellati 2007). Ideally, a social HRI system requires no expert operator or extensive training of the user (Feil-Seifer and Matarić 2005). The majority of social HRI research focuses on the design of *fully autonomous* systems to perform rehabilitation tasks for older adults and children with autism (Chan and Nejat 2012; Dautenhahn and Werry 2002; Hansen, Bak, and Risager 2012; Louie et al. 2014; Louie, Despond, and Nejat 2015; Tapus, Ţăpuş, and Matarić 2009).

Dautenhahn and Werry (2002) are the only researchers who have investigated the effects of the level of autonomy of a robot on social HRI. They studied the influence of autonomy on the engagement of children with autism. Children with autism were given the opportunity to interact with a noninteractive toy truck and the autonomous mobile robot Labo-1, which was similar in appearance to the truck. The autonomous robot was programmed to avoid obstacles, follow children, and generate speech during following (robot follows child) or chasing (child follows robot) games. Child eye gaze from videos taken of the interactions were coded to determine their engagement toward the toy and the robot. Results of the study showed that the duration of eye gaze toward the autonomous robot was greater than toward the passive toy.

HRI Interface and Types of Information Exchange

There are two important dimensions to address when designing an HRI interface for a robot taking part in social HRI: the modes of interaction and the personality of the robot. A robot's modes of interaction are the individual means in which a robot communicates its intentions, and a robot's personality defines how a robot acts under different conditions utilizing the different modes of communication.

The mobile robot Pearl was designed to motivate older adult users during exercise routines (Goetz and Kiesler 2002). A study was conducted to investigate the effect the personality of the robot had on user compliance with the robot's advice, as well as user perceptions of the robot. Healthy adult participants either interacted with a robot displaying playful behaviors or interacted with a robot displaying serious behaviors during an exercise activity. Participants were led by Pearl (with either personality) through a series of breathing and stretching routines and were then asked by the robot to make up their own routine. The participants then rated the robot's personality using a customized questionnaire that measured user perceptions of robot agreeableness, conscientiousness, extraversion, neuroticism, openness to new experiences, and intellect. Compliance was also measured during postinteraction analysis of video-recorded interactions to determine how long users performed their routine. For both personality conditions, the robot was found to be extraverted, agreeable, and conscientious. The playful robot was rated more positively than the serious robot. Perceptions of intellect decreased over trials (personality had no effect). Overall, participants complied more with the serious robot.

The humanoid Nao robot was designed to provide in-home social assistance, such as notifications and reminders to older adults (Cuijpers et al. 2011). The robot provided notifications and reminders for: (1) phone calls; (2) medical emergencies; and (3) physical exercises. The influence of the approach behavior of the robot on user perceptions was investigated. Healthy adult participants were provided the notifications and reminders used by Nao using three different approach behaviors: (1) the robot followed a participant; (2) the robot intercepted a participant as the participant was walking; and (3) the robot went to a participant's anticipated destination and waited for the participant. After the participants interacted with the Nao robot, they completed the Godspeed questionnaire to measure their perceptions of the robot for each of the approach conditions under the different contexts. Results showed that approach behavior did not affect participants' perceptions on the animacy, anthropomorphism, perceived intelligence, perceived safety, likability, and appropriateness of the robot.

A study with older adults at a retirement home was conducted to investigate user perceptions toward different modes of interaction with the robot exercise coach Bandit (Figure 2.3) (Fasola and Matarić 2011). Older adults interacted with both the virtual (i.e., a simulation of the robot) and the physically embodied robot during exercise sessions. After participants interacted with both types of the robot, they completed a customized questionnaire that investigated their perceptions of enjoyment, usefulness, helpfulness, and social presence. Results of the study showed that,

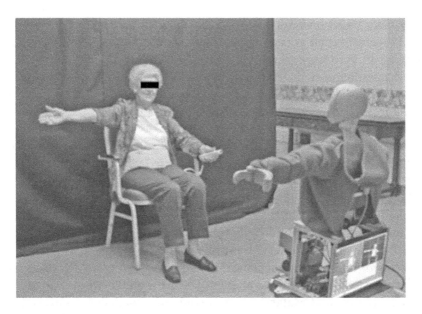

Figure 2.3 Bandit coaching an older adult through an exercise session. (From Fasola, J., and Matarić, M. J. 2013. Socially assistive robot exercise coach: Motivating older adults to engage in physical exercise. *Experimental Robotics*, 88: 463–479. © Springer.)

overall, the older adults preferred interacting with the physically embodied robot over the virtual robot and found it more enjoyable, useful, and helpful. Furthermore, the participants felt a greater sense of social presence toward the physical robot than the virtual robot.

Adaptation, Training, and Learning

Adaptation, training, and learning have been incorporated into social robots designed for use by older adults to improve user acceptance (Sheba et al. 2012), moods (Wada et al. 2003), enjoyment (Fasola and Matarić 2010), and rehabilitation task performance (Chan and Nejat 2012; Tapus, Ţăpuş, and Matarić 2009). A handful of these studies explicitly investigated the effects adapting robot behaviors and task difficulty as well as providing user training on a robot had on the HRI metrics for older adult users (Fasola and Matarić 2010; Sheba et al. 2012; Wada et al. 2003).

The seal-like robot Paro's adaptive behaviors were investigated to determine if they improved user moods and interest during animal-assisted therapy (Wada et al. 2003). For three weeks, healthy older adult participants from a health service facility either interacted with a placebo Paro that executed defined simple motions or an intelligent Paro that learned robot behaviors that were preferred by the older adults (i.e., adapting its behaviors based on positive reinforcement such as stroking or negative reinforcement such as beating provided by older adults). Familiarity and interest in Paro were measured once a week with a short 5-point Likert scale questionnaire. In addition, moods of older adults were measured using the Profile of Mood States (POMS) questionnaire and a self-reported scale from 1 to 20 (1 being most positive and 20 being most negative) before and after interacting with Paro for three weeks. Results of the study showed that older adults who interacted with the placebo Paro did not lose interest in the robot while those who interacted with the intelligent Paro lost interest in the robot. The researchers postulated that the reason older adults lost interest in the intelligent Paro was because its reactions were unpredictable.

The anthropomorphic mobile robot Bandit (Figure 2.3) was designed to adapt the difficulty of a button-pressing memory game to improve user enjoyment and task performance during physical therapy for poststoke rehabilitation and cognitive therapy for older adults with Alzheimer's disease (Fasola and Matarić 2010). A study was conducted to investigate the effects adapting game difficulty had on user enjoyment, frustration, and task performance. University students participated in the button-pressing memory game facilitated by the robot under two different conditions: (1) the robot did not explicitly motivate the participant to improve performance on the task and increased the difficulty level of the game at a constant rate; and (2) the robot praised the participant for completing a task and adapted the difficulty level of the game based on user performance. After participating in the games, participants were asked to rank the robot conditions based on enjoyableness, frustration, and challenge and were asked questions on whether the robot conditions improved motivation. Results of the study showed that participants found the constantly increasing difficulty condition more frustrating and challenging. Furthermore, user enjoyment was highly correlated with participant performance.

A dog-like therapeutic robot ERIC was used to study acceptance of the robot after older adults were trained on it (Sheba et al. 2012). Older adult participants with cognitive impairments interacted with the robot during physiotherapy training before and after being trained on the robot's capabilities by one of the researchers. The acceptance score was then calculated by determining: (1) the time to initiate interaction with the robot by a participant; (2) total time a participant interacted with a robot during a session; (3) time needed for the robot to react to environment states; and (4) total number of erroneous behaviors exhibited by the robot during the interaction. Results showed that when users were trained on the robot's capabilities before they interacted with it, they had higher acceptance.

Aesthetics
The aesthetics of a socially assistive robot play a key role in its assistive effectiveness (Tapus, Matarić, and Scassellati 2007). This is because people will often attribute intentions, goals, emotions, and personalities to simple machines with life-like movements or form, which in turn can affect how humans interact with such robotic systems (Reeves and Nass 1996). Studies have already demonstrated that modifying the aesthetics (e.g., human-likeness and face shape) of a socially assistive robot can affect users' desire to interact with the robot (DiSalvo et al. 2002; Goetz, Kiesler, and Powers 2003; Robins, Dautenhahn, and Dubowski 2006; Zhang et al. 2010).

Different robot appearances were investigated to study what types of appearances encouraged interactions between a child with autism and a robot (Robins, Dautenhahn, and Dubowski 2006). Children with autism were provided with an opportunity to interact with the following: (1) a 45-cm tall doll with "pretty" girls' clothing and a detailed human-like face; (2) the same doll with a plain and robotic appearance; (3) a life-size plain and featureless "robot" that was a mime artist behaving as a robot; and (4) a robot with human-like appearance (i.e., the mime artist himself). The children's interactions with the robots were coded for eye gaze (directed at the robot), touch (touching the robot), imitation behavior (imitation of robot movements), and proximity (approaching the robot and staying close to the robot). Results of the study showed that the children gazed, touched, and moved closer to the plain and featureless life-size robot than the life-size human-like robot. They also socially interacted more with the plain-looking life-size robot and ignored the life-size human-like robot. Similar findings occurred with the small humanoid doll: children showed preference for interaction with the robot with a plain and robotic appearance over the doll with pretty clothing.

A study with older adult participants from a retirement home was conducted with a PeopleBot robot to investigate the participants' perceptions and attitudes regarding the facial features of a medicine delivery robot (Zhang et al. 2010). The robot had one of three different anthropomorphic features when delivering medicine to the participants: a simple face mask with cameras for eyes (Figure 2.4), voice capabilities via a speech synthesizer, or a touch display for user interactivity. Participant perceptions of the robot features were measured using a customized perceived anthropomorphism questionnaire, and participant emotional

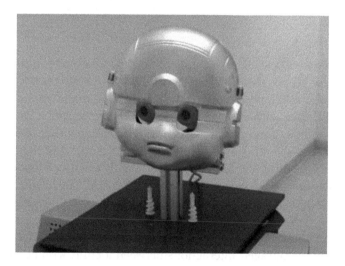

Figure 2.4 Human-like face configuration for the PeopleBot robot with a simple face mask and cameras for eyes. (From Zhang, T., Kaber, D. B., Zhu, B., Swangnetr, M., Mosaly, P., and Hodge, L. 2010. Service robot feature design effects on user perceptions and emotional responses. *Intelligent Service Robotics*, 3(2): 73–88. © Springer.)

responses were measured using the SAM questionnaire. Results of the study showed that human-like features such as a face and voice promoted positive emotional responses based on the SAM questionnaire. Furthermore, when features became more human-like, user perceptions of anthropomorphism increased based on the perceived anthropomorphism questionnaire.

Facial features of the Pearl robot that contributed to perceptions of human-likeness were investigated (DiSalvo et al. 2002). Participants were presented with 48 images of different robot heads and were asked to rate each head on a scale from 1 (not very human-like) to 5 (very human-like). Each robot head was categorized based on the presence of eyes, ears, nose, mouth, eyelids, eyebrows, height/width ratio of the face, percentage of various facial regions (forehead, chin, and other facial features) size of the eyes, distance between the eyes, and width of the mouth. Statistical analysis was then performed to identify the relationship between participant perceptions of robot human-likeness and the robot facial features. Results showed that the presence of eyelids, nose, and mouth increased the perceptions of human-likeness the most. The total number of facial features also increased perceptions of human-likeness. Furthermore, the larger the ratio between the width and height of the robot head, the less human-like it was perceived.

Length of Exposure

Social HRI is a new emerging field with limited studies conducted to date on investigating the length of exposure to a robot. Currently, only Wada et al. (2002) has studied the effects of this principle; older adults' moods were measured during experiments performed with the Paro robot. Older adult participants with and without dementia interacted with Paro over a 5-week period. A questionnaire modified from the POMS questionnaire was administered to the participants each week before and after the interactions with Paro to measure any changes in moods. Furthermore, the number of times the older adults touched or spoke to the robot were counted during postinteraction analysis of the video-recorded interactions, and comments from nursing staff were gathered utilizing open-ended questions regarding the interactions. Results of the study showed that participants spoke more to Paro and touched it for longer periods of time in the fifth week compared to the second week. However, in the fifth week, older adults' moods did not improve as much (baseline was moods measured at the start of the week) as in the second week after interacting with Paro.

Physical HRI

Level of Autonomy

The main motivation for robots undertaking physical HRI is to help users restore normal functionality to their limbs and to assist users with the completion of activities of daily living using technologies such as wheelchairs, assistive manipulators, and prosthetics (Maciejasz et al. 2014). From the therapist's point of view, rehabilitation robots should be designed to be as autonomous as possible to minimize the time the therapist needs to dedicate to each session and user. From the user's point of view, a robot's level of autonomy should vary with the user's recovery stage, and the robot should avoid providing too much assistance. A user's initiative has been shown to significantly improve recovery results by restoring and developing the neurological ability to coordinate the correct muscle groups in performing an action (Maciejasz et al. 2014). In addition, implicit learning tends to be important in improving recovery time, and overly instructing or aiding a user may cause reduced recovery results due to reduced patient attention (Patton, Smal, and Rymer 2008). There needs to be a balance between the user and robot autonomy levels. This is done to maintain the user's motivation and involvement in the activity without putting too much workload on the user, thus maintaining a high level of ease of use and comfort.

Dijkers et al. (1991) explored patient and staff acceptance of a robotic arm autonomously performing occupational therapy as an aide to a therapist in treating elderly stroke patients. The robotic arm autonomously moved to various locations and gave a seated participant a short period of time to reach and touch a pad attached to the robot's **end-effector** before moving to the next location. The participants were then asked to fill out a customized questionnaire asking the following: (1) Did you like this treatment? (2) Did you feel it was helpful? (3) Was this boring? and (4) Was it confusing to use? The study also showed that participants were displeased in its inability to adapt the difficulty level of the rehabilitation to participants with higher levels of **mobility**.

Colombo et al. (2007) examined the correlation between autonomy and patient motivation measures in robotic rehabilitation for stroke patients with upper limb impairments. The study examined the effect of robotic intervention by an arm exoskeleton (Chapter 6) on user experience. Two exoskeleton arms were used: (1) a 1 degree of freedom (DOF) wrist actuator; and (2) a 2-DOF elbow-shoulder actuators (Figure 2.5). Each robot was used with a participant who had the corresponding impairments. All participants were required to perform trajectory following with their

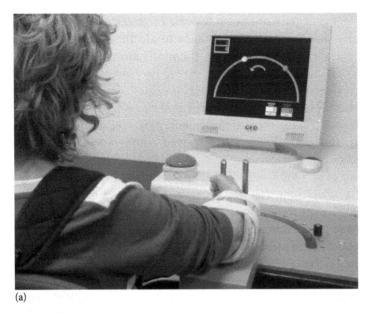

(a)

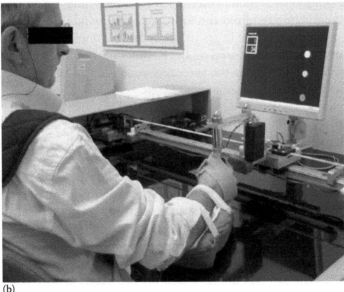

(b)

Figure 2.5 Stroke patients performing arm rehabilitation tasks with robot exoskeleton arms that have (a) a 1-DOF wrist actuator or (b) a 2-DOF elbow-shoulder actuator. (From Colombo, R., Pisano, F., Mazzone, A., Delconte, C., Micera, S., Carrozza, M. C., Dario, P., and Minuco, G. 2007. Design strategies to improve patient motivation during robot-aided rehabilitation. *Journal of Neuroengineering and Rehabilitation*, 4(3): 1–12.)

robot. If a participant did not actively try to track the trajectory, the robot would increase the level of assistance to aid the participant. After completing each session with a robot, the motivation of each participant was evaluated using the IMI questionnaire to measure: (1) interest/enjoyment; (2) perceived competence; (3) effort; (4) value/usefulness; and (5) pressure and tension. The less autonomy provided by each robotic arm, the higher the ratings were for interest/enjoyment, perceived usefulness, and effort; however, they were lower for perceived competence, and pressure and tension.

Parikh et al. (2005) explored the usability of different levels of autonomy of a wheelchair. Healthy participants entered navigation goals into the wheelchair through a visual interface and performed navigation tasks using three different control modes: (1) manual; (2) semiautonomous; and (3) autonomous (Parikh et al. 2004). The control modes were evaluated based on: (1) the task completion time; (2) the number of user commands; (3) a cognitive complexity rating based on answering math questions; and (4) the NASA-TLX questionnaire. Participants completed the task fastest with the autonomous mode and slowest with the semiautonomous mode. The manual mode required the most user commands. The autonomous mode performed the best in terms of cognitive complexity, and the other modes did equally well. Based on the NASA-TLX results, participants felt less in control when using the autonomous mode and felt it was easier to use the wheelchair as autonomy increased.

Carlson and Demiris (2012) compared a manual and semiautonomous joystick-controlled wheelchair in terms of ease of use and user safety. Healthy participants used the wheelchair to drive in two different modes in an office: (1) manual; and (2) semiautonomous. The following measurements were used: (1) the completion time; (2) the number of collisions; (3) the reaction time in responding to a personal computer (PC) tablet, which periodically lit up, by clicking on the screen; and (4) a customized ease-of-use questionnaire. The manual mode resulted in a shorter mean completion time and had more collisions. The participants also responded slower to the tablet using the manual mode compared to the semiautonomous mode. Based on the questionnaire results, the semiautonomous mode made maneuvering easier and it was easier to use while performing the PC tablet reaction task; it required less concentration to drive than in the manual mode. However, the semiautonomous mode conformed less to participant expectations and felt less natural than the manual mode.

Tsui and Yanco (2007) investigated the effects of level of autonomy on ease of use and user acceptance of an autonomous robotic arm mounted on a wheelchair. Healthy participants moved the robotic arm to where they considered it to be "sufficiently close" to a desired object using two techniques: (1) manually controlling the robotic arm with a joystick; and (2) using a joystick to select the object location on a visual display for the robotic arm to autonomously move to the corresponding location. The following measurements were used to determine ease of use and user acceptance: (1) task completion time; (2) number of failures; (3) distance the arm stopped from the object; and (4) number of clicks executed. Using manual control, the participants took more joystick inputs and longer to finish the task, had fewer failures and a greater degree of arm accuracy compared to the second technique. Participants completed a customized likability questionnaire, and the results showed more participants preferred the manual control due to increased accuracy.

HRI Interface and Types of Information Exchange
Numerous types of HRI interfaces and types of information exchange have been studied in physical HRI. The studies discussed below have focused on how different interaction modes affected user acceptance, effort, and motivation.

The haptic force feedback glove MRAGES, developed to provide robotic poststroke therapy, was investigated to determine user acceptance (Winter and Bouzit 2007). The glove was attached to a robotic arm exoskeleton. To use the robot, the participant inserted his or her right arm into the exoskeleton and the right hand into the glove. Healthy adults participated in a study to measure participants' ability to feel distinctive differences in force feedback levels, as well as their acceptance of the robotic system. In the study, a force level was exerted through the glove, and the participant was asked to identify and compare the force with previous applied forces. A customized comfort level questionnaire was administered using a 5-point scale and yes/no responses. The questions and their corresponding results were as follows: (1) user comfort level ($\mu = 3.7$); (2) appropriateness of force level ($\mu = 3.7$); (3) usability of the exoskeleton and glove ($\mu = 4.4$); (4) adequacy of finger workspace (100% yes rate); (5) constriction of finger motion (71% yes rate); and (6) constriction of arm workspace (0% yes rate). The glove performed well for comfort and appropriateness of the force and did well for usability. The majority of users reported the workspace was adequate and did not constrain their movements.

Adams and David (2013) developed a Lego car robot for children with **cerebral palsy** in wheelchairs. The children performed measurement tasks using three different techniques: (1) controlling the Lego robot attached with a ruler and pen; (2) explaining to a teacher the steps required to perform the task; and (3) directing the teacher to physically perform the task. The measurement tasks performed were drawing and measuring a line, and measuring the length of a shape (e.g., a parallelogram). Teachers not involved in the study rated each of the three techniques by answering the question: How well does the participant portray his or her level of understanding about the concept being discussed (answered using a 5-point Likert scale)? On average, teachers rated that participants portrayed greater understanding when using the Lego robot than with the other two techniques.

A new user interface for the MANUS robotic arm, which attaches to a wheelchair and is controlled by a joypad, was investigated to determine the physical and cognitive load experienced by wheelchair users with impaired upper limbs (Tijsma, Liefhebber, and Herder 2005a). Studies examined two different control input techniques. The first technique had the participant use a double flick-up motion with the joypad to select the menu on a screen mounted on the wheelchair (Tijsma, Liefhebber, and Herder 2005b). Once the menu was selected, the participant used the joypad to select one of four modes: (1) drinking mode; (2) folding mode; (3) joint mode; or (4) Cartesian mode. Depending on the selected mode, the robotic arm would move accordingly when given an input from the joypad. In the second technique, the menu could be selected with only a single flick, and the mode could be set with a single flick. The two techniques were studied by having healthy adults perform a series of tasks. During the study, the number of mode switches was recorded. After the study, the Rating Scale of Mental Effort (RSME) questionnaire was administered to participants; questions were asked to assess the amount of mental effort the participants exerted. The results showed that the new interface feature had better functionality and usability than the old interface, had a significantly reduced number of joypad flicks required to complete each task, and scored better on the RSME, signifying lower cognitive and physical load.

Min et al. (2002) compared using a head-mounted interface with a shoulder-mounted interface for controlling a wheelchair in terms of ease of use, user acceptance, and user safety. Participants drove the wheelchair through a corridor. Task completion time and number of collisions were measured. On average, participants finished the task more quickly with the shoulder interface, and both techniques had the same number of collisions. In a customized user satisfaction questionnaire, participants ranked the head interface as more satisfying in terms of wearability and design, and less satisfying in terms of workload and accuracy than the shoulder interface.

Tsui et al. (2008) studied the effect of using different interfaces for controlling a wheelchair-mounted arm on user acceptance and ease of use. Participants selected a target object for the arm to grip using four different interfaces: (1) touching the desired object on a touch screen; (2) moving a cursor to the desired object's location on a visual display using a joystick and then pressing a button to confirm selection; (3) using directional buttons on the touch screen to center the image frame on the desired object and then pressing a button to confirm selection; and (4) using a joystick to center the image frame on the desired object on a visual display and then pressing a button to confirm selection. The object selection time was measured, and the authors provided their own rating of attentiveness and the need for prompting. On average, touching the desired object on the touch screen was fastest in terms of object selection time, and moving a cursor to the desired object's location on a visual display using a joystick was the slowest in terms of object selection time. On average, the authors rated that using a joystick to center the image frame on the desired object on a visual display had the highest attentiveness level, and moving a cursor to the desired object's location on a visual display had the lowest attentiveness level. The authors ranked using directional buttons on the touch screen to center the image frame on the desired object as needing the most prompting, and touching the desired object on a touch screen as needing the least prompting. Results from a customized user likability questionnaire showed that the participants most liked moving a cursor to the desired object's location on a visual display using a joystick, and least liked using a joystick to center the image frame on the desired object on a visual display.

Shiomi et al. (2015) studied the influence of social interactions in autonomous wheelchairs on perceived ease of use, perceived enjoyment, and user attitudes. Elderly participants used a wheelchair with different navigation techniques: (1) a simple technique that moved at a medium speed with no social behaviors; (2) a social technique that greeted the participant, talked about the location (e.g., "We are about to navigate in a narrow hallway"), introduced the location (e.g., "We are entering the dining room"), and set its speed to a preferred speed of either low, medium, or high based on the participant's preference as acquired before the experiment; and (3) a caregiver pushing the wheelchair at a medium speed and discussing the locations the same as in technique 2. After using the three types of techniques, participants completed a questionnaire and rated the social technique as the easiest to use and to make a request with, and the most enjoyable. The social technique and caregiver technique both ranked highest in terms of comfort.

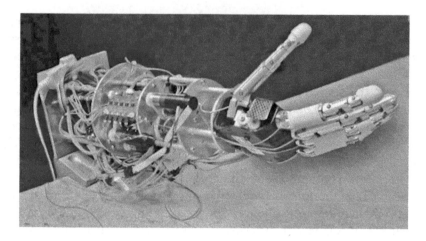

Figure 2.6 Robotic hand prosthesis, Pisa-hand. (From Rosen, B., Ehrsson, H. H., Antfolk, C., Cipriani, C., Sebelius, F., and Lundborg, G. 2009. Referral of sensation to an advanced humanoid robotic hand prosthesis. *Scandinavian Journal of Plastic and Reconstructive Surgery and Hand Surgery*, 43(5): 260–266. © Taylor & Francis.)

Rosen et al. (2009) investigated sensor transfer for a robotic prosthetic hand (Figure 2.6). A finger on the prosthetic hand was brushed at the same time as a participant's stump. In the experiments, only the prosthetic hand was visible to the participants. In a questionnaire adapted from the work of Botvinick and Cohen (1998), the participants positively rated the following statements regarding sensor transfer: (1) I felt the touch of the brush on the prosthesis; (2) it seemed that the brush on the prosthesis generated the touch I felt; and (3) I felt as if the prosthesis was my hand.

Marasco et al. (2011) developed a sensory feedback interface for linking a prosthetic arm to the cutaneous sensory nerves of a missing limb. The prosthetic arm worn by participants was touched by a person, and haptic feedback was provided to the reinnervated nerve endings on the residual limb to propagate the touching sensation. The same questionnaire was used as in the work of Rosen et al. (2009). The results were positive for each question.

Adaptation, Training, and Learning
For physical HRI scenarios, rehabilitation robots can adapt to a user to improve user comfort (Kawamoto and Sankai 2002), as well as user recovery (Shirzad and Van der Loos 2015). Kawamoto and Sankai (2002) studied the effects of different types of control methods for adapting a user's impaired gait to a healthy gait during walking rehabilitation. The study was

conducted with a healthy adult using the Hybrid Assistive Leg 3 (HAL-3) system, an electromyography-based lower limb exoskeleton that assists elderly and gait-impaired participants with walking. During the study, floor reaction force on the foot was used to measure discomfort. Three control techniques were tested while the participant was wearing the exoskeleton: (1) the participant walking without any assistance from the exoskeleton; (2) the participant walking with physical assistance from the exoskeleton to reduce the participant's physical effort; and (3) the participant walking with physical assistance from the exoskeleton where the exoskeleton adapted the participant's gait to account for real-time floor reaction force (FRF) measurements. It was shown that the third technique, which directly accounted for the FRF, reduced the participant's discomfort more than the other two techniques.

Shirzad and Van der Loos (2015) studied the effects of machine learning techniques on the acceptance of a robotic manipulandum for stroke patients. A participant manipulated the robotic end-effector to move a shape on a screen to a specified location. The robot introduced different levels of error between the motion of the gripper and the motion of the shape to adjust the level of difficulty of the therapy. A therapy session comprised several training blocks; each training block specified a difficulty level as well as a destination for the shape. Healthy participants were divided into two groups. One group received training blocks based on a machine learning technique trained to select difficulty levels that were challenging for the user, but still within the user's capabilities. The other group received training blocks of random difficulty levels. The techniques were evaluated by measuring the participant's experience and motivation. The SAM questionnaire was administered to the participants, as was a customized postexperiment questionnaire that combined questions from the NASA-TLX, the Godspeed questionnaire, and the User Engagement Scale. The SAM questionnaire focused on participant task satisfaction and attractiveness throughout the duration of the therapy. The customized questionnaire measured: (1) mental demand; (2) physical demand; (3) task performance; (4) perceived effort; (5) frustration; (6) usefulness; (7) dominance; (8) engagement; (9) willingness to continue; (10) motivation; (11) satisfaction; and (12) attentiveness. The results showed that participant engagement improved when performing exercises at an optimal difficulty level as determined by the machine learning technique. It was also shown that engagement during the exercise can increase the amount of time spent actively participating in the therapy and hence improve overall therapy recovery speed and recovery amount.

Zondervan et al. (2015) studied the use of video games in improving training of a user in controlling a wheelchair with a joystick. Therapists used a training method in which new users played video games with the joystick to teach them to use a wheelchair. The video games were played at a stationary monitor or with an onboard laptop attached to their wheelchair (Figure 2.7a). The therapists compared this training technique with their traditional training technique of having the user drive the wheelchair around (Figure 2.7b). The two techniques were evaluated by the therapists using a questionnaire in which they rated: (1) dimensions; (2) weight; (3) ease in adjusting; (4) safety; (5) durability; (6) ease of use; (7) comfort; and (8) effectiveness. The video game technique was rated higher in terms of ease in adjusting, safety, durability, comfort, and effectiveness and lower in terms of weight than the traditional technique. Both techniques were rated equally in terms of dimensions and ease of use.

Morales et al. (2013) studied the effect of different wheelchair navigation techniques on user comfort. Healthy participants sat in a wheelchair as it navigated through a corridor using two navigation techniques: (1) a comfortable path algorithm based on the user's preferred velocity and safety distance from walls; and (2) a shortest-path algorithm. In a customized questionnaire, participants rated the two trajectories in terms

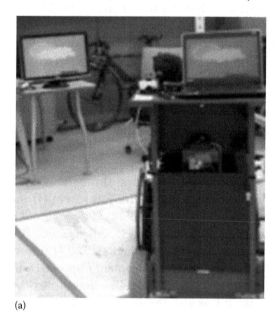

(a)

Figure 2.7 Participant training with video games using a stationary monitor (a).

(Continued)

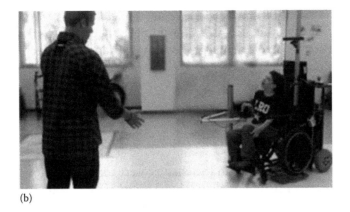

(b)

Figure 2.7 (Continued) Participant training with the traditional training technique of driving a wheelchair around (b). (From Zondervan, D. K., Secoli, R., Darling, A. M., Farris, J., Furumasu, J., and Reinkensmeyer, D. J. 2015. Design and evaluation of the Kinect-Wheelchair Interface Controlled (KWIC) **smart wheelchair** for pediatric powered mobility training. *Assistive Technology,* 27(3): 183–192. © Taylor & Francis.)

of comfort. The results verified that the comfortable trajectory was rated more comfortable than the shortest-path trajectory.

Sawabe et al. (2015) developed a velocity control technique for a fully autonomous wheelchair. The velocity control technique adjusted the velocity of the wheelchair based on behavior-dependent observability (BDO), where BDO was defined as the ratio between the visible and the traversable area. Healthy participants sat in a wheelchair as it navigated a corridor using four different control modes: (1) constant velocity with no BDO control; (2) maintaining BDO above 60%; (3) maintaining BDO above 80%; and (4) maintaining BDO above 90%. The measurement used to determine the participant's stress level was the ratio of low-frequency heart rates to high-frequency heart rates (LF/HF). It was shown that increased use of BDO, on average, resulted in a reduction in the participant's measured stress level during the navigation.

Length of Exposure
For physical HRI scenarios, length of exposure influences the user's overall experience. Kronreif et al. (2007) studied how varying duration of interaction affects ease of use of a remote-controlled pick-and-place robot, PlayROB. Children used PlayROB to play with Lego blocks in a specified area. The following measures were used: (1) duration of playing session; (2) number of Lego blocks used; (3) number of different types of Lego blocks used; (4) time required for Lego block placement (blocks/min);

and (5) utilization of the area (%). It was found that, as session duration increased, there was an increase in the number of Lego blocks used, a more uniform distribution of each Lego block type being used, a decrease in the number of Lego blocks placed per minute, and an increase in utilization of the area.

Discussion

The HRI studies presented in the chapter were for a variety of rehabilitation scenarios consisting of physical and social HRI. One of the predominant themes for both social and physical HRI is that users expect robots to adapt the level of difficulty of the rehabilitation task to their own specific capabilities. This adaptation is important for improving user engagement as well as user perceptions in terms of enjoyment and usefulness. For social HRI, the aesthetics of a robot influenced user acceptance and perceptions of a robot, but the particular desired features were dependent on the intended user population. HRI design in rehabilitation robots has focused on specific application areas or a demographically specific group. Therefore, conclusions cannot be easily generalized; currently, there is still no general consensus on the best HRI practices.

Future Directions

Human–robot interaction for rehabilitation robotics is an emerging field and research to date has primarily focused on the incorporation of HRI principles within the design of the robotic systems themselves. With respect to length of exposure, mainly short-term studies have been conducted. One of the important future directions for social and physical HRI will be to investigate the impact of long-term exposure and use of rehabilitation robots.

Currently, the majority of robots are implemented in one-on-one interaction scenarios. Therefore, the incorporation of these robotic systems in different interaction structures to maximize their use should also be investigated, including teams of multiple robots working together to simultaneously provide rehabilitation care to multiple users; multiple robots working together with therapists to provide care to individual or groups of users; and a robot independently providing care to multiple users at the same time. Consequently, it will be necessary to investigate the effective design of such interaction structures.

Most of the currently available research has focused on the development of rehabilitation robots targeted toward specific user groups without aiming for general consensus regarding the best practices to implement HRI principles. Therefore, significantly more research is needed to create such a body of knowledge.

STUDY QUESTIONS

1. Which existing research area did HRI branch from?
2. What are the two main goals of applying HRI to rehabilitation robots?
3. What two types of HRI do rehabilitation robots engage in?
4. Name and define each of the six HRI design principles.
5. Name the three modalities used for HRI interfaces.
6. Which HRI metrics have been used in social HRI scenarios with rehabilitation robots? In physical HRI scenarios?
7. When should the Godspeed questionnaire be used instead of the Almere model?
8. What is the NASA-TLX used for?
9. What is the difference between engagement and compliance?
10. Name and describe the two measures used to determine engagement.
11. Name and describe the two measures used to determine compliance.
12. Explain an HRI study with respect to the design principles and metrics used.
13. What physical features on a robot have children with autism preferred?
14. Excessive amounts of assistance from physical rehabilitation robots can cause what effect?
15. List four safety considerations for robotic wheelchairs.

References

Adams, J. A. 2002. Critical considerations for human–robot interface development. *Proceedings of the AAAI Fall Symposium*, November 3, 1–8.

Adams, K., and David, B. L. 2013. Methods of manipulation for children with severe disabilities to do hands-on math activities: Robot, directing, guiding. Presented at the RESNA Conference, Bellevue, WA, June 20–24, 1–4.

Alonso-Mora, J., Gohl, P., Watson, S., Siegwart, R., and Beardsley, P. 2014. Shared control of autonomous vehicles based on velocity space optimization. *IEEE International Conference in Robotics and Automation (ICRA)*, May 31–June 7, 1639–1645.

Alqasemi, R., and Dubey, R. 2007. Maximizing manipulation capabilities for people with disabilities using a 9-DOF wheelchair-mounted robotic arm system. *IEEE International Conference in Rehabilitation Robotics*, June 13–15, 212–221.

Bartneck, C., Kanda, T., Mubin, O., and Al Mahmud, A. 2009. Does the design of a robot influence its animacy and perceived intelligence? *International Journal of Social Robotics*, 1(2): 195–204.

Bartneck, C., Kulic, D., Croft, E., and Zoghbi, S. 2009. Measurement instruments for the anthropomorphism, animacy, likeability, perceived intelligence, and perceived safety of robots. *International Journal of Social Robotics*, 1(1): 71–81.

Beer, J., Fisk, A. D., and Rogers, W. A. 2014. Toward a framework for levels of robot autonomy in human–robot interaction. *Journal of Human–Robot Interaction*, 3(2): 74–99.

Bellman, R. D., Holgate, M. A., and Sugar, T. G. 2008. SPARKy 3: Design of an active robotic ankle prosthesis with two actuated degrees of freedom using regenerative kinetics. *IEEE/RAS/EMBS International Conference in Biomedical Robotics and Biomechatronics*, October 19–22, 511–516.

Bevilacqua, R., Cesta, A., Cortellessa, G., Macchione, A., Orlandini, A., and Tiberio, L. May 2014. Telepresence robot at home: A long-term case study. *Ambient Assisted Living*, 73–85.

Birch, G. E. 1993. Development and methodology for the formal evaluation of the Neil Squire Foundation robotic-assistive appliance. *Robotica*, 11(6): 529–534.

Botvinick, M., and Cohen, J. 1998. Rubber hands "feel" touch that eyes see. *Nature*, 391(6669): 756.

Bradley, M. M., and Lang, P. J. 1994. Measuring emotion: The self-assessment manikin and the semantic differential. *Journal of Behavior Therapy and Experimental Psychiatry*, 25(1): 49–59.

Buhler, C., Hoelper, R., Hoyer, H., and Humann, W. 1995. Autonomous robot technology for advanced wheelchair and robotic aids for people with disabilities. *Robotics and Autonomous Systems*, 14(2): 213–222.

Burke, J. L., Murphy, R. R., Rogers, E., Lumelsky, V. J., and Scholtz, J. 2004. Final report for the DARPA/NSF interdisciplinary study on human–robot interaction. *IEEE Transactions on Systems, Man, and Cybernetics, Part C (Applications and Reviews)*, 34(2): 103–112.

Burke, J. W., McNeill, M. D. J., Charles, D. K., Morrow, P. J., Crosbie, J. H., and McDonough, S. M. 2010. Designing engaging, playable games for rehabilitation. *Proceedings of the 8th International Conference on Disability, Virtual Reality and Associated Technologies*, Vina del Mar/Valparaiso, Chile, August 31–September 2, 195–201.

Carlson, T., and Demiris, Y. 2012. Collaborative control for a robotic wheelchair: Evaluation of performance, attention, and workload. *IEEE Transactions on Systems, Man, and Cybernetics, Part B: Cybernetics*, 42(3): 876–888.

Castellano, G., Leite, I., Pereira, A., Martinho, C., Paiva, A., and McOwan, P. W. 2012. Detecting engagement in HRI: An exploration of social and task-based context. *ASE/IEEE International Conference on Social Computing and ASE/IEEE International Conference on Privacy, Security, Risk and Trust*, September 3–5, 421–428.

Chan, J., and Nejat, G. 2012. Social intelligence for a robot engaging people in cognitive training activities. *International Journal of Advanced Robotic Systems*, 9(1): 1–13.

Chao, C., and Thomaz, A. L. 2010. Turn taking for human–robot interaction. *AAAI Fall Symposium: Dialog with Robots*, November 11–13, 132–134.

Chen, S., Kazi, Z., Foulds, R., and Chester, D. 1994. Multi-modal direction of a robot by individuals with a significant disability. *Proceedings of the 4th International Conference on Rehabilitation Robotics*, June 14–16, 55–64.

Chen, T. L., and Kemp, C. C. 2010. Lead me by the hand: Evaluation of a direct physical interface for nursing assistant robots. *Proceedings of the 5th ACM/ IEEE International Conference on Human–Robot Interaction*, March 2–5, 367–374.

Colombo, R., Pisano, F., Mazzone, A., Delconte, C., Micera, S., Carrozza, M. C., Dario, P. et al. 2007. Design strategies to improve patient motivation during robot-aided rehabilitation. *Journal of Neuroengineering and Rehabilitation*, 4(3): 1–12.

Cuijpers, R. H., Bruna, M. T., Ham, J. R. C., and Torta, E. 2011. Attitude towards robots depends on interaction but not on anticipatory behaviour. *Proceedings of the International Conference on Social Robotics*, 7072(1): 163–172.

Culmer, P. R., Jackson, A. E., Makower, S., Richardson, R., Cozens, J. A., Levesley, M. C., and Bhakta, B. B. 2010. A control strategy for upper limb robotic rehabilitation with a dual robot system. *IEEE/ASME Transactions on Mechatronics*, 14(4): 575–585.

Dautenhahn, K., and Werry, I. 2002. A quantitative technique for analysing robot-human interactions. *IEEE International Conference on Intelligent Robots and Systems*, 2: 1132–1138.

Davis, F. D. 1993. User acceptance of information technology: System characteristics, user perceptions and behavioral impacts. *International Journal of Man-Machine Studies*, 38(3): 475–487.

Dedic, R., and Dindo, H. 2011. SmartLeg: An intelligent active robotic prosthesis for lower-limb amputees. *IEEE International Symposium in Information, Communication and Automation Technologies (ICAT)*, October, 1–7.

Dellon, B., and Matsuoka, Y. 2007. Prosthetics, exoskeletons, and rehabilitation. *IEEE Robotics and Automation Magazine*, 14(1): 30–34.

Derry, M., and Argall, B. 2013. Automated doorway detection for assistive shared-control wheelchairs. *IEEE International Conference in Robotics and Automation (ICRA)*, May 6–10, 1254–1259.

Dijkers, M. P., deBear, P. C., Erlandson, R. F., Kristy, K., Geer, D. M., and Nichols, A. 1991. Patient and staff acceptance of robotic technology in occupational therapy: A pilot study. *Journal of Rehabilitation Research and Development*, 28(2): 33–44.

DiSalvo, C. F., Gemperle, F., Forlizzi, J., and Kiesler, S. 2002. All robots are not created equal: The design and perception of humanoid robot heads. *ACM Conference on Designing Interactive Systems: Processes, Practices, Methods, and Techniques*, 321–326. doi:http://dx.doi.org/10.1145/778712.778756.

Dovat, L., Lambercy, O., Gassert, R., Maeder, T., Milner, T., Leong, T. C., and Burdet, E. 2008. HandCARE: A cable-actuated rehabilitation system to train hand function after stroke. *IEEE Transactions on Neural Systems and Rehabilitation Engineering*, 16(6): 582–591.

Duffy, B. R. 2003. Anthropomorphism and the social robot. *Robotics and Autonomous Systems*, 42(3): 177–190.

English, B. A., and Howard, A. M. 2014. Engagement study of an integrated rehabilitation robotic tablet-based gaming system. *IEEE Workshop on Advanced Robotics and Its Social Impacts (ARSO)*, September 11–13, 14–19.

Epley, N., Waytz, A., and Cacioppo, J. T. 2007. On seeing human: A three-factor theory of anthropomorphism. *Psychological Review*, 114(4): 864–886.

Fasola, J., and Matarić, M. 2010. Robot motivator: Increasing user enjoyment and performance on a physical/cognitive task. *IEEE International Conference on Development and Learning*, August 18–21, 274–279.

Fasola, J., and Matarić, M. 2011. *Comparing Physical and Virtual Embodiment in a Socially Assistive Robot Exercise Coach for the Elderly*. Los Angeles: Center for Robotics and Embedded Systems, Technical Report CRES-11-00.

Fasola, J., and Matarić, M. J. 2013. Socially assistive robot exercise coach: Motivating older adults to engage in physical exercise. *Experimental Robotics*, 88: 463–479.

Feil-Seifer, D., and Matarić, M. J. 2005. Defining socially assistive robotics. *International Conference on Rehabilitation Robotics*, July, 465–468.

Feil-Seifer, D., and Matarić, M. 2008. Robot-assisted therapy for children with autism spectrum disorders. *Proceedings of the 7th International Conference on Interaction Design and Children*, 49–52. doi:http://dx.doi.org/10.1145/1463689.1463716.

Fleischer, C., Kondak, K., Wege, A., and Kossyk, I. 2009. Research on exoskeletons at the TU Berlin. In *Advances in Robotics Research*, T. Kroger and F. M. Wahl, eds. Berlin: Springer-Verlag, 335–346.

Fong, T., Nourbakhsh, I., and Dautenhahn, K. 2003. A survey of socially interactive robots. *Robotics and Autonomous Systems*, 42(3): 143–166.

Furusho, J., Koyanagi, K., Imada, Y., Fujii, Y., Nakanishi, K., Domen, K., Miyakoshi, K. et al. 2005. A 3-D rehabilitation system for upper limbs developed in a 5-year NEDO project and its clinical testing. *IEEE International Conference on Rehabilitation Robotics (ICORR)*, June 28–July 1, 53–56.

Gassert, R., Dovat, L., Lambercy, O., Ruffieux, Y., Chapuis, D., Ganesh, G., Burdet, E. et al. 2006. A 2-DOF fMRI compatible haptic interface to investigate the neural control of arm movements. *Proceedings of the IEEE International Conference on Robotics and Automation*, June, 3825–3831.

Gerlich, L., Parsons, B. N., White, A. S., Prior, S., and Warner, P. 2007. Gesture recognition for control of rehabilitation robots. *Cognition, Technology, & Work*, 9(4): 189–207.

Goetz, J., and Kiesler, S. 2002. Cooperation with a robotic assistant. *ACM Extended Abstracts on Human Factors in Computing Systems*, April 20–25, 578–579.

Goetz, J., Kiesler, S., and Powers, A. 2003. Matching robot appearance and behavior to tasks to improve human–robot cooperation. *Proceedings of the 12th IEEE International Workshop on Robot and Human Interactive Communication (ROMAN)*, October 31–November 2, 55–60.

Goodrich, M. A., and Schultz, A. C. 2007. Human–robot interaction: A survey. *Foundations and Trends in Human-Computer Interaction*, 1(3): 203–275.

Gopura, R. A. R. C., and Kiguchi, K. 2009. Mechanical designs of active upper-limb exoskeleton robots: State-of-the-art and design difficulties. *IEEE International Conference on Rehabilitation Robotics (ICORR)*, July, 178–187.

Hansen, S. T., Bak, T., and Risager, C. 2012. An adaptive game algorithm for an autonomous, mobile robot—A real world study with elderly users. *IEEE International Symposium on Robot and Human Interactive Communication*, September 9–13, 892–897.

Hargrove, L. J., Simon, A. M., Young, A. J., Lipschutz, R. D., Finucane, S. B., Smith, D. G., and Kuiken, T. A. 2013. Robotic leg control with EMG decoding in an amputee with nerve transfers. *The New England Journal of Medicine*, 369(13): 1237–1242.

Hart, S. G., and Staveland, L. E. 1988. Development of NASA-TLX (Task Load Index): Results of empirical and theoretical research. *Advances in Psychology*, 52(1): 139–183.

Heerink, M., Kröse, B., Evers, V., and Wielinga, B. 2010. Assessing acceptance of assistive social agent technology by older adults: The Almere model. *International Journal of Social Robotics*, 2(4): 361–375.

Hitt, J., Sugar, T., Holgate, M., Bellman, R., and Hollander, K. 2009. Robotic transtibial prosthesis with biomechanical energy regeneration. *Industrial Robot*, 36(5): 441–447.

Huttenrauch, H., and Eklundh, K. S. 2002. Fetch-and-carry with CERO: Observations from a long-term user study with a service robot. *Proceedings of 11th IEEE International Workshop on Robot and Human Interactive Communication*, September 27, 158–163.

Jain, S., and Argall, B. 2014. Automated perception of safe docking locations with alignment information for assistive wheelchairs. *IEEE/RSJ International Conference in Intelligent Robots and Systems (IROS)*, September 14–18, 4997–5002.

Jiang, N., Vujaklija, I., Rehbaum, H., Graimann, B., and Farina, D. 2014. Is accurate mapping of EMG signals on kinematics needed for precise online myoelectric control? *IEEE Transactions on Neural Systems and Rehabilitation Engineering*, 22(3): 549–558.

Johnson, M. J., Van der Loos, H. M., Burgar, C. G., Shor, P., and Leifer L. J. 2005. Experimental results using force-feedback cueing in robot-assisted stroke therapy. *IEEE Transactions on Neural Systems and Rehabilitation Engineering*, 13(3): 335–348.

Junius, K., Cherelle, P., Brackx, B., Geeroms, J., Schepers, T., Vanderborght, B., and Lefeber, D. 2013. On the use of adaptable compliant actuators in prosthetics, rehabilitation and assistive robotics. *IEEE Workshop in Robot Motion and Control (RoMoCo)*, July 3–5, 1–6.

Kanda, T., and Ishiguro, H. 2013. Novelty effect. *Human–Robot Interaction in Social Robotics*, 49–50.

Kanda, T., Hirano, T., Eaton, D., and Ishiguro, H. 2004. Interactive robots as social partners and peer tutors for children: A field trial. *Journal of Human-Computer Interaction*, 19(1): 61–84.

Kang, K. I., Freedman, S., Matarić, M. J., Cunningham, M. J., and Lopez, B. 2005. A hands-off physical therapy assistance robot for cardiac patients. *IEEE International Conference on Rehabilitation Robotics (ICORR)*, June 28–July 1, 337–340.

Kawamoto, H., and Sankai, Y. 2002. Comfortable power assist control method for walking aid by HAL-3. *IEEE International Conference on Systems, Man and Cybernetics*, 4(6): 1–6.

Klein, J., Spencer, S., Allington, J., Bobrow, J. E., and Reinkensmeyer, D. J. 2010. Optimization of a parallel shoulder mechanism to achieve a high-force, low-mass, robotic arm exoskeleton. *IEEE Transactions on Robotics*, 26(4): 710–715.

Koenig, A., Omlin, X., Zimmerli, L., Sapa, M., and Krewer, C. 2011. Psychological state estimation from physiological recordings during robot-assisted gait rehabilitation. *Journal of Rehabilitation Research and Development*, 48(4): 367–385.

Krebs, H. I., Hogan, N., Aisen, M. L., and Volpe, B. T. 1998. Robot-aided neurorehabilitation. *IEEE Transactions on Rehabilitation Engineering*, 6(1): 75–87.

Kronreif, G., Prazak, B., Kornfeld, M., Hochgatterer, A., and Furst, M. 2007. Robot assistant "PlayROB"—User trials and results. *IEEE International Workshop on Robot and Human Interactive Communication (ROMAN)*, August 26–29, 113–117.

Lin, M., and Song, K. 2014. Design and experimental study of a shared-controlled omnidirectional mobile platform. *IEEE International Conference in System, Man and Cybernetics (SMC)*, October 5–8, 3579–3584.

Lopes, A. C., Pires, G., and Nunes, U. 2013. Assisted navigation for a brain-actuated intelligent wheelchair. *Robotics and Autonomous Systems*, 61(3): 245–258.

Louie, W. G., Despond, F., and Nejat, G. 2015. Social robot learning from demonstration to facilitate a group activity for older adults. *IEEE International Conference on Intelligent Robots and Systems Workshop on Bridging User Needs to Deployed Applications of Service Robots*, September 28–October 3, 1–6.

Louie, W. G., McColl, D., and Nejat, G. 2014. Acceptance and attitudes toward a humanlike socially assistive robot by older adults. *Assistive Technology*, 26(3): 140–150.

Louie, W. G., Li, J., Vaquero, T., and Nejat, G. 2014. A focus group study on the design considerations and impressions of a socially assistive robot for long-term care. *IEEE International Symposium on Robot and Human Interactive Communication (RO-MAN)*, August 25–29, 237–242.

Louie, W. G., Vaquero, T., Nejat, G., and Beck, J. C. 2014. An autonomous assistive robot for planning, scheduling and facilitating multi-user activities. *IEEE International Conference in Robotics and Automation (ICRA)*, May 31–June 7, 5292–5298.

Maciejasz, P., Eschweiler, J., Gerlach-Hahn, K., Jansen-Troy, A., and Leonhardt, S. 2014. A survey on robotic devices for upper limb rehabilitation. *Journal of Neuroengineering and Rehabilitation*, 11(3): 1–29.

Mandel, C., Huebner, K., and Vierhuff, T. 2005. Towards an autonomous wheelchair: Cognitive aspects in service robotics. *IEEE International Conference Towards Autonomous Robotic Systems (TAROS)*, September 12–14, 165–172.

Marasco, P. D., Kim, K., Colgate, J. E., Peshkin, M. A., and Kuiken, T. A. 2011. Robotic touch shifts perception of embodiment to a prosthesis in targeted reinnervation amputees. *Brain*, 134(3): 747–758.

Marchal-Crespo, L., and Reinkensmeyer, D. J. 2009. Review of control strategies for robotic movement training after neurologic injury. *Journal of Neuroengineering and Rehabilitation*, 6(20): 1–15.

Matarić, M. J., Eriksson, J., Feil-Seifer, D. J., and Winstein, C. J. 2007. Socially assistive robotics for post-stroke rehabilitation. *Journal of NeuroEngineering and Rehabilitation*, 4(5): 1–9.

McColl, D., Louie, W. G., and Nejat, G. 2013. Brian 2.1: A socially assistive robot for the elderly and cognitively impaired. *IEEE Robotics & Automation Magazine*, 20(1): 74–83.

McColl, D., and Nejat, G. 2013. Meal-time with a socially assistive robot and older adults at a long-term care facility. Special Issue on HRI System Studies, *Journal of Human Robot Interaction*, 2(1): 152–171.

Melnikow, J., and Kiefe, C. 1994. Patient compliance and medical research. *Journal of General Internal Medicine*, 9(2): 96–105.

Min, J., Lee, K., Lim, S., and Kwon, D. 2002. Human-friendly interfaces of wheelchair robotic system for handicapped persons. *IEEE/RSJ International Conference in Intelligent Robots and Systems (IROS)*, 2(1): 1505–1510.

Morales, R., Badesa, F. J., García-Aracil, N., Sabater, J. M., and Pérez-Vidal, C. 2011. Pneumatic robotic systems for upper limb rehabilitation. *Medical & Biological Engineering & Computing*, 49(1): 1145–1156.

Morales, Y., Kallakuri, N., Shinozawa, K., Miyashita, T., and Hagita, N. 2013. Human-comfortable navigation for an autonomous robotic wheelchair. *IEEE Conference in Intelligent Robots and Systems (IROS)*, November 3–7, 2737–2743.

Norman, D. A. 2013. *The Design of Everyday Things*. Revised and expanded ed. New York: Basic books.

Novak, D., Nagle, A., Keller, U., and Riener, R. 2014. Increasing motivation in robot-aided arm rehabilitation with competitive and cooperative gameplay. *Journal of Neuroengineering and Rehabilitation*, 11(64): 1–15.

Palankar, M., Laurentis, K. J., Alqasemi, R., Veras, E., Dubey, R., Arbel, Y., and Donchin, E. 2009. Control of a 9-DoF wheelchair-mounted robotic arm system using a P300 brain computer interface: Initial experiments. *IEEE International Conference in Robotics and Biomimetics*, February 22–25, 348–353.

Parikh, S. P., Grassi, V., Kumar, V., and Okamoto, J. 2004. Incorporating user inputs in motion planning for a smart wheelchair. *IEEE International Conference in Robotics and Automation (ICRA)*, April 26–May 1, 2043–2048.

Parikh, S. P., Grassi, V., Kumar, V., and Okamoto, J. 2005. Usability study of a control framework for an intelligent wheelchair. *IEEE International Conference in Robotics and Automation (ICRA)*, April 18–22, 4745–4750.

Patton, J., Smal, S. L., and Rymer, W. Z. 2008. Functional restoration for the stroke survivor: Informing the efforts of engineers. *Topics in Stroke Rehabilitation*, 15(6): 521–541.

Pires, G., Araujo, R., Nunes, U., and Almeida, A. T. 1998. RobChair—A powered wheelchair using a behaviour-based navigation. *IEEE International Workshop in Advanced Motion Control (AMC)*, January, 536–541.

Reeves, B., and Nass, C. 1996. *How People Treat Computers, Television, and New Media Like Real People and Places*. Stanford, CA: CSLI, and Cambridge, U.K.: Cambridge University Press, 19–36.

Robins, B., Dautenhahn, K., and Dubowski, J. 2006. Does appearance matter in the interaction of children with autism with a humanoid robot? *Interaction Studies*, 7(3), 509–542.

Rosati, G., Rodà, A., Avanzini, F., and Masiero, S. 2013. On the role of auditory feedback in robot-assisted movement training after stroke: Review of the literature. *Computational Intelligence and Neuroscience*, 1(11): 1–15.

Rosen, B., Ehrsson, H. H., Antfolk, C., Cipriani, C., Sebelius, F., and Lundborg, G. 2009. Referral of sensation to an advanced humanoid robotic hand prosthesis. *Scandinavian Journal of Plastic and Reconstructive Surgery and Hand Surgery*, 43(5): 260–266.

Rosenstock, I. M. 1975. Patients' compliance with health regimens. *Journal of the American Medical Association*, 234(4): 402–403.

Ryan, R. M. 1982. Control and information in the intrapersonal sphere: An extension of cognitive evaluation theory. *Journal of Personality and Social Psychology*, 43(3): 450–461.

Sawabe, T., Kanbara, M., Ukita, N., Ikeda, T., Saiki, L. Y. M., Watanabe, A., and Hagita, N. 2015. Comfortable autonomous navigation based on collision prediction in blind occluded regions. *IEEE International Conference in Vehicular Electronics and Safety (ICVES)*, November 5–7, 75–80.

Schiele, A. 2009. Ergonomics of exoskeletons: Subjective performance metrics. *IEEE/RSJ International Conference on Intelligent Robots and Systems*, October 10–15, 480–485.

Schrock, P., Farelo, F., Alqasemi, R., and Dubey, R. 2009. Design, simulation and testing of a new modular wheelchair mounted robotic arm to perform activities of daily living. *IEEE International Conference in Rehabilitation Robotics*, June 23–26, 518–523.

Sheba, J. K., Elora, M. R., and García, E. A. M. 2012. Easiness of acceptance metric for effective human robot interactions in therapeutic pet robots. *IEEE Conference on Industrial Electronics and Applications*, July 18–20, 150–155.

Sheridan, T. B. 1992. *Telerobotics, Automation, and Human Supervisory Control.* Cambridge, MA: MIT Press.

Sheridan, T. B., and Verplank, W. L. 1978. *Human and Computer Control of Undersea Teleoperators.* Cambridge, MA: Man-Machine Systems Laboratory, Massachusetts Institute of Technology.

Shiomi, M., Iio, T., Kamei, K., Sharma, C., and Hagita, N. 2015. Effectiveness of social behaviors for autonomous wheelchair robot to support elderly people in Japan. *PLoS One*, 10(5): 1–15.

Shirzad, N., and Van der Loos, H. F. 2015. Evaluating the user experience of exercising reaching motions with a robot that predicts desired movement difficulty. *Journal of Motor Behavior*, 48(1): 31–46.

Song, W., Lee, H., and Bien, Z. 1999. KARES: Intelligent wheelchair-mounted robotic arm system using vision and force sensor. *Robotics and Autonomous Systems*, 28(1): 83–94.

Steinfeld, A., Fong, T., Kaber, D., Lewis, M., Scholtz, J., Schultz, A., and Goodrich, M. 2006. Common metrics for human–robot interaction. *Proceedings of the 1st ACM SIGCHI/SIGART Conference on Human–Robot Interaction*, March 2–3, 33–40.

Taha, T., Miro, J., and Dissanayake, G. 2008. POMDP-based long-term user intention prediction for wheelchair navigation. *IEEE International Conference in Robotics and Automation (ICRA)*, June, 3920–3925.

Tapus, A., Matarić, M. J., and Scassellati, B. 2007. Socially assistive robotics [grand challenges of robotics]. *IEEE Robotics & Automation Magazine*, 14(1): 35–42.

Tapus, A., Țăpuș, C., and Matarić, M. J. 2009. The use of socially assistive robots in the design of intelligent cognitive therapies for people with dementia. *IEEE International Conference on Rehabilitation Robotics (ICORR)*, June 23–26, 924–929.

Tijsma, H. A., Liefhebber, F., and Herder, J. L. 2005a. Evaluation of new user interface features for the MANUS robot arm. *IEEE International Conference on Rehabilitation Robotics*, January, 258–263.

Tijsma, H. A., Liefhebber, F., and Herder, J. L. 2005b. A framework of interface improvements for designing new user interfaces for the MANUS robot arm. *IEEE International Conference on Rehabilitation Robotics*, January, 235–240.

Toth, A., Fazekas, G., Arz, G., Jurak, M., and Horvath, M. 2005. Passive robotic movement therapy of the spastic hemiparetic arm with REHAROB: Report of the first clinical test and the follow-up system improvement. *IEEE International Conference on Rehabilitation Robotics (ICORR)*, June 28–July 1, 127–130.

Tsui, K., and Yanco, H. A. 2007. Simplifying wheelchair mounted robotic arm control with a visual interface. *AAAI Spring Symposium: Multidisciplinary Collaboration for Socially Assistive Robotics*, January, 97–102.

Tsui, K., Yanco, H., Kontak, D., and Beliveau, L. 2008. Development and evaluation of a flexible interface for a wheelchair mounted robotic arm. *IEEE International Conference in Human Robot Interaction*, March 12–15, 105–112.

Urdiales, C., Perez, E. J., Peinado, G., Fdez-Carmona, M., Peula, J. M., Annicchiarico, R., Sandoval, F. et al. 2013. On the construction of a skill-based wheelchair navigation profile. *IEEE Transactions on Neural Systems and Rehabilitation Engineering*, 21(6): 917–927.

Vaquero, T., Nejat, G., and Beck, J. C. 2014. Planning and scheduling single and multi-person activities in retirement home settings for a group of robots. *Proceedings of the ICAPS Workshop on Planning and Robotics*, June 21–26, 1–10.

Van der Linde, R. Q., and Lammertse, P. 2003. HapticMaster—A generic force controlled robot for human interaction. *Industrial Robot*, 30(6): 515–524.

Van der Loos, H. F. M. 1995. VA/Stanford rehabilitation robotics research and development program: Lessons learned in the application of robotics technology to the field of rehabilitation. *IEEE Transactions on Rehabilitation Engineering*, 3(1): 46–55.

Van der Loos, H. F. M., Wagner, J. J., Smaby, N., Chang, K., Madrigal, O., Leifer, L. J., and Khatib, O. 1999. ProVAR assistive robot system architecture. *IEEE International Conference in Robotics and Automation*, 1(1): 741–746.

Volosyak, I., Ivlev, O., and Gräser, A. 2005. Rehabilitation Robot FRIEND II—The general concept and current implementation. *IEEE International Conference on Rehabilitation Robots*, June 28–July 1, 540–544.

Wada, K., Shibata, T., Saito, T., and Tanie, K. 2002. Analysis of factors that bring mental effects to elderly people in robot assisted activity. *IEEE/RSJ International Conference on Intelligent Robots and Systems*, 2(1): 1152–1157.

Wada, K., Shibata, T., Saito, T., and Tanie, K. 2003. Psychological and social effects of robot assisted activity to elderly people who stay at a health service facility for the aged. *IEEE International Conference on Robotics and Automation (ICRA)*, 3(1): 3996–4001.

Wang, H., and Liu, X. P. 2014. Adaptive shared control for a novel mobile assistive robot. *IEEE/ASME Transactions in Mechatronics*, 19(6): 1725–1736.

Winter, H., and Bouzit, M. 2007. Use of magnetorheological fluid in a force feedback glove. *IEEE Transactions on Neural Systems and Rehabilitation Engineering*, 15(1): 2–8.

Yanco, H. A. 1998. Wheelesley: A robotic wheelchair system: Indoor navigation and user interface. *Assistive Technology and Artificial Intelligence*, 1458: 256–268.

Zhang, T., Kaber, D. B., Zhu, B., Swangnetr, M., Mosaly, P., and Hodge, L. 2010. Service robot feature design effects on user perceptions and emotional responses. *Intelligent Service Robotics*, 3(2): 73–88.

Zimmerli, L., Krewer, C., Gassert, R., Müller, F., Riener, R., and Lünenburger, L. (2012). Validation of a mechanism to balance exercise difficulty in robot-assisted upper-extremity rehabilitation after stroke. *Journal of Neuroengineering and Rehabilitation*, 9(6): 1–13.

Zondervan, D. K., Secoli, R., Darling, A. M., Farris, J., Furumasu, J., and Reinkensmeyer, D. J. 2015. Design and evaluation of the Kinect-Wheelchair Interface Controlled (KWIC) smart wheelchair for pediatric powered mobility training. *Assistive Technology*, 27(3): 183–192.

3

Assistive Robotic Manipulators

Arthur Blom and Harry Stuyt

Contents

Learning Objectives

After completing this chapter, readers will be able to

1. Define an **assistive robotic manipulator** (ARM) and describe its differences for industrial and service robots.
2. Identify potential end users and the added value of an ARM.
3. Describe the basic requirements for an ARM in relation to the needs of potential end users.
4. Explain the functions of an ARM.
5. List possible uses of an ARM as an **augmentative manipulation** assistive technology.
6. List commercially available ARMs and their main features and limitations.

Principles of Assistive Robotic Manipulators

Working Definition of Assistive Robotic Arms

A robotic manipulator is a set of rigid links connected by actuated joints. The most common joints are revolute joints, allowing adjacent links to turn around them. The number of joints in a robotic manipulator usually determines the number of degrees of freedom (DOF) of the manipulator, that is, the number of independent variables that needs to be specified to locate all parts of the manipulator (Craig 2005). The higher the number of DOF, the higher the flexibility in positioning the end-effector of the manipulator (i.e., the device attached to the manipulator wrist; examples in this chapter are a spoon, a cup bearing a forearm, or a gripper). The set of all positions and orientations that the end-effector can attain is called the workspace of a given manipulator. Many robotic manipulators have been designed for industrial purposes. These applications typically require high speed and high accuracy. Many industrial robots are also required to handle heavy payloads. Because of these high speeds, high accelerations, and heavy payload capabilities, you can find most industrial robots behind a fence because it is not considered safe for humans to be close to them. This would be a problem for our application: We want the robot to be near a human to assist that person. Therefore, we need to have another group of robotic manipulators, the so-called assistive robotic manipulators (ARMs). ARMs are designed to interact with humans in a safe manner. This will of course give the robotic manipulator some restriction with respect to speed and force and require some special sensors or other measures to guarantee the safety of interactions with humans.

Another important difference between (most) industrial robots and (most) ARMs is the way they are controlled. Most industrial robots are set up at a fixed position and a given (structured) environment. Within this environment, the robot can perform its task. The robot, again in general, is following the instructions coming from a program, following the same sequences over and over again. For several ARMs, the location in space is changing continuously (e.g., mounted on a wheelchair), and the environment is, in general, unstructured. A wheelchair-mounted robot can be used one time as a feeder, making repetitive movements from the plate to the mouth, and the same robot is used to pick up a glass for drinking. Neither will the plate nor the glass ever be at the same spot. The shape of the glass might also change. Usually, the human is in the control loop, meaning that the user has control over at least some of the manipulator's

DOF (e.g., the user is able to move the manipulator end-effector in the Cartesian space with the help of a joystick that allows for up/down and left/right movements, although the actual joint angles are controlled by the robot to hold the end-effector orientation fixed).

Assistive robotic manipulators can be seen as augmentative and alternative manipulation tools for people with upper limb physical impairments. Their goal is to provide these persons an alternative way of manipulating objects in their environment. They differ from the robotic prosthesis described in Chapter 4 because they're not attached to the person's body. The fact that joints should be actuated by motors is critical in the definition of a robotic manipulator.

This chapter addresses robotic manipulators with at least 6 DOF. This number of DOF is the minimum required to be able to position and orient arbitrarily an object in three-dimensional (3-D) space. When describing the movement of the robot end-effector, we usually do it in reference to an inertial frame located at the base of the robot with the x and y axes on the plane where the robot sits and with the z axis pointing up. Rotations about the x, y, and z axes are usually termed roll, pitch, and yaw movements, respectively. Six DOF are required for an ARM to be able to perform relatively complex tasks. Imagine that you have a full glass of water on a table. You want a robot to pick up the glass and bring it to your mouth without spilling so you can start drinking. Table 3.1 lists the robot joint actions necessary to accomplish this task. This typical application would not be possible for any robot with less than 6 DOF.

Although 6 DOF are enough to position and orient the cup, some movements require more DOF. Suppose you have a robot holding a glass of water at the same position and orientation in space but with different joint

TABLE 3.1 Required DOF for Drinking

	Action	Robot Joint Actions	Required DOF
1	Robot holding a glass	Starting point	
2	Robot lifts glass	z-axis movement up and simultaneously movement of gripper down (pitch) to keep glass horizontal	z + pitch
3	Move glass to user	x-axis and y-axis movement toward the user and simultaneous rotation of the gripper on the horizontal plane (yaw) to keep the same gripper orientation	x, y + yaw
4	Start drinking	z-axis movement and roll of gripper	z + roll

configurations (see Figure 3.1). to go from the "elbow-up" to the "elbow-down" configuration, while keeping the glass of water in exactly the same position, an extra DOF is necessary. In fact, a human arm has 7 DOF (Figure 3.2), which enables us to move our elbow up and down while keeping our wrist in the same position. It can be shown that, except for some singular points in the robotic manipulator workspace, a given position and orientation of the end-effector of a 6-DOF manipulator can be achieved at least by two joint configurations. An extra DOF allows moving from one configuration to another while keeping the end-effector orientation. With a 7-DOF manipulator, there are an infinite number of possible joint angles that achieve the same position and orientation of the end-effector.

Industrial robots mostly have dedicated end-effectors for dedicated tasks, often with an end-effector exchange option. Because rehabilitation robots have to perform many different tasks and be able to pick up and hold many different objects with different shapes, dedicated end-effectors are not an option. We are looking more toward a "universal" gripper. This gripper may not be the ideal solution for every task; but it must do the job.

The human hand is effective for multipurpose tasks, so it makes sense to give it a closer look. Most of us use all five of our fingers unconsciously, but imagine what you can do with only three fingers or even with only two fingers. You will soon find out that most of the tasks can be done by two fingers only. Many current ARMs have grippers as end-effectors that emulate the functioning of the human hand. Opening and closing a gripper is not considered as an extra DOF (Poole 1989).

In summary, our definition of an ARM is as follows: any robotic arm that is not body bound with a minimum of 6 DOF and a gripper, which is safe to interact with humans, especially humans with special needs or a disability, and can assist with several activities under the control of the user.

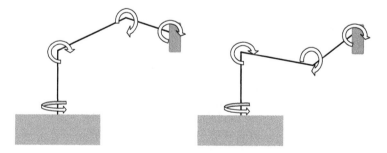

Figure 3.1   Joint configurations: "elbow" up and down.

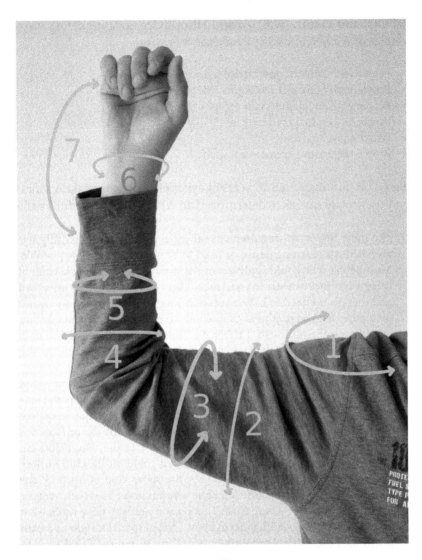

Figure 3.2 The 7 DOF of the human arm.

Who Is the End User?

Based on the definition of an ARM, we can now describe the potential end user. In general an end user would be *anyone who has no or limited arm or hand function*. A formal classification of limitations in arm or hand functions can be found in the International Classification of Functioning,

Disability, and Health (ICF) (World Health Organization 2001). Typical examples of ARM end users include the following:

- People with amyotrophic lateral sclerosis (ALS);
- People with muscular dystrophy (MD);
- People with spinal muscular atrophy (SMA);
- People with spinal cord injuries (SCIs);
- Stroke survivors; and
- People with strong tremors/spasticity.

Based on our more than 25 years of experience, we can make a short list of end-user requirements to determine if an ARM could be useful for them:

1. The most important requirement for an end user to successfully use an ARM is the strong desire or need to be as independent as possible. Most people who could apply for an ARM already have a whole team of caregivers. Those caregivers will most likely do anything they are asked and there is no need to have a robot. It might also be easier and faster for a potential end user to ask somebody to perform a certain task than performing the task with a robot. So, only the desire or need to do a task independently or to be alone for a certain amount of time during the day gives enough motivation to actually use an ARM.

2. Potential end users should have enough cognitive skills to do some kind of path planning. This sounds complicated, but we are doing path planning unconsciously every second. How do we pick up a mug of coffee? We need to decide how to approach the mug: from the top or from the front or from the side. Do we turn the handle of the mug before we lift it or while we lift it. We anticipate that it could hit the chin or nose during drinking. All these actions require some kind of unconscious path planning. Now, imagine someone who has never used their arms or hasn't used them for a long time. That person needs to tell a robot what to do and how to do it. That needs some level of spatial insight and path planning. Research has been conducted (Kim, Wang, and Behal 2012) to partially or fully eliminate the need of human path planning by adding cameras to the robot and creating a library of objects and tasks. As far as we know, this study has been completed, but has never been implemented in any commercially available ARM.

3. As discussed in further sections, most ARMs will be controlled by input devices having fewer control signals than the ARM's DOF. This means some menu structure has to be created to access all possible movements of the ARM. Although a lot can be done with visual or audio feedback for menu structures, good cognitive skills are important in learning and understanding the several menus.

4. Potential end users should have the ability to control the robot, that is, assessing the current state of the robot and providing the appropriate commands (input signals) for the robot to perform the desired task.

5. The end user must have some vision. The end user should be able to see what the ARM is doing and where it is going and be able to stop in case of a potential collision. A camera or other sensor could help the user, but it will be difficult to fully eliminate human vision, at least with the current available technology.

6. The ARM needs some kind of power source. This could come from the mains or a battery. If the mains are being used, we are compromising the potential mobility of an ARM, whereas with a battery, the robot can be used anywhere and even be integrated on a mobile platform. Typical end users are using a powered wheelchair for mobility. The battery of these chairs is a good power source for ARMs.

What to Expect from the ARM: What Should It Do?

As we have seen from our definition of an ARM, it should be capable of grasping and handling objects (cf. Figure 3.3). This ability is fundamental

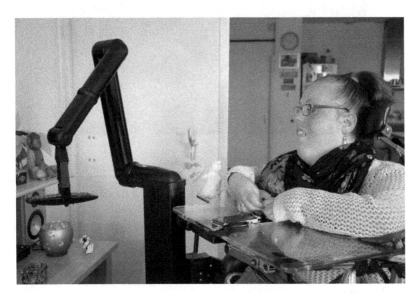

Figure 3.3 End user with ARM picking up remote controller.

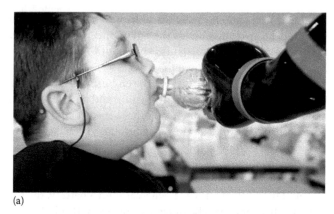

(a)

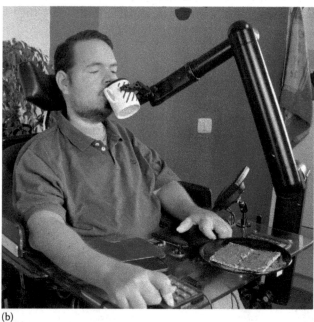

(b)

Figure 3.4 Drinking examples with different ARMs: (a) drinking water with the JACO robot and (b) drinking coffee with the *i*ARM robot.

to perform activities of daily living (ADLs). Some typical ADLs (as illustrated in Figure 3.4) are as follows:

- Bathing and showering;
- Dressing;
- Self-feeding and -drinking (dehydration is a huge risk when being alone without someone to help);

- Performing personal hygiene and care (including combing hair, brushing teeth);
- Performing toilet hygiene (getting to the toilet, cleaning oneself, and getting back up);
- Doing housework;
- Preparing meals;
- Shopping; and
- Using the telephone or other form of communication.

Because we have defined our potential end users as typical persons with a drive to be as independent as possible, we need ARMs that are able to assist in the majority of the ADL tasks and be able to help with at least eating and drinking.

Also, an ARM can help a person perform work-related tasks. Typical examples are light office work (e.g., taking a file from a cabinet, taking paper out of the printer, opening/closing doors, starting a computer, or picking something off the floor). The last category to consider is recreational or socially related activities (e.g., painting, playing games, going to a pub, photography, bird watching). Table 3.2 provides an overview of ICF categories and activities that can be accomplished with the use of an ARM by people with severe physical disabilities (Gelderblom et al. 2004).

To be able to assist a person in the activities mentioned, ARMs should satisfy a number of technical requirements. These are considered in the following list:

1. *Lifting capabilities*: Lifting a person out of bed requires more lifting capabilities of an ARM compared to lifting a glass of water.
2. *Accuracy*: Putting a USB stick into a computer requires more accuracy of the ARM compared to pressing a button to call for the elevator.
3. *Speed*: Throwing a ball to play with your dog requires different speed and acceleration profiles than putting food in your mouth.
4. *Gripper*: Picking up a football requires a different gripper than picking up a mobile phone.
5. *Number of grippers*: For some tasks, it is more convenient to have two hands, such as opening a bottle. For other tasks, one hand is enough, such as opening a door.
6. *Complex tasks*: Consider the ADL task of undressing. Now, try the following: You sit on a chair and use just one arm and one hand to undress. Did you succeed? How long did it take you? As you most likely experienced, undressing can be considered a complex task, especially when you cannot move any part of your body to help. Toileting is even more complex: You have the combination of (partially) undressing and

TABLE 3.2   ADL and ICF Combined for ARM Users

ICF ID	ICF Category	ICF Description	Supported by Commercially Available ARMs
d360	Using communication devices and techniques	Using devices, techniques, and other means for the purposes of communicating, such as calling a friend on the telephone	Yes.
d430	Lifting and carrying objects	Raising an object or taking something from one place to another, such as when lifting a cup or carrying a child from one room to another	Yes, for small objects only.
d440	Fine hand use	Performing the coordinated actions of handling objects, picking up, manipulating, and releasing them using one's hand, fingers, and thumb, such as required to lift coins off a table or turn a dial or knob	Yes.
d445	Hand and arm use	Performing the coordinated actions required to move objects or to manipulate them by using hands and arms, such as when turning door handles or throwing or catching an object	To some extent. Throwing and catching is not possible.
d520	Caring for body parts	Looking after those parts of the body, such as skin, face, teeth, scalp, nails, and genitals, that require more than washing and drying	To some extent. For some activities, special tools are required. For example, shaving is only safe with an electric razor.
d540	Dressing	Carrying out the coordinated actions and tasks of putting on and taking off clothes and footwear in sequence and in keeping with climatic and social conditions, such as by putting on, adjusting, and removing shirts, skirts, blouses, pants, undergarments, saris, kimono, tights, hats, gloves, coats, shoes, boots, sandals, and slippers	Hardly.

(Continued)

TABLE 3.2 (CONTINUED) ADL and ICF Combined for ARM Users

ICF ID	ICF Category	ICF Description	Supported by Commercially Available ARMs
d550	Eating	Carrying out the coordinated tasks and actions of eating food that has been served: bringing it to the mouth and consuming it in culturally acceptable ways, cutting or breaking food into pieces, opening bottles and cans, using eating implements, having meals, feasting or dining	To some extent. Eating is possible; opening bottles and cans is hardly possible.
d560	Drinking	Taking hold of a drink, bringing it to the mouth, and consuming the drink in culturally acceptable ways; mixing, stirring, and pouring liquids for drinking; opening bottles and cans; drinking through a straw or drinking running water, such as from a tap or a spring; feeding from the breast	Yes: drinking is possible; opening bottles and cans is hardly possible.
d620	Acquisition of goods and services	Selecting, procuring, and transporting all goods and services required for daily living, such as selecting, procuring, transporting, and storing food, drink, clothing, cleaning materials, fuel, household items, utensils, cooking ware, domestic appliances and tools; procuring utilities and other household services	Yes, for small items only.
d630	Preparing meals	Planning, organizing, cooking, and serving simple and complex meals for oneself and others, such as by making a menu, selecting edible food and drink, getting together ingredients for preparing meals, cooking with heat and preparing cold foods and drinks, and serving the food	Preparation can be done. Cooking with heat is considered too dangerous.

(Continued)

TABLE 3.2 (CONTINUED)   ADL and ICF Combined for ARM Users

ICF ID	ICF Category	ICF Description	Supported by Commercially Available ARMs
d640	Doing housework	Managing a household by cleaning the house, washing clothes, using household appliances, storing food and disposing of garbage, such as by sweeping, mopping, washing counters, walls, and other surfaces; collecting and disposing of household garbage; tidying rooms, closets, and drawers; collecting, washing, drying, folding, and ironing clothes; cleaning footwear; using brooms, brushes, and vacuum cleaners; using washing machines, dryers, and irons	Only a subset of relatively simple tasks like collecting and disposing of household garbage; tidying rooms; collecting, washing, drying clothes; using washing machines, dryers.
d650	Caring for household objects	Maintaining and repairing household and other personal objects, including house and contents, clothes, vehicles and assistive devices, and caring for plants and animals, such as painting or wallpapering rooms, fixing furniture, repairing plumbing, ensuring the proper working order of vehicles, watering plants, grooming and feeding pets and domestic animals	Only a subset, such as watering plants, grooming and feeding pets and domestic animals.
d660	Assisting others	Assisting household members and others with their learning, communicating, self-care, or movement within the house or outside; being concerned about the well-being of household members and others	Yes.

transferring from wheelchair to toilet. What does this require from our robot? Consider all the complex movements in combination with the lifting capabilities.

7. *Environment*: When the ARM is mounted to a powered wheelchair, the ARM could be not only inside the house but also outside in hot summer or cold winter conditions, in the rain or on a sandy beach. What should we consider as normal conditions?

8. *Weight and dimensions*: Given the required ADL tasks, what requirements do we have with respect to weight of the robot and length of the arm? Most industrial robots weigh from tens to hundreds of kilograms. Usually, they have huge control cabinets. These are impractical for mounting to a wheelchair. The weight of an ARM should be as low as possible. The dimensions of the ARM should be chosen in such a way that the ARM is as compact as possible, but still allows the end user to grab something from the floor or to take something out of a cabinet. These weight and length constraints also provide direction in terms of material selection and design.

How to Perform Tasks

Another important issue to consider regarding ARMs is the way that they can be controlled by the user to perform tasks. This includes the input devices, the menu structures, and different modes of control.

Input Devices
For industrial robots, there are several different input devices

- Input coordinates via computer
- Control panels
- Several kinds of (solid, but heavy) joysticks

People with disabilities in their arms/fingers would in general not be able to control a robot with one of these devices.

For our application, we could consider a joystick that can provide many independent control signals, like those used for many games (e.g., Xbox® or PlayStation®). The higher the number of independent control signals, the more movements of the ARM can be combined (e.g., moving the end-effector in the 3-D space while controlling its orientation). However, joysticks that generate many control signals are more difficult to handle, especially for people who have problems with their arms/hands. For our target group, the following input devices are usually considered:

- Two control signal mini-joysticks that are hand operated or can be controlled by the mouth, chin, or feet;
- Mini-keypads (e.g., the keypad may contain direction keys that make the robot move up/down and left/right);
- Wheelchair joysticks, which usually have features that make them accessible to persons with fine-motor impairments;

- Touch screens;
- Microlight switches; and
- Personal computer (PC) control (e.g., the user controls the ARM through software running in the computer).

Other input devices may be considered, although they require special attention:

- Eye-tracking control: A disadvantage of eye-tracking control is that an end user needs to look both at a screen and at the end-effector.
- Voice control: This is generally not useful for giving nondiscrete commands. Switching a light "on" or "off" is relatively safe to implement with voice. For something that involves movement, safety is important. You could implement "up," but how is this movement stopped when the robot does not "hear" the stop command correctly? This would mean you need to implement an extra safety feature. You could use voice to select commands, but have a (microlight) switch to actually initiate the movement. Once you release the switch, the ARM must stop.
- Brain- or body-robot interface: This is still in an early stage of implementation. Currently, these input devices require a high degree of concentration by the user and are thus tiring.

Combinations of these controls can be effective for individual end users; therefore, ARMs should be able to support some or all of these input devices.

Menu Structures

Many input devices do not provide simultaneous control of all ARM DOF. Consider the example of a 6-DOF robot with an analog mini-joystick as an input device. This joystick has been specially designed for people with minimal finger movements and limited finger force, providing two analog control signals.* Are we able to control all ARM DOF? When we include a gripper with two fingers that can be opened and closed, we have six plus one joints, moving in two directions. To control these joints, we need seven different analog control signals. The solution for controlling such an ARM with a joystick with two control signals is the use of menu structures such as the one in Figure 3.5. One of the control signals is used to move from one option to the other, each option corresponding to a robot joint. The other control signal is used to move the joint corresponding to the active joint. Some kind of feedback, visual or auditory, to tell the end user which

---

* An analog signal can take any value within a certain range.

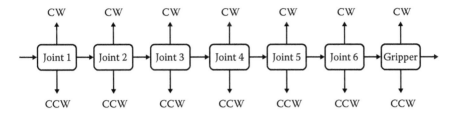

Figure 3.5 Basic example of controlling a 6-DOF robot and gripper with a joystick.

joint has been selected is usually incorporated. Similar solutions where a control signal is used to scan between the different joints can be created for joysticks providing more than two control signals, n-button keypads, single switches, or a combination of these.

However, controlling one joint at a time does not allow for the robot to perform more complex tasks, such as picking up a glass of water. In fact, this requires the simultaneous control of several joints of the robot in such a way that the gripper remains horizontal during the complete movement. To achieve this with an input device that generates fewer control signals than the DOF of the ARM, different control modes are required.

Joint versus Cartesian Control
Controlling each of the ARM joints directly may be easy to implement but does not provide a practical control method to the user. In fact, some training is necessary to be able to map the joint angles to the x-y-z position of the end-effector. Computing the Cartesian position of a manipulator end-effector from the joint angles (i.e., mapping the joint space to the Cartesian space) is known as the **forward kinematics** of a manipulator (Craig 2005). For a user, it would be more practical to directly control the x-y-z position of the end-effector, that is, to control the ARM end-effector directly in the Cartesian space. This involves solving the **inverse kinematics** (Craig 2005) of the ARM, a task that is left to the ARM control electronics.

In Cartesian space, we can tell the gripper to go straight up by making a translation parallel to the z axis. The orientation of the gripper remains unchanged. A menu structure implementing ARM control in Cartesian space with a joystick with two control signals is shown in Figure 3.6.

Velocity Control
Some input devices only provide on/off control signals. With these, it is not possible to control the speed; it is only possible to activate/deactivate

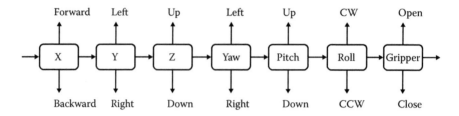

Figure 3.6 Menu structure for controlling a 6-DOF robot and gripper with a joystick with two control signals in Cartesian space.

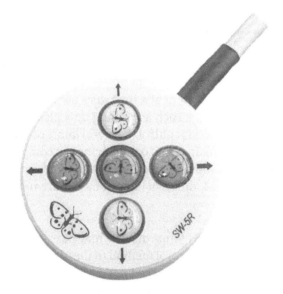

Figure 3.7 Example of an assistive keypad with five single switches.

the movement in a given direction. This can also be addressed using a menu structure. Consider, for example, the problem of controlling a 6-DOF ARM with a gripper in Cartesian space using a small keypad with five single switches (Figure 3.7). The menu structure in Figure 3.8 provides a solution to the problem.

Position Feedback

To implement the control methods described, it is necessary for the ARM electronics to know the joint angles exactly. One way is to measure the angle of each joint with respect to a reference, such as by counting the number of the joint motor rotations. However, with this method, it is necessary to have a way of measuring the initial position of the robot. For

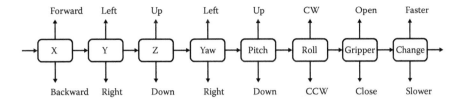

Figure 3.8 Menu structure to control a 6-DOF robot and gripper with five single switches.

industrial robots, it is common that they perform a calibration sequence when the robot is turned on. Each joint is moved slowly in a certain direction until it hits an end switch. At that moment, the position is known for that joint. This is typically a process that takes some time. Adopting such a method for assistive robotic arms would therefore not be practical.

Another solution is to perform a one-time factory calibration and then put a brake on all joints such that the joints cannot be rotated when the robot is turned off; thus, the previous joint angle measurement will still correspond to the joint position after turning it on. One can also measure the absolute angle of the joint using a potentiometer mounted to each joint or other absolute encoders.

Serviceability

We mentioned that ARM end users would like to be as independent as possible. This means that they will utilize the ARM on a daily basis to perform several tasks that rely on a perfect working ARM. Moreover, many people with ARMs are known to be alone or to have a working spouse. They are on their own for a large part of the day. This means that the ARM has to be reliable. But, just like any other piece of equipment, it could malfunction. Most problems are cable-related problems, such as a damaged wire. For these end users, it is extremely important that a broken ARM can be repaired/serviced as soon as possible. This requires not only a special design in terms of serviceability (e.g., a modular design, ease of mounting/demounting of the ARM and its components) but also a dealer network with professional service engineers.

Safety and Norms

Safety is a key issue with assistive robotic arms. ARMs are usually capable of relatively fast movements and of exerting relatively large forces. How do we prevent the robot from hurting someone or damaging something? This concern is especially important given that most of the end users are almost defenseless.

Consider a practical example: To feed himself, a user puts a fork in the ARM's gripper and picks up some food with this fork. Now, he can bring the fork to his mouth. How do we prevent the user from hurting himself with the fork? We cannot say "don't get near your face" because that would not make sense. How is this dilemma solved? The first approach is to instruct the user on how to perform the activity with the ARM, which is not necessarily in the same way the person would be doing the activity with a natural arm. For example, end users can be told not to use sharp objects like knives, forks, needles, and so on with the ARM. If they want to eat, a spoon can be used. Also, end users can be taught not to enter the spoon into the mouth. The spoon could be placed just before the mouth and then the end user would move his neck or body to eat from the spoon. This would solve some of the safety issues.

However, safety measures should be implemented in the ARM. The robot should be equipped with sensors (e.g., force sensors, cameras, tactile sensors) to provide automatic feedback on the robot operation. For example, the force exerted by the robot end-effector can be measured and kept within a safety limit. This countermeasure solves some safety issues when the robot is applying force to an object. But, the robot should also be able to handle some external forces. Suppose someone is leaning on the robot. Forces on a joint can then easily reach 100 N. In this case, either the controller can give a warning and stop trying to keep the robot in this position or a countermeasure can be taken from the mechanical construction of the robot, applying slip clutches to the joints. Slip clutches will prevent too much force from being applied to a joint. When the force to a joint is higher than the maximum allowed value, the clutch will slip.

The 2014 standard "Robots and Robotic Devices—Safety Requirements for Personal Care Robots," (International Organization for Standardization [ISO] 13482) provides more information on safety considerations for ARMs (please refer to Chapter 1).

Acceptance Aspects

Media usually picture assistive robots as a panacea that will solve all problems of our aging society. On the other extreme, many movies show robots coming to life and killing people. These two opposing scenarios make people hesitate about using an ARM.

Another barrier to the acceptance of ARMs is the fact that some care-givers (e.g., parents) don't believe it is socially acceptable and feel guilty about replacing their loving caregiving by something as cold and heartless as a robot. Some caregivers may even fear losing their jobs.

Social isolation arising from the independence provided by an ARM can also be a concern. This should be counterbalanced with the fact that a more independent end user has more choices on where to be and with whom, giving him or her more social possibilities in the end.

One factor that is important with respect to ARM acceptance is that, in general, no one wants to look different (see Chapter 10). So, again gener-ally speaking, people in a wheelchair want to look as "normal" as possible. Adding a robot to the wheelchair does not help with this appearance.

Also, a saying often heard is: "This is not going to work for my (client/son/daughter)." This comment is made without consulting the potential end user. An open mind, without prejudice and putting the end user at the center of the process, could help arriving at a good decision (please refer to the Human Activity Assistive Technology [HAAT] model briefly described in Chapter 1).

Assessment Aspects

Buying a robot cannot be compared to anything else. There are many factors to be considered. Some have been mentioned because they also inform the design characteristics of an ARM. The following list provides a brief overview of what should be considered when equating the acquisi-tion of an ARM:

- *End-user characteristics*: Does the end user have enough drive to be as independent as possible? Does the end user have enough cognitive skills to effectively use the ARM?
- *Research on available ARMs*: What are their capabilities? How can they be objectively compared? What is the availability?
- *Research on the companies behind the different ARMS*: What are their service level and skills? What do I expect?
- *Input devices*: What input devices are available that I can actually use? Can I try this before I decide to buy this robot?
- *ARM mounting*: What are the mounting possibilities of the ARM (where and how)? Can anyone do this mounting, or does it need to be done by a dealer? And, if so, do I lose my wheelchair for a certain amount of time?

Assessment for an ARM, as for any other assistive technology, should be done by a team, including

- The end user;
- An occupational therapist for helping with setting targets, training, and guidance in the initial period;
- The caregiver for general support and creating possibilities to achieve the goals of the end user; and
- A wheelchair technician to obtain local support for wheelchair integration or minor troubleshooting.

Financial Aspects

The market for assistive robotics will by nature be a niche market. Inherently, this means low volumes and therefore relatively high(er) prices. Most individuals will not have enough financial resources to purchase an ARM individually and need to find some kind of funding. Important arguments for applying funding could be found in quantitative financial arguments like return on investment and hard-to-measure qualitative arguments such as quality of life. The following section provides a critical review of studies that have evaluated several aspects of ARM use, including associated cost savings, user acceptance, and design.

Critical Review of the Technology Available

In the past two decades, a growing body of research has addressed the development, use, and evaluation of ARMs. However, only a few ARMs have moved beyond the stages of development and testing into commercially available prototypes. In the United States alone, approximately 150,000 people with disabilities could benefit from using an ARM, including people with conditions such as MD, SCI, and ALS, among others (Laffont et al. 2009). Further, in a U.K.-based survey conducted by Prior (1990) and colleagues of people with severe physical disabilities, 84% of participants ($N = 50$) said they would consider buying an ARM, provided that it was within their means. In addition, participants in the survey indicated that reaching, stretching, and gripping were involved in the top task that they would like to be able to do but could not due to their disability. These results indicate the potential of ARMs to increase independence and functioning among people with physical disabilities. Further, they indicate that perceived usability of the technology (in principle) and intention to use may not be the main causes of such low success rates of these technologies in the market.

High cost, ergonomic design flaws, difficulty in control, and failure to engage people with disabilities in the design process are some of the factors that contribute to low rates of technology transfer (Prior 1990). Commercially available ARMs, such as JACO® (by Kinova, Canada, http://www.kinovarobotics.com/) and the *i*ARM® (by Exact Dynamics, the Netherlands, http://www.exactdynamics.nl) currently range between U.S.$28,000 and U.S.$50,000. Table 3.3 provides an overview of the technical characteristics of these ARMs. As a way to increase the cost-effectiveness of these technologies, several studies have analyzed the cost savings associated with increased independence resulting from the use of ARMs by people with severe physical disabilities (Gelderblom et al. 2007; Römer, Stuyt, and Peters 2005). Römer and colleagues (2005) estimated that approximately 7,000 to 18,000 euros per year can be saved for each user in costs associated with ADL assistants. Additional indirect cost savings can result from increased opportunities for employment for ARM users (Römer, Stuyt, and Peters 2005). Other laboratories have focused on

TABLE 3.3   Characteristics of the Commercially Available JACO and *i*ARM

Characteristic	*i*ARM	JACO
Manufacturer	Exact Dynamics	Kinova Technology
Weight	9 kg	5 kg
Weight limit	1.5 kg	1.5 kg (45 cm), 1.0 kg (90 cm)
Reach	90 + 20 cm (lift unit)	90 cm
Maximum speed	15 cm/s	15 cm/s
Degrees of freedom (DOF)	7, including gripper; 8 with lift unit	7, including gripper
Hand	2 fingers	3 fingers
Finger force	20 N	7 N
Control possibilities	Several power wheelchair interfaces, keypad, joystick (digital or analog), single switches, game pad, computer	Several power wheelchair interfaces, mini-joystick, three-axis joystick, button controls, game pad, computer
Power	24-V DC/3 A (maximum)	24-V DC/1.5 A

Source: Adapted from Chung, C. S., and Cooper, R. A. 2012. "Literature review of wheelchair-mounted robotic manipulation: user interface and end-user evaluation." Proceedings of the 12th Annual RESNA Conference, Baltimore.

developing low-cost ARMs. For example, KATIA (by Carbon Robotics, United States, http://www.carbon.ai/) is a highly versatile ARM; its creators hope to launch the prototype soon.

Control interfaces are also an important factor when it comes to usability of the technology. As shown in Table 3.3, off the shelf, the MANUS *i*ARM can be controlled through the same control system that operated the power wheelchair, a keypad, a joystick (digital or analog), single switches, a game pad, or a computer. The JACO ARM can also be controlled through the power wheelchair control system, using a (mini- or three-axis) joystick, a game pad, or button controls or through a computer. These interfaces have been shown to be adequate for people with physical disabilities and potential users. For example, in a study of 34 wheelchair user participants, Maheu and colleagues (2011) found that wheelchair users perceived the JACO's interface as easy to use and were able to perform all the basic movements as well as six different ADLs.

Although current control interfaces allow clients with different needs physical access to the ARM, they may not be intuitive for some clients, and they require certain cognitive skills (e.g., sequencing, memory, spatial reasoning, timing) (Tsui et al. 2008). Thus, current research efforts have focused on developing alternative control interfaces that can better serve the unique needs of clients. For example, Athanasiou, Chawla, and Leichtnam (2006) have developed and compared three alternative control interfaces for the MANUS, designed for people with muscular dystrophy. Their three proposed interfaces included an infrared sensory open cube with motion sensors and a probe; a 6-DOF pen-shaped stylus device with joints that match the ARM's joints; and finally a Logitech® mouse. The mouse alternative was found to be the superior option due to its low cost, wide availability, light weight, and safety. This option was also the most intuitive for users given their wide exposure to mouse control.

Further, Tsui and colleagues (2008) developed a flexible multimodal control interface for the *i*ARM. The interface can be slightly adjusted to different access methods (touch screen or joystick), has flexible options for image capturing (moving or fixed camera mounted on the robot), and allows users to directly select objects in the environment to which the arm then reacts (e.g., reaching or grasping). Sui and colleagues tested the interface with eight participants who had different severe physical disabilities and were wheelchair users. They found that participants performed better when using the moving camera coupled with the touch screen option ($p < .05$) than with the moving camera coupled with the joystick. Similarly, participants performed better when using the fixed camera and joystick than when using the moving camera and joystick. Further, participants indicated greater preference for the fixed camera with joystick interface. The preference for joystick over touch screen may be due to the fact that the touch screen required an element of abstraction between real-life objects and the images captured by the camera, which was a barrier for some users.

More recently, Kim and colleagues (2010) compared two modes of *i*ARM control: manual versus autonomous. In the manual mode, participants directly controlled the Cartesian 3-D positioning of the robot and the orientation of the gripper. In the autonomous mode, participants clicked on the image of the object of interest displayed on a screen, acquired through a mounted camera. The robot would then move toward the object and grab it. The autonomous mode was found to enable users to perform tasks more efficiently, faster, and with less effort. However, participants preferred the manual model, which gave them greater control over the task.

Tijsma, Liefhebber, and Herder (2005) compared the control of MANUS through a joypad with the control through a touch screen. This control scheme significantly lowered the cognitive and physical load placed on the user. The joypad interface is discussed in detail in Chapter 2.

In spite of the current design and cost-related barriers on the use of ARMs, those that have reached the market are currently enhancing independence and function for people with physical disabilities. As early as 1990, Bach, Zeelenberg, and Winter (1990) followed six participants with Duchenne muscular dystrophy as they used an ARM for 6 to 72 months. Increasing times of daily use of the ARM were shown to reduce caregiving time required, indicating increased independence. Similarly, Römer and colleagues (2004) compared 13 long-term ARM users (more than 4 years of use) and 21 non-ARM users with similar levels of impairment. They found that with a 2-hour daily use average, ARM users performed 40% more ADLs than the nonuser group. In their study, Maheu and colleagues (2011) found that 48% to 79% of participants thought the JACO arm enabled them to be "very able" to perform ADLs that a caregiver typically performed for them. Further, the study showed that ARMs could potentially reduce caregiving time by 41% for these participants.

A critical note has to be made: Although many end users are happy with their ARMs, it is only a subset of ADL tasks that can be performed. Neither of the robots can help you with dressing, toileting, or transferring, for example. The last column of Table 3.2 provides an overview of the activities currently supported by commercially available ARMs.

In summary, ARMs provide increased independence for people with physical disabilities, reduce caregiving time, and can be cost-effective if accounting for additional income resulting from increased independence and opportunities for employment and reduced costs in caregiving. However, developers and researchers are faced with numerous challenges pertaining to improved interfaces that are more intuitive and user friendly and are less cognitively demanding. Client-centered research is a critical factor for the industry to overcome these challenges. By involving potential users in all stages of the design and development, such obstacles may be mitigated. Commercially available ARMs can also benefit from ongoing developments in new user interfaces, making the input signals to the robots (even more) intuitive and eventually reducing the time needed to perform a task.

Future Directions

The focus of future development is on the following:

- New input devices (like brain- or body-robot interfaces);
- Vision and force feedback;
- **Impedance control**, imposing a desired dynamic to the interaction between the robot end-effector and the object being manipulated instead of directly controlling the exerted forces or the end-effector position (Hogan 1985);
- ARMs with 7 DOF instead of 6 DOF; and
- Five-finger hands and gripper developments.

So far, ARM systems are being developed especially for persons with no or limited arm or hand function. This is a relatively low-volume market that may not be interesting for many companies. It might be more effective to make ARM systems that also have potential in industrial environments where service robots are required.

Another research approach is to reduce the cost of ARMs so the ARM is financially attractive for end users, for charity organizations, for insurance companies, and so on. New technologies such as 3-D printing might help solve this problem (MacCurdy et al. 2016).

A good example of using mainstream technology available for physically challenged people is the use of a smartphone as a human–robot interface (HRI). Some HRIs, such as joysticks, keypads, single switches, or special displays especially designed for persons with disabilities, could be replaced by a general-purpose smartphone (Pathak et al. 2015), which saves costs. Other technologies that are in a research stage of development will become commercially available sooner or later. When, for example, brain- or body-robot interfaces become mainstream, it will certainly improve the HRI technology and save costs.

Currently, the mechanical and the electronic adaptation of an ARM to a powered wheelchair and the implementation in the wheelchair control system are also costly. Newly available technology such as Bluetooth and Wi-Fi make wireless integration possible, which saves costs because less electrical wiring/adaptation is needed. Safety issues (e.g., electrical interference, vulnerability to ARM control by others) are part of the risk analysis during design. Standardization of how an ARM should be fitted or integrated at a power wheelchair (e.g., 24-V outlets, mounting holes, electronic control integration) could also help market ARMs, making them more cost-effective "plug-and-play" devices.

Public health and insurance companies' policies are of paramount importance for persons with disabilities because these policies usually provide limited resources; thus, it might be difficult for these persons to acquire expensive assistive technologies such as an ARM without financial support. It is our opinion and experience that the development or improvement of acceptance of ARM systems in a public health system is as challenging or even more challenging than product development. There are some front-runner nations, but even in most Western highly developed countries, ARMs are not part of any health insurance or other funding system.

STUDY QUESTIONS

1. What differentiates an ARM from other robots?
2. Draw a picture of a 5-DOF robot with two fingers.
3. What do we mean by inverse kinematics?
4. Instead of other assistive solutions for ADLs, when will an ARM become a potential assistive device for someone with physical impairments?
5. Why will an ARM not suit people who only have physical impairments of their upper limbs (people who don't need a power wheelchair)?
6. Write a motivation or funding request letter (maximum 50 words) for an ARM application for a person who might have a need for it.
7. Why would people with physical impairments not apply for an ARM?
8. Write at least five things an end user could use the ARM for that are not mentioned in this chapter.
9. Imagine you are going to develop the next ARM. How are you going to start, and what are the most important aspects to focus on?
10. In your opinion, what obstructs the acceptance of ARMs?

References

Athanasiou, P., Chawla, N., and Leichtnam, E. 2006. "Assistive robotic manipulator interface." *Proceedings of the IEEE 32nd Annual Northeast Bioengineering Conference*, Easton, PA, April 1–2, pp. 171–172.

Bach, J. R., Zeelenberg, A. P., and Winter, C. 1990. "Wheelchair-mounted robot manipulators: Long term use by patients with Duchenne muscular dystrophy." *American Journal of Physical Medicine & Rehabilitation* 69(2): 55.

Chung, C. S., and Cooper, R. A. 2012. "Literature review of wheelchair-mounted robotic manipulation: User interface and end-user evaluation." Proceedings of the 12th Annual RESNA Conference, Baltimore.

Craig, J. J. 2005. *Introduction to Robotics: Mechanics and Control*. 3rd ed. Upper Saddle River, NJ: Pearson Education.

Gelderblom, G. J., Willen, A., Cremers, G. B., and de Witte, L. 2004. *Manus & Co. Een onderzoek naar voorwaarden voor doelmatige verstrekking van een robotmanipulator. Eindrapport.* iRv.

Hogan, N. 1985. "Impedance control: An approach to manipulation: Part I, part II, part III." *ASME Journal of Dynamic Systems, Measurement, and Control* 107(1): 1–24.

International Organization for Standardization (ISO). *ISO 13482 International Standard: Robots and Robotic Devices—Safety Requirements for Personal Care Robots*. Geneva: ISO, 2014.

Kim, D. J., Hazlett, B., Godfrey, H., Rucks, G., McNally, T., Portee, D., Bricout, J. et al 2010. "On the relationship between autonomy, performance, and satisfaction: Lessons from a three-week user study with post-SCI patients using a smart 6DOF assistive robotic manipulator." Proceedings of the IEEE International Conference on Robotics and Automation (ICRA), Anchorage, May 3–8, pp. 217–222.

Kim, D. J., Wang, Z., and Behal, A. 2012. "Motion segmentation and control design for UCF-MANUS—An intelligent assistive robotic manipulator." *IEEE/ASME Transactions on Mechatronics* 17(5): 936–948.

Laffont, I., Biard, N., Chalubert, G., Delahoche, L., Marhic, B., Boyer, F. C., and Leroux, C. 2009. "Evaluation of a graphic interface to control a robotic grasping arm: A multicenter study." *Archives of Physical Medicine and Rehabilitation* 90(10): 1740–1748.

MacCurdy, R., Katzschmann, R., Kim, Y., and Rus, D. 2016. "Printable hydraulics: A method for fabricating robots by 3D co-printing solids and liquids." Proceedings of the IEEE International Conference on Robotics and Automation (ICRA), Stockholm, May 16–21.

Maheu, V., Frappier, J., Archambault, P. S., and Routhier, F. 2011. "Evaluation of the JACO robotic arm: Clinico-economic study for powered wheelchair users with upper-extremity disabilities." Proceedings of the IEEE International Conference on Rehabilitation Robotics (ICORR), Zurich, June 27–July 1, pp. 1–5.

Pathak, M. K., Khan, J., Koul, A., Kalane, R., and Varshney, R. 2015. "Robot control design using Android smartphone." *Journal of Business Management and Economics* 3(2): 31–33.

Poole, H. 1989. "Fundamentals of Robotics Engineering." Springer: the Netherlands.

Prior, S. 1990. "A survey of potential users of an electric wheelchair mounted robotic arm." Proceedings of the 13th Annual RESNA Conference, Washington, DC, June, pp. 297–298.

Römer, G. W., Stuyt, H., and Peters, B. 2005. "Cost-savings and economic benefits due to the assistive robotic manipulator (ARM)." Proceedings of the IEEE 9th International Conference on Rehabilitation Robotics (ICORR), Chicago, June 28–July 1, pp. 201–204.

Römer, G. W., Stuyt, H., Peters, G., and Woerden, K. V. 2004. "14 processes for obtaining a 'Manus' (ARM) robot within the Netherlands." *Advances in Rehabilitation Robotics* 306: 221–230.

Tijsma, H. A., Liefhebber, F., and Herder, J. L. 2005. "Evaluation of new user interface features for the MANUS robot arm." Proceedings of the IEEE International Conference on Rehabilitation Robotics (ICORR), Chicago, June 28–July 1, pp. 258–263.

Tsui, K., Yanco, H., Kontak, D., and Beliveau, L. 2008. "Development and evaluation of a flexible interface for a wheelchair mounted robotic arm." Proceedings of the 3rd International Conference on HumanRobot Interaction (HRI), Amsterdam, March 12–15.

World Health Organization. 2001. *International Classification of Functioning, Disability and Health (ICF)*. Geneva: WHO.

4

Upper and Lower Limb Robotic Prostheses

Patrick M. Pilarski and Jacqueline S. Hebert

Contents

Learning Objectives

After completing this chapter, readers will be able to

1. Describe the challenges and benefits of rehabilitation robots that are directly mounted to the human body in the case of limb amputation to assist the user in daily life.
2. List the different components of upper and lower limb prosthetic devices, describe how these components are integrated with the human body to form a functional unit, and explain how user intent is used to direct the motion of prosthetic limbs.
3. Explain how prosthetic devices are used in clinical practice, including insights into user acceptance and **embodiment**, and measures used to assess prosthesis use.
4. Demonstrate high-level understanding of next-generation prosthetic technologies that are not yet seeing regular clinical application. These include advanced control paradigms, robotic devices with numerous controllable joints and actuators, novel brain-body-machine interfaces for prosthetic control, and new surgical innovations to more effectively merge prosthetic devices with the human body.

Introduction

Robotic technology helps persons undergoing rehabilitation to recover lost abilities. Robotic technology also has an important, persistent role in replacing lost abilities that cannot be recovered or mitigating the impact of that loss on a long-term basis. One special example of a rehabilitation robot that replaces lost function is the *robotic prosthesis*: a robotic device that is attached to a patient's body throughout daily life to replace the functions of the patient's missing limb (Figures 4.1 and 4.2). Robotic prostheses consist of battery-powered, motorized components with movements that are user initiated, typically by way of muscle signals (termed *myoelectric control*) but also in some cases by external switches. This is in contrast to traditional body-powered hook-and-cable harness prostheses that mechanically couple proximal motion of the body (i.e., shoulder or chest) to the excursion of a cable that physically "pulls" or actuates the motion of a prosthetic joint. Advanced robotic prostheses tend to be more anthropomorphic in appearance, often simulating motions and common grip patterns of the human hand.

Robotic prostheses differ from other assistive rehabilitation robots in the way that they directly interact with the human body and the way that they must interpret user intent. To greater or lesser degrees, robotic

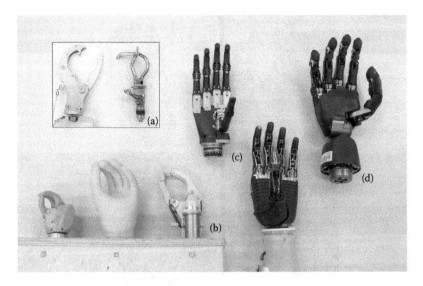

Figure 4.1   An example of electromechanical and mechanical prosthetic hands: (a) common nonrobotic, body-powered grippers; (b) clinically available single-actuator robotic grippers; (c) clinically available robotic grippers with multiple grasp patterns and fingers that can flex and extend independently; (d) research prosthetic hand and wrist with diverse sensor systems, three-axis wrist motion, and dexterous finger and thumb actuation.

prostheses must become the body part they intend to replace. This physical, long-term connection between a human and his or her robotic device is a challenging setting for technical development and a powerful area for improving the lives of people who have lost limbs due to injury, illness, or other complications. Robotic prostheses currently see regular clinical prescription and daily use, and there are a large number of prosthesis manufacturers worldwide producing robotic prostheses. At the same time, new robotic prostheses are being developed that may be able to closely approximate and someday even exceed the abilities of a patient's lost biological limb.

Principles

The ultimate goal of a robotic prosthesis is to completely and seamlessly replace the form, function, and abilities lost due to limb amputation (Castellini et al. 2014; Olson 2014; Williams 2011; Zuo and Childress 1985). In other words, the objective of a robotic prosthesis is commonly considered to be returning the

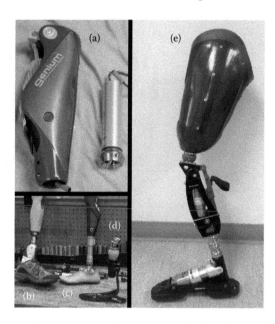

Figure 4.2   An example of lower limb electromechanical and mechanical prostheses: (a) disassembled microprocessor-controlled robotic prosthetic leg; a clinical prosthetics workbench demonstrating (b) an assembled prosthetic knee and ankle robot, (c) an assembled knee-only prosthesis, and (d) a purely mechanical, nonrobotic prosthetic foot; and (e) a fully assembled lower limb robotic prosthesis with **socket**.

user to the same condition as prior to losing the limb. Importantly, this restoration must be done without creating additional burden or inconvenience to the user beyond what they would have had in using their nonamputated limb (Williams 2011). No current prosthesis achieves this grand goal, but progress is being made toward restoring individual aspects or functions of a lost limb and reducing the mental and physical effort that devices require of their users. In particular, a significant amount of research and development has been done to improve the *form* and *functionality* of prostheses, the ease of *control* for prosthetic users, and more recently the quality of *feedback* that can be delivered from the device to its user (Castellini et al. 2014; Peerdeman et al. 2011; Scheme and Englehart 2011; Williams 2011). These three principles of function, control, and feedback come together to support the user in incorporating a prosthesis as part of daily life and ideally as part of his or her own body—termed *user embodiment* (Longo et al. 2008). The following four sections describe these core principles and how they come together to create useful prosthetic technology.

Form and Function

Form and function are often the first aspects that spring to mind when discussing a prosthetic device. *Form* includes how the different parts of the device are configured, how they relate to each other, the material used in the construction of the prosthesis, and the cosmetic appearance of these parts (such as color and texture). For example, a prosthesis could be formed from a fiberglass or plastic base that is painted to match the color of the user's skin, with metal parts concealed under cosmetic rubber liners to simulate the look of regular human tissue. Alternately, a device might be fabricated from black carbon fiber with visible motors and some exposed metal parts or highlighted technology. Some prostheses are painted with custom artwork. Others are sculpted to exactly match the shape and appearance of a user's nonamputated limb. While form may vary greatly, it is dictated in a large part by the functional and social needs of the user.

Often, there is a trade-off between appearance and usability. The most functional terminal device is often still regarded to be the hook shape form due to the provision of clear lines of sight to the user and ability to provide fine-motor pinch, compared to the more anthropomorphic-appearing powered hands. With the advent of newer multigrip powered hands with multiple grasp patterns, the functional gap is closing, but nonetheless the vast majority of hands have a mechanical robotic appearance rather than a cosmetic one. For this reason, some patients may prefer a passive device with better **cosmesis** over one with robotic appearance and function. Form also includes the quality of movement, for example, the smoothness or rate of change of a device's moving parts; it is considered desirable for a prosthesis not to move in mechanical or unnatural ways (Childress 1992; Weir 2004).

Function describes what the device can accomplish: the abilities that the device is able to confer or the different degrees of control that it affords for the user. Simple examples of function include the number of joints or powered actuators used in a device, the maximum strength of any of these actuators, and the length of time a device can be used without replacing or recharging its battery. More general examples of function include the number of grasp types available to a user of a robotic hand, the capacity of the robotic hand to hold a cup of coffee without it slipping from the user's grasp, or the ability of the robotic ankle of a lower limb prosthesis to flex appropriately while walking up stairs. The functionality of a prosthesis is governed by design and chosen based on the needs of the user and the recommendations of the clinical practitioners prescribing the user's device.

For lower limb prostheses, the clear functional goal is stable weight bearing and propulsion for mobility. Over basic level surfaces, this can be achieved with the simplest prosthetic devices, but the degree to which the prosthesis can accommodate for the challenges of daily mobility can vary dramatically. Robotic lower limb prostheses strive to replace functionality over the widest range of conditions, allowing stability and mobility over a variety of terrains, including inclines, declines, and uneven ground, and for ascending and descending stairs. For upper limb function, the end goals are much more diverse and dependent on each user. In the absence of ability to completely replace the function and form of a normal human hand and arm, users must prioritize between features such as durability, grasp function, cosmesis, and weight. For example, only a small portion of powered upper (and lower) limb devices are waterproof, so working in wet environments would preclude many component choices in comparison to working in an office setting.

As one example of functional needs, users of forearm prostheses reported a desire for their device to have multiple selectable wrist movements and grasping patterns to suit common situations of daily life (Peerdeman et al. 2011). Further, they desired the simultaneous control of more than one of these functions at any given time—for example, the ability to both bend their wrist and close their hand in a pinching motion to pick up a small object. Finally, users and clinicians recommended that devices have no noticeable delay between the time when a user intends to execute a motion through muscle contraction and the time that the user sees the effect of the prosthetic joint motion. While initial reports have suggested that a delay of 300 ms may be acceptable to users, more recent reports suggest an ideal delay as low as 100 to 125 ms (Peerdeman et al. 2011).

Because of the weight and power demands of each powered actuator deployed within a robotic prosthesis, function is also limited by factors such as the type and nature of the user's amputation, the length and shape of the residual limb, how the prosthesis may be secured to the user's body, and other physical properties. As described in the section that follows, the functionality of a prosthesis is also intimately connected to how its user will be controlling the various functions of the device.

Control

Control is defined here as the aspect of a prosthesis that links user intent to the motion and operation of prosthetic functions. User intent cannot in practice be recorded directly (or in many cases even clearly defined). However, it is possible to record a number of signals from the human body that, taken together, form a first approximation of how a user intends to use the prosthesis or how the user wishes the prosthesis to behave. These signals can take the form of electrical activity recorded from the muscles of the residual limb, contact forces in a socket, manual or mechanical switches, or other biometric recordings. In addition to signals actively delivered to the prosthesis by the user, a prosthesis may passively record signals relating to the user, the prosthesis, and their environment.

Control of a robotic prosthesis can therefore be thought of as the process of mapping recorded signals to the motion of one or more prosthetic actuators or functions. Depending on the nature and number of signals that can be recorded and the number of functions the user wishes to control, control can be straightforward or in other cases can be extremely challenging for both users and prosthesis designers (Micera, Carpaneto, and Raspopovic 2010; Parker, Englehart, and Hudgins 2006; Scheme and Englehart 2011). A user's capacity to generate control commands is often a major limiting factor in directing the form and function of their prosthesis.

In many cases, especially in upper limb prostheses, the number of prosthetic functions that are possible to implement within a device are much greater in number than the number of clear, unique signals that can be recorded from the user's body. For example, with an amputation in the upper arm or at the shoulder, it may only be possible to record different muscle command signals from one or two regions of a user's residual limb. At the same time, it would be desirable to give the user control over a robotic elbow, a wrist that flexes and rotates, and a hand with multiple grasp patterns. The more biological function a user has lost, the more function is required from the robotic device (Parker, Englehart, and Hudgins 2006; Scheme and Englehart 2011; Williams 2011). However, due to the nature of the amputation, the user often does not have the ability to provide clear information about his or her control intent to the prosthetic device, leading to frustration and abandonment (Biddiss and Chau 2007a,b; Castellini et al. 2014; Parker, Englehart, and Hudgins 2006).

As core principles of effective prosthetic control, it is therefore important that

- The functions of a prosthetic device are readily accessible to the user;
- The burden of control does not outweigh the benefits of the implemented form and function and does not negatively impair other user abilities;
- Shifting between the multiple capabilities of a device is swift and seamless for the user;

- There be minimal delays between a user sending a command to the device and having the device respond to their command; and
- Use of the device as a whole is as intuitive and natural as possible.

These principles are evident in the usability requirements noted by patients, clinicians, and rehabilitation staff in a number of classical surveys (e.g., Biddiss and Chau 2007a,b; Childress 1992; Oskoei and Hu 2007; Peerdeman et al. 2011; Weir 2004). In addition, autonomy of some basic functions has been noted as a further desirable property of a prosthetic control approach. For example, in a task such as grasping an object, it may be desirable for a user to initiate the action but to have the prosthesis complete or maintain the movement or position without the direct attention of the user (Peerdeman et al. 2011). Current systems that automatically detect and prevent objects slipping from a user's grasp are one example of this paradigm. Artificial reflexes, as reviewed by Weir (2004), are another example of additional autonomy on the part of the control system, as are recent demonstrations of control interface reorganization (i.e., a prosthesis adaptively changing how the user selects functions), semiautonomous grasp selection, and grasp preshaping (i.e., a prosthesis selecting hand postures and their apertures for the user) (Castellini et al. 2014). Simultaneous control of multiple functions is considered to be an important objective for effective control approaches. It has also been argued that, to be intuitive, control should mirror a user's original neuromuscular control as closely as possible in terms of the arrangement of control channels and the timing of signals flowing between the user and the user's device (Peerdeman et al. 2011).

Feedback

The flow of signals from a prosthetic user to his or her device allows a device to perform motions that enact the intent of the user. However, as in conventional control systems in machines of all kinds, the use of a robotic prosthesis is challenging or impossible for a user without a complementary channel of information flowing from the device back to the user. This information to the user, termed *feedback*, is a critical part of effective prosthesis control.

In its simplest form, feedback is provided to the user as a by-product of the form and regular operation of the robotic prosthesis. Users are able to see and hear how their limb is moving and interacting with other objects. Vibration, torque, or impact forces to the limb are transmitted through the chassis of the device to the interface with the user's body. These mechanical sensations are well known to be an important way for users to interpret the operation of their prosthetic device, even when they are not looking at it. Similarly, the sound, vibration, and movement of all the actuators within a limb are conveyed to the user through the chassis and have been reported to be one of the most important components of feedback for users of commercially available limb systems (Lundborg and Rosen 2001). At present, the majority of available prosthetic technologies use intrinsic signals from the device to the user as their only form of feedback—sensation is not explicitly recorded and transmitted from a robotic prosthesis to the user. For lower limb robotic prostheses, vibrations, sounds, and impacts often provide a significant percentage of the information that a user needs to skillfully locomote; for upper limb prostheses, users often desire more information about what their prosthesis is feeling and how it is operating.

One limitation of the simple forms of feedback noted is that they do not capture the full range of sensations that might be accessible to a biological limb; thus, the type of feedback signals that help provide dexterous, natural control of an artificial arm and hand is missing. For example, in many cases it would be desirable for users to receive feedback about temperature, texture, the motion or position of the limb in space (proprioception and kinesthesia), and even damage or pain. These modalities are not typically present in commercially available devices but are the subject of significant research and development. Communicating the full range of perceptual information from a device back to the human is considered to be a significant remaining challenge for closing the loop between a user and a robotic prosthesis.

Some approaches to closing this loop aim to link actual actions of the device to specific sensations delivered to the user's body that are perceived by a user in the same way as the information that was recorded by the robot (e.g., the user perceives the robot's contact with other objects as touch or its proximity to a flame as heat). This feedback can be provided in ways that are matched or nonmatched in form and physiology (Antfolk et al. 2013; Schofield et al. 2014). True physiologically matched sensations would have the patient perceive the sensation on the robot arm as the exact same sensation on their now-amputated biological limb—that is, the patient perceives pressure on the robot's index finger as pressure on his or her missing index finger. An alternative approach that leverages the body and brain's ability to adapt is substitution, which delivers sensation to the body in forms other than the way they were recorded (nonphysiologically matched sensations). For example, force of contact with an object may be reported to the user by vibration in the socket of the limb or at another location on his or her body. In either case, physiologically matched or unmatched feedback, the intent is for the user to understand aspects of the operation of the device not otherwise readily perceivable through the user's direct physical attachment to the device. The device is actively, as opposed to passively, transmitting information to the user.

Because a robotic prosthesis has internal information relating to its actuators, power system, sensors, and control system, devices may also provide a user feedback about things not directly relating to the physical interactions of the prosthesis with the environment. It is important to communicate information to the user about the operation of the prosthesis itself, for example, communicating to the user which functions or modes the user is currently operating or signaling to the user that the battery is getting low. These forms of information must be communicated in a way that the user immediately knows what they mean and in a way that is not distracting or irritating during constant use. Wireless links to external devices such as a smartphone or tablet are also possible ways for users to receive different forms of information about their prosthesis, its operation, and the kinds of signals it is perceiving from the user's body (e.g., plots of the muscle activity signals being recorded in the socket or a schematic of the configuration of grasps that the user can currently select during their use of the device).

With these examples in mind, we can readily identify that the core principles of feedback and control of robotic prostheses are in fact similar to those of human-to-human communication and also to those of machine-to-machine communication—for example, information theory, communication theory, classical cybernetics, and a large body of work dating back to researchers such as Harry Nyquist, Ralph Hartley, Claude Shannon, Norbert Wiener, and Alan Turing. Signals should be clear and interpretable, contain an amount of information that is appropriate to their complexity, and readily preserve the intent of the sender on its interpretation by the receiver. Moreover, different signals need to be distinguishable as unique for the control system to understand that each signal has a different meaning (as well described in a mathematical sense by Shannon 1948). Practically, this means that the feedback delivered from a robotic prosthesis should

- Not be too detailed or complex for the user to understand and be presented in a way that it can indeed be understood (clarity and interpretability);
- Be delivered at a rate that is appropriate for the physical interface with the user (frequency, timing, and timeliness);

- Capture the most useful or important aspects of the information being recorded by the prosthesis (saliency); and
- Optimize how the modes of sensation recorded from the robot are matched to the perceptual information perceived by the human body (perceptual alignment or matching).

Embodiment

The sense of ownership of the different parts of one's body is essential for navigating the world around us and for successful interactions with other objects and people. *Embodiment* is a term used to describe awareness of what makes up our own body. Interestingly, we can be tricked into thinking that an external object, such as an artificial hand, is our own hand. Similarly, when we use a tool, we sense that it becomes a part or an extension of our body. In both of these cases, we can say that the object becomes "embodied." Limb ownership in healthy populations can be manipulated through illusory embodiment of a rubber hand.

A landmark study by Botvinick and Cohen (1998) first demonstrated the rubber hand illusion. In this protocol, the subject's arm is hidden from view behind a screen, and a rubber model of the same arm is placed on the table in front of the subject. The subject is instructed to fixate on the rubber limb, while two small paintbrushes simultaneously stroke the rubber hand and the subject's hidden hand. Within minutes, subjects report that they feel the touch on the rubber hand, not their hidden hand, as if their arm has embodied the rubber arm (Botvinick 2004). Hallmarks of embodiment include a sense of *ownership, location*, and *agency* of the rubber hand as rated by questionnaires; an autonomic arousal to threat when measuring skin conductance response; and proprioceptive drift where the participant's own hand is felt to disappear and be physically located in the position of the rubber hand (Armel and Ramachandran 2003; Longo et al. 2008), suggesting that the rubber hand actively displaces the actual hand, rather than merely being mistaken for it.

This embodiment phenomenon is of great interest for those who have lost a limb. It has been suggested that use of a prosthesis after limb amputation may be most related to the integration of the prosthesis into the individual's body schema (Gallagher 1986), and embodiment is generally considered to be a central factor in how well a user accepts his or her device. Clearly, form and function will affect how the user perceives his or her prosthetic limb and be influenced by how closely the operation of the limb matches the intent. Control affects how swiftly and accurately the user's intent is communicated to the prosthesis and brought to life. Feedback further closes the loop and allows the user to feel sensations and situations encountered by their robotic prosthesis. Taken together, these aspects lay the groundwork for embodiment. To have a user fully embody their prosthetic device as their own limb is perhaps the most important goal of prosthetic design, regardless of the level of complexity or functionality provided by the device. As such, a core principle of robotic prosthesis design is to make choices in form, function, control, and feedback that support a user's successful embodiment of his or her device.

Evidence from Armel and Ramachandran (2003), Botvinick and Cohen (1998), Ehrsson et al. (2008), Longo et al. (2008), and Tsakiris and Haggard (2005) suggested that the sense of body self-identification or body schema is intrinsically linked with cutaneous touch. Studies of embodiment after limb amputation have supported the contention that this illusion can be robustly applied using prosthetic limbs. The embodiment illusion was demonstrated in transradial (lower arm) amputees with cutaneous mapping (Ehrsson et al. 2008), in which questionnaires, skin conductance response, and temperature regulation all shifted toward the artificial hand. Marasco et al. (2011) measured embodiment using questionnaires and physiological temperature measurements to show that a prosthetic device that provided a physiologically appropriate sense of cutaneous touch could drive a shift in perception toward incorporation of the device into the self-image of the amputee. They created an artificial sense of touch for a prosthetic limb by coupling a pressure sensor on the hand through a robotic simulator to surgically redirected cutaneous sensory nerves that once served the lost limb. The results suggested that providing physiological and anatomically appropriate direct sensory feedback for a prosthetic limb created a more vivid illusion of embodiment, enough to elicit an involuntary physiological change in temperature regulation. Other studies using a sensory substitution paradigm with vibrotactile stimulation to induce the rubber hand illusion (D'Alonzo, Clemente, and Cipriani 2015) have also shown strong embodiment responses. Results from these studies give insight into how to improve the embodiment of robotic limbs for amputees by incorporating active feedback, which might lead to greater acceptance of the robotic prosthesis.

Critical Review of the Technology Available

Robotic prostheses have been in development for decades and have to date seen extensive use in the daily life of people with amputations (Childress

1992; Zuo and Olson 2014). There are numerous companies worldwide supplying prosthetic components and complete prosthetic solutions for individual patients. These devices are therefore considered to be at the highest technology readiness level (TRL), TRL 9, as defined in Chapter 1. Historically, these prosthetic components have tended to be "one size fits all" based on ideal engineering specifications. As a result, modern prostheses are modular in nature—they are formed from a range of possible technological components that must be skillfully combined to address the needs of a specific person. As such, the sections that follow present a high-level overview of the main components of a prosthetic robot: actuators, chassis, and power; the socket; signal acquisition; and the control and interface system (Figures 4.1 through 4.3). Each section presents the currently available technology that relates to the described component

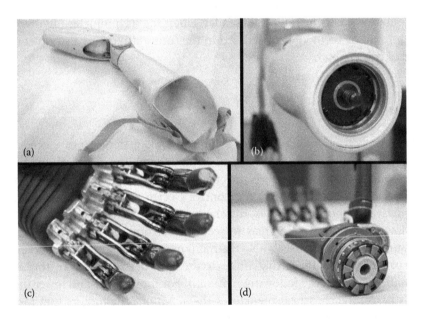

Figure 4.3 Examples of prosthetic chassis, actuators, interconnects, power, and socket systems. (a) Assembled prosthesis with a powered elbow attached to a socket and harness; power system and battery are visible in the hollow to the left of the actuator. (b) Interconnect system at the terminal end of the forearm of the prosthesis, connecting power and control signals to a robotic hand. (c) Small actuators and linkages that move the individual fingers of a robotic hand to provide multiple grasp patterns for the user. (d) A different robotic hand, also capable of multiple grasp patterns; interconnect on the displayed end mates with interconnect shown in (b).

and details how the technology interacts with the other components of a prosthetic limb.

The pace of commercial development of robotic prostheses is rapid. Prosthetic systems are highly modular, and new solutions are constantly being developed to the point of prescription for patients. Therefore, where possible, we avoid reference to specific commercial products or models. Information on robotic modules, specifications, and components is readily available from the catalogs of prosthetic manufacturers. However, exceptions are made to this policy when an emerging technology is only available from a single source or when mentioning a supplier or manufacturer is required for clarity. The intent of this section is to give the reader a clear understanding of the modern technological components of a robotic prosthesis—that is, commercially available products and solutions (defined as TRL 8–9)—and comprehension of how these components can be combined into a unified whole to support the daily life needs of patients with amputations. For the interested reader, emerging technologies (defined as TRL 7 and below) will be discussed in the future directions section at the end of this chapter.

Actuators, Chassis, and Power

The physical parts of prostheses can be broken down into electrical, mechanical, and electromechanical components. The main mechanical component of the prosthesis is the chassis: the shell that encloses the moving parts, the power system, the control electronics, and the computing hardware. In most prostheses, the chassis is a rigid exterior that is mostly hollow inside to provide areas to secure electromechanical components (Figure 4.3a). The chassis is also the main point of contact for the *socket*—the part of the prosthesis that affixes to the body of a user with an amputation (described in the following material). For most upper and lower limb prostheses, the chassis also encloses the *actuators*: the motors that move parts of the chassis with respect to the user's body.

In many cases that involve more proximal amputations (those closer to the body's center), the chassis of a robotic prosthesis is also modular, such that a user or his or her prosthetist can remove more distal components (those farther from the body's center) in a straightforward way. For example, with an upper limb arm-and-hand system, the prosthetic hand, wrist, and elbow are potentially independent modules and connect together at the wrist by way of a locking mechanism. Power and information are shared between these connected components via electrical contacts present in mating ends of any interlocking parts. For example, metal contacts on the surface of a standard electrical and mechanical locking mechanism at the proximal end of a robotic hand chassis mate with a similar arrangement of metal contacts on the distal end of a robotic elbow and forearm chassis (Figures 4.3b, d). The exact design of the interface between chassis modules is typically specific to each manufacturer, although efforts have been made to standardize interfaces for physical and electrical connection of components (Sutton et al. 2011).

Actuators provide the forces needed to move the different parts of the robotic prosthesis (Figures 4.3a, c). They must be robust, generate forces that allow the user to be able to perform daily life tasks, and be efficient in their use of power. Depending on the joint that is being powered by an actuator, the size and type of motor vary. Actuation of individual fingers in a prosthetic hand is readily done by a series of small actuators at the base of a finger or in the palm of the hand (Figures 4.1 and 4.3c). Larger actuators are used in joints such as the knee, elbow, or wrist (Figure 4.3a). For the most part, direct current (DC) motors remain the standard source of actuation, as well reviewed with technical clarity by Weir (2004). Specifically with regard to prosthetic hands, models are now available that allow more than two dozen different grasp patterns through actuators for each finger, with either a manually movable thumb or powered thumb opposition (Belter et al. 2013).

The chassis further provides a housing for the batteries that power the actuators and control hardware (Figure 4.3a). These batteries can be removable, such that they can be interchanged during extended periods of use, or they can be permanently mounted within the chassis such that a prosthesis must be directly connected to charging electronics via a plug on its exterior surface (Weir 2004). Batteries range in type, but in recent years older nickel-cadmium (Ni-Cad) and nickel-metal hydride (Ni-MH) models have been replaced with lithium (Li) and lithium polymer (Li-Po) equivalents that have better charging properties, smaller size and weight, and more charge-carrying capacity (Weir 2004).

Important considerations when designing the chassis and its internal components are robustness during daily use and weight. These two considerations are often in opposition: Stronger and more durable chassis are heavier and more bulky for a user. To be accepted by users, a chassis with all power and actuators installed should be significantly lighter than a biological arm, as the lack of direct skeletal attachment makes the prosthesis feel heavier due to soft tissue motion between the socket and limb. Importantly, as the number of actuators within a prosthesis increases, so does the battery demand and the weight of the device. As such, a great amount of design has gone into the shape, size, and materials of prosthetic chassis.

Efforts are ongoing to reduce the size and weight of prescribed prostheses while not compromising the functionality of these systems. Commercially available chassis and actuator configurations are designed to be worn by children, and many new robotic hands come in both a small and a large size to better suit a range of individuals.

Sockets, Harnessing, and Attachment to the Body

The socket is the foundation of the prosthesis and acts as the main structural interface between the prosthetic components and the remaining bone and soft tissue (Figure 4.3a). Generally, a poor-fitting socket will almost universally lead to rejection of the device, regardless of the potential functionality of the components and control system. The standard clinical method of attaching a prosthetic device to the user requires a socket and interface between the residual limb and the prosthetic components, with some form of suspension to hold the prosthesis in place either through socket design or by adding harnessing and straps. The socket is typically a rigid laminated material that is custom molded to the body, with an interface against the skin, such as a flexible thermoplastic material or various types of liners that distribute forces across the soft tissue, reduce friction, and in some cases provide suspension (e.g., pelite or gel liners such as silicone, urethane, or thermoplastic elastomer). As a general principle, areas of the residual limb that can withstand pressure (muscle and soft tissue) are loaded or compressed to ensure secure suspension of the prosthesis and to reduce excess movement between the socket and the user's residual limb. Areas that cannot withstand pressure, such as bony prominences, scar tissue, and neuromas, are relieved to avoid pain and skin breakdown.

The secondary role of the socket as the main communication transmitter between the user and the terminal components should not be overlooked. In the upper limb, the electrodes for the muscle control signals are encased in the socket and must maintain adequate and consistent contact over the muscle sites. In addition, in both upper and lower limb sockets, indirect feedback clues regarding the state of the prosthesis are provided through vibration and torque felt on the residual limb, based on the activity and position of the prosthesis. The more intimate the fit of the prosthetic socket, the more likely the user will incorporate these feedback clues into his or her awareness of the function of the prosthesis.

Lower limb sockets must be fashioned to transmit the load of the entire body during gait and are designed to accomplish this through reliance on weight bearing occurring through specific load-tolerant areas (i.e., the patellar tendon and tibial flares for amputation below the knee and the ischial tuberosity for amputation above the knee). With newer materials such as polyurethane and elastomer liners, the traditional designs have been able to move more toward a "total weight-bearing" approach in which the forces are transmitted hydrostatically throughout the entire residual limb. Suspension is often provided through suction, sleeves, or a locking pin in the end of the liner to avoid the need for belts and cuffs, which were historically required prior to suction methods of suspension using newer materials. The more proximal the limb loss, the more extensive the socket and suspension system generally must be to secure the weight of the prosthesis to the body and allow adequate control.

In the upper limb, bearing axial loads are less of a concern as the major challenge becomes one of maintaining suspension or preventing slippage of the socket when carrying loads or moving the arm. In addition, the socket must be designed with consideration not to restrict the available degrees of movement of the more proximal joints. For below-elbow levels of amputation, bony prominences can often be used for suspension by contouring around the elbow, but for more proximal levels in the upper arm, harnessing and strapping across the contralateral shoulder and trunk are almost universally required. Newer designs, such as high compression or high-low alternating compression (Alley et al. 2011), and adjustable sockets using pneumatic inflation air bladders have been described (Resnik 2014) to try to avoid the requirement for harnessing.

In even the most advanced socket designs, as the bony residuum is not directly secured to the prosthesis, rotation and movement of the limb in relationship to the socket typically occur to some degree. Problems with loss of socket fit and poor suspension can be magnified with limb atrophy, changes in limb volume throughout the day, or physical load on the limb. Importantly, this loss of suspension or a loose socket often leads to the patient reporting "heaviness" of the device, when in fact if motion is eliminated and better suspension achieved, the weight of the device will feel less. In the upper limb myoelectric device, slipping of the prosthesis or lack of contact will create poor control not only due to poor mechanical coupling of the device to the limb but also due to shifting of muscle electrodes, creating inconsistent contact of the control sensors to the muscle sites.

In summary, advances in materials such as gel liners have significantly improved socket comfort and skin condition and offered additional suspension methods. Newer socket designs that focus on stabilizing the limb for effective transmission of forces are an improvement on traditional sock-and-harness fittings. However, ongoing work to improve these factors is required as the socket remains the key to comfort, wear time, control, and acceptability for advanced prosthetic users.

Signal Acquisition and Myoelectric Recording

How user intent is communicated to the robotic prosthesis is important and is a key element informing the design of the robot. As discussed previously, user intent is approximated by the signals that are recorded from the user and state information that is maintained within the control system of the device. These signals can take many forms—mechanical, electrical, or combinations of the two—and can be recorded in a variety of ways (Fougner et al. 2012). As a simple example, manual switches, touch pads, linear transducers, and buttons are commonly used to change control options or inform the movement of prostheses. However, the dominant method for reading a user's intent during the control of a robotic prosthesis is a tech nique called *electromyographic* (EMG) *recording*: the sampling of electrical signals generated by muscle tissue in the user's residual limb or adjacent regions (Micera 2010; Oskoei and Hu 2007; Parker 2006; Scheme and Englehart 2011). This process of using these signals in the control of a robotic prosthesis is called *myoelectric control*.

Myoelectric recording for the control of prostheses has been pursued since as early as the 1940s (Childress 1985) and has matured to the point of widespread use in commercial prostheses (TRL 9). Sampling of EMG signals is typically done at the *surface* of the skin (denoted sEMG), and specifically through contact between the skin of the residual limb and a series of metal electrodes embedded within the socket of the prosthesis. These electrodes measure small changes in electrical potential generated by the muscle tissue located directly beneath them in the socket. As small units of muscle tissue, termed *motor units*, are recruited during muscle contraction, they contribute to consistent changes in the electrical properties of a specific muscle group or part of a muscle (Micera, Carpaneto, and Raspopovic 2010; Parker, Englehart, and Hudgins 2006). Muscle contractions can be detected through the increased amplitude and differing frequency components of electrical signals recorded at the skin above the muscle. Electrodes are thus placed and oriented within a socket to best acquire clear signals from relevant muscle groups while minimizing the amount of cross talk received from neighboring muscles (as described in detail by Micera, Carpaneto, and Raspopovic 2010; Oskoei and Hu 2007; Parker, Englehart, and Hudgins 2006; Weir 2004; and others).

In practical application, there is limited real estate within a prosthetic socket for recording, and the exact location and type of electrodes placed within the socket has to be carefully considered to maximize the number of clear channels of information that can be recorded from the user. To aid in this placement process, electrodes are sold in different shapes and sizes that can be mounted to socket liners or to the hard wall of a socket. Furthermore, electrodes can be positioned side by side in a single hard case or arranged remotely at the end of short leads that form differential pairs with a dedicated reference electrode, single points with a common electrode for reference, or a range of alternate configurations to suit specific circumstances (Micera, Carpaneto, and Raspopovic 2010). For example, in the case of a user with a transhumeral (upper arm) amputation and the desire to control a prosthetic elbow actuator, EMG electrodes might be placed in differential pairs over the biceps and triceps of the user's residual limb; this could take the form of two small metal domes protruding from the inside of the socket. For the case of a transradial (lower arm) amputation, electrodes are placed around the interior of the socket to make contact at the flexor and extensor muscles of the user's residual forearm.

Sampled myoelectric signals are amplified, filtered, and processed by the electronics housed within the prosthetic chassis, such that they can be readily used to inform prosthesis control (as described in more detail in material that follows). Some electrodes conduct this amplification and filtering at the point of recording to better reduce the amount of noise in the signals, while others rely primarily on amplification and filtering by electrical components at another point in the prosthetic chassis. Recorded signals may be rectified and conditioned or left unfiltered, depending on the needs of a particular manufacturer's actuators and control systems. Electrodes are connected to other electrical hardware within the chassis via shielded electrical cables.

In summary, myoelectric recording is an effective, widely used method for reading user control intent from voluntary contractions of the user's muscle tissue. EMG recording technology is designed and deployed to maximize the number of distinct myoelectric signals that can be sampled from a user's residual limb. Prosthetists configure the socket, chassis, number of actuators, and internal hardware of a robotic prosthesis to best utilize the information contained in these myoelectric signals. However, there remains room for improvement in myoelectric recording, as evidenced by a large body of ongoing work in industry and academia.

Examples include new electrodes with different conduction properties and sockets with dense arrays of recording electrodes (Daley et al.
2012; Tkach et al. 2012) that promise to greatly enhance the effectiveness
and resiliency of myoelectric control once they see widespread clinical
deployment.

Control Systems and Interfaces

The control system is the principal means of linking signals recorded
from the user to the control actions to be performed by the user's robotic
device (Figure 4.4). As reviewed by Micera, Carpaneto, and Raspopovic
(2010), Parker, Englehart, and Hudgins (2006), and more recently by
Scheme and Engelhart (2011), a range of methods and approaches exists
for developing a control system to transform the signals provided by a user
into precise motor commands for a robotic limb (Figure 4.4). In practical application, these range from simple routines in hardware and software that map input signals to output commands using straightforward

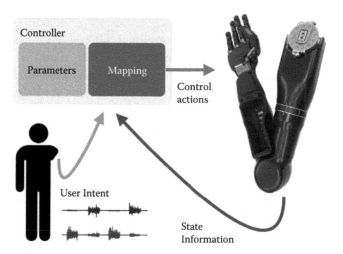

Figure 4.4 Control interactions between a user and the user's prosthetic device.
User intent is measured from the body, for example, using myoelectric recording (labeled "User Intent"). These signals are passed to a control system, in many
cases along with information from the robot's actuators and state (labeled "State
Information"). Informed by electrical and software parameter settings and calibration values, the control system forms a mapping from these input signals to
control actions for the robotic limb.

mathematical relationships, to approaches that use machine learning and advanced statistical techniques to map a series of complex myoelectric patterns onto a range of discrete motions. This section focuses on upper limb applications, as practically speaking, no current available systems provide myoelectric-powered control for the lower limb outside the research laboratory. Most current commercial lower limb prostheses (e.g., Figure 4.2) are indirectly, passively controlled by alignment with respect to the ground-reaction force and momentum through proximal joint motion (hip or knee). The most advanced lower limb prostheses use internal torque and accelerometer sensors with a computer control algorithm to control stance phase resistance and passive prosthetic joint motion. A few more recent powered components also provide active powered motion, controlled based on motion, position, and velocity sensors rather than direct muscle signals (Sup, Varol, and Goldfarb 2011).

For upper limb robotic devices, in the simplest case each commercial robotic module or actuator accepts one or more myoelectric signals as input (via wires that connect the module to the electrodes mounted in the user's socket) and proportionally or discretely maps these analog signals in a predefined way to the movement of the module's respective joints. A prosthetist is able to manually change the amplification of the signals to match the quality and intensity of signals that can be provided by the user or configure the other internal control parameters of the device itself. In more recent systems, a robotic prosthesis will provide a wireless or wired interface to a mobile device or computer that gives access to some or all of its control parameters, such that they can be tuned by a user or a prosthetist. In practice, the initial calibration and tuning of the control system for a robotic prosthesis is done by a prosthetist trained in the setup of a given prosthetic component. The user is then trained on the use of the new control approach and related robotic technology through sessions with occupational and physical therapists. This training is crucial for a number of reasons, but as it relates to control, it helps the user provide myoelectric signals that can more readily be interpreted by the control system of the prosthesis. As such, there is often an iterative in-clinic process of training and calibration focused on improving control for the user (Resnik et al. 2012).

As a user-centered example, some modern multifunction robotic hands allow users to connect to the device with a smartphone and modify the way that they select grasp patterns and even customize the grips available during daily use. However, in all commercial cases, the low-level control of actuators and the related parameters is not presented to the user, and

control typically relies on hardware and software proprietary to the manufacturer of each prosthetic component.

More advanced control options have only recently become available to
prosthetic users, in the form of *pattern recognition* (TRL 8–9). In contrast to the approach described previously, where a series of electrodes are
mapped by the prosthetist in a fixed way to the input control channels of
prosthetic components, pattern recognition uses statistical machine learning approaches to automatically form a mapping from input signals to output motion on a robotic prosthesis (Micera, Carpaneto, and Raspopovic
2010; Scheme and Englehart 2011). In essence, a control system is given
the task of perceiving the pattern of signals being recorded from a set of
electrodes at any given movement and learning how to match this pattern
with a user-specified movement of the attached robotic actuators. Then,
when a user later presents one of the learned patterns of myoelectric activity, the control system is able to detect the pattern and generate the appropriate movement. This mapping can be formed using machine learning
algorithms such as linear discriminant analysis, support vector machines,
or other well-established classification methods (Castellini et al. 2014).
A significant amount of research has been conducted to determine the
correct way to train such a classifier and how best to provide myoelectric information to the classifier in the form of processed time, frequency,
and time-space features (Castellini et al. 2014; Micera, Carpaneto, and
Raspopovic 2010; Scheme and Englehart 2011).

The only currently commercially available example of pattern recognition is Complete Control (Coapt LLC); in this control solution, all electrodes in a socket are fed into a single pattern recognition module, which
then provides output signals to a set of downstream actuators. The pattern
recognition hardware and software form an intermediary between the
electrodes and actuators of a number of other manufacturers. To use the
system, the user presses a training button mounted on the chassis of the prosthesis. Under the control of the pattern recognition module, the prosthesis
then automatically generates a set of motions that the user must copy by
flexing residual muscles in the way the user thinks is most appropriate for
the given motion. The pattern recognition system records a set of training examples wherein each motion is linked to multiple examples of the
corresponding myoelectric patterns as provided by the user and computes
a mapping from EMG input signals to output control signals. After training, control is returned to the user. Multiple movements can be learned
and effected in this way, without detailed calibration by a prosthetist,
and the user is in control of retraining the control system in response to
day-by-day and moment-by-moment changes in the user's myoelectric

signals. Training of the pattern recognition systems is straightforward and brief. In Figure 4.4, the training of the pattern recognition system can be thought of as changing the mapping block from input signals to output control actions.

Recent control approaches based on machine learning represent an important paradigm shift in technology for robotic prostheses—prosthetic control systems are now able to play an active role in adapting to their user and the way a person's signals and patterns of use change outside the clinic (Castellini et al. 2014; Pilarski, Dawson et al. 2013). In particular, advanced control approaches such as pattern recognition are decreasing the time that it takes for users to be able to control a new robotic prosthesis and increasing the number of accessible prosthetic functions available to a user. However, in upper limb prostheses, whether with conventional control or pattern recognition, users are presently still limited to controlling a single actuator or motion at a time or, in promising cases, performing two simultaneous movements. A significant amount of work is required and ongoing to provide users with fluid, natural, and simultaneous control of large numbers of actuators (Castellini et al. 2014).

Critical Review of the Available Utilization Protocols

The goal of prescribing a robotic prosthesis is to provide a functional replacement for the lost limb that the user wears on a daily basis. Lower limb prosthetic users typically don their prosthesis every morning as part of their dressing routine and wear it throughout the day, with occasional breaks for comfort or to adjust socket fit as limb volume can change throughout the day. At night, they must clean and air the limb and the prosthetic interface to maintain hygiene and skin condition. Externally powered components often must be charged throughout the night. For the upper limb, constant use for a full day is less common, as patients can manage with one-handed function at home, so typically the prosthesis is used when out of the house or for specific tasks that require bimanual function.

Choosing the right prosthesis requires that the clinician understands the needs and goals of the patient, the environment in which the prosthesis will be used, and the required tasks. In addition, psychological adjustment to amputation includes learning to incorporate the prosthesis into the individual's body image as well as function, so appearance is an important factor for some. For the lower limb, a patient must have a minimum level of strength and ability to weight bear in the remaining limb to allow adequate prosthetic function, as well as proximal joint (hip or knee) range and strength to drive the prosthesis. For the upper limb, shoulder and contralateral arm function are important factors to evaluate, as is condition of the residual limb. Most limb anomalies, such as scarring, grafted skin tissue, and bony prominences, can be adequately managed with today's technology and advanced interfaces, but daily inspection of the residual limb and meticulous skin care are essential to maintain limb health and must be incorporated into the daily routine.

Training to use a prosthesis is an essential factor in success, as prosthetic provision alone does not equate to restoration of function (Dawson, Carey, and Fahimi 2011). Gait training typically progresses through graduated weight bearing and reduction of gait aids as the user learns to trust the prosthesis and the limb accommodates to the new forces being transmitted through the socket, which must be guided by a therapist experienced in lower limb prosthetics. This is particularly true for advanced microprocessor and powered robotic components, which act and respond in very different ways than traditional prostheses. For the upper limb, training for myoelectric control can often start prior to provision of the prosthesis, through teaching the user to activate and strengthen existing muscle signal control signals. This can be as simple as visualization techniques by which the user imagines phantom limb movements and voluntarily activates remaining muscles or can use virtual reality or table-mounted robotic arms to practice myoelectric control using affixed EMG electrodes (Dawson, Carey, and Fahimi 2011). During this process, the prosthetist establishes the location of the most efficient and separable control signals and manufactures the socket with the electrodes placed in the optimal locations on the interior of the socket. Once the socket is fit to the user, control training using the robotic prosthesis continues, starting with simple tasks (hand open/close control), progressing to more complex multijoint tasks, and eventually moving to coordinated bimanual tasks simulating performance of activities of daily living (ADL). The user is also encouraged to try new tasks at home and then problem solve any difficulties encountered with the therapist. This process can take several weeks to months to achieve expert control of the system and is typically directed by the occupational therapist. Close coordination between an interdisciplinary team (prosthetist, therapist, physiatrist) is ideal throughout prosthetic fitting and training to ensure all potential issues are addressed to maximize function and create a successful outcome for the patient.

Upper Limb Robotic Prostheses

Myoelectric prostheses have a long history of development but generally have been available for widespread clinical use since the late 1970s (Childress 1985). There are no definitive criteria for which devices to fit to which patient, but in general several factors are considered for each individual, such as function, comfort, cosmesis, reliability, and cost. Myoelectric devices are more expensive and heavier and require more maintenance than body-powered prostheses; however, they have the advantages of requiring less harnessing, allowing greater range of motion and functional range of the terminal device; having a more natural control scheme; and having better cosmetic appearance.

Over the years, several studies have shown varying rates of rejection of electrically powered prostheses, from 25% (Biddiss 2007b) up to 50% in some studies (Silcox et al. 1993; Wright, Hagan, and Wood 1995). Heavy weight, low durability, slow response, and lack of sensory feedback are often stated as limiting factors (Biddiss 2007a). However, some studies, such as one in injured workers, showed 83% acceptance of electrically powered prostheses (Millstein, Heger, and Hunter 1986) and that many workers used more than one type of prosthesis to meet all their functional needs.

With the more recent advances in multifunction grip hands, patterns of use may be changing. As more options are available for hands to provide more functional grasp patterns, users can use the myoelectric prostheses for a wider range of activities. In the clinic, the sooner the amputee is fit with a prosthesis, the better the long-term acceptance of the device. Usage patterns and acceptance in general are highest for transradial amputation levels versus higher levels of amputation, as the complexity of the system increases with multiple components. Often, hybrid prostheses with a combination of body-powered and myoelectric components are prescribed for higher-level amputations to minimize weight, cost, and complexity of operation. Critical factors for acceptance often are the ease of donning and doffing the prosthesis and the robustness and reliability of control. For this reason, recent advancements, such as interface liners with embedded electrodes and pattern recognition with onboard calibration, may improve long-term acceptance due to greater reliability and less effort to don and adjust myoelectric sites.

Lower Limb Robotic Prostheses

Lower limb prostheses are more commonly accepted and used for greater hours during the day due to the need to restore functional ambulation. Prescription of prosthetic components is typically based on assessment of an individual's functional ambulatory potential. For example, an individual expected to only be ambulatory in the household or over level surfaces using gait aids at one cadence is not expected to benefit from a cadence-responsive hydraulic knee, and in fact the increased weight may be a detriment. As functional ability increases to the point of community ambulation at varying cadences, the advantages of advanced components become more evident. Of particular importance is the ability of most microprocessor-controlled knees to provide resistance to involuntary stance phase knee flexion by altering resistance based on real-time input, which is thought to reduce risk of falls. Reported advantages of advanced prosthetic knees include improved balance and more normalized gait pattern (Kaufman et al. 2007); a subjective impression of improved ability to navigate uneven terrain, slopes, and inclines; and possibly less cognitive load required during ambulation (Williams et al. 2006).

Powered lower limb robotic prostheses are unique in that they are designed to generate powered movements rather than rely on passive variable dampening of microprocessor knees. This provides a specific advantage in movements, such as from sit to stand and stair ascent (Lawson et al. 2013). This is hoped to reduce the requirements of the proximal joints and contralateral limb to generate the additional power required to compensate for the loss of anatomic knee power, thereby normalizing the biomechanics of gait (Goldfarb, Lawson, and Shultz 2013). The major barriers to accessing this technology are cost and acceptance of funding agencies. Ongoing work is required to document the potential benefits of these advanced technologies through appropriate metrics and economic analyses.

Review of User Studies, Outcomes, and Clinical Evidence

Acceptance, Use Cases, and Clinical Successes

Upper Limb

Development of advanced upper limb technology has been dramatic in the last decade, but parallel improvements in clinical usage and success have not been thoroughly documented yet. As noted, rates of abandonment in the past have been reported to be from 25% to 50% (Biddiss and Chau 2007a,b), with concerns over poor control, limited dexterity, discomfort, poor durability, weight, cost, and limited sensory feedback commonly cited as reasons for rejection (Atkins 1996; Biddiss and Chau 2007a,b). It is presumed that those who continue to use their prosthesis do so because they have attained a level of control that improves their function, although cosmesis may also play a role. In general, this is an understudied area, and the rates of acceptance may change with more recent technological advances. This has led to increasing focus on a "user-centered" approach to design and development (Resnik 2011). Usability research has only recently incorporated end users in the device development stages in an attempt to overcome barriers to clinical use and meet the needs of consumers. From an ergonomic human factors approach, this would seem an essential component in the deployment of robotic prostheses, for which usability hinges on acceptable human interaction with the device.

An additional challenge is lack of agreement on the best methods of measuring clinical success in the application of robotic technology. Substantial work has been done by the working group on Upper Limb Prosthetic Outcome Measures (ULPOM) (Hill et al. 2009). They recommended the use of the World Health Organization's (2001) International Classification of Functioning, Disability, and Health (ICF) as a framework for selection of outcome measures. However, a clear limitation of existing metrics is that no one measure covers the range of potential outcomes of interest; therefore, a range of metrics covering the elements of the ICF is advised, including measurement of body structure and function (performance of the prosthesis), activity (carrying out tasks), and participation (use of the prosthesis in real-life situations). In addition, standard metrics were developed for standard technology and basic function and do not always take into account the types of improvement expected with advanced robotic devices that add dexterity and feedback. The measurement of higher cognitive functions, such as embodiment and cognitive load/visual attention, are not traditionally considered as prosthetic outcomes but need to be incorporated into future assessments of effectiveness of robotic devices from a human-machine interaction perspective. This will be especially important as strides are made in neural machine interfacing, improved communication protocols, and other advances in limb attachment (detailed in the material that follows) that improve the function of advanced devices past research settings into the clinical environment.

Lower Limb

Similar concerns over lower limb functional outcome metrics exist, with many standard mobility tests focusing on assessment of basic levels of function. A comprehensive review of lower limb prosthetic outcomes was published by Condie, Scott, and Treweek in 2006, which was updated and catalogued according to ICF elements in 2009 (Deathe et al. 2009; Hebert et al. 2009), and was most recently reviewed from a clinical perspective (Heinemann et al. 2014). In general, most metrics evaluate basic mobility and have significant ceiling effects, inadequately addressing potential advantages of more complex advanced prostheses. More advanced metrics for higher-level function have been introduced with less functional ceiling effect (Gailey et al. 2013), but to truly discern the differences with advanced components, most researchers rely on detailed biomechanical/gait analysis evaluations versus global mobility metrics. The most advanced microprocessor and power knees claim to have significant beneficial effects on improving stability and ability to navigate uneven terrain and stairs, reducing compensatory gait strategies and lessening cognitive load in having to control the prosthesis; however, existing metrics do not capture these mostly qualitative findings (Orendurff 2013). It is clear that more sensitive metrics will need to be developed to detect these more subtle effects of advanced components.

Remaining Barriers to Patient Acceptance

As reviewed in a number of recent publications, and noted previously, there are remaining barriers to the acceptance and consistent use of prescribed myoelectric prostheses (Atkins, Heard, and Donovan 1996; Biddiss and Chau 2007; Micera, Carpaneto, and Raspopovic 2010; Peerdeman et al. 2011; Resnik 2012; Scheme and Englehart 2011). Coarsely grouped, these barriers have been found to relate to the functionality of the robotic prosthesis, the amount of feedback users receive from their device, the complexity of the control interface, comfort, durability, and the appearance of their device.

By way of examples from a study by Peerdeman et al. of forearm prosthesis users (2011), grasp execution time for hand prostheses remains too slow for many users (~1 second); while force-based control and velocity-based control, as opposed to positional control, have been listed as desirable control properties, their execution for precise user manipulation in practice is still lacking. Further, users report that their devices often do not have the right number or type of functions (e.g., lack of a movable wrist on a forearm prosthesis or lack of individual finger control); they desire more actuation. However, when multiple functions are supplied, they are at present not always easy for users to access. In many cases where multiple functions are present, users often disregard or cannot access already-present functionality due to the complexity of the control interface. Commercially available pattern recognition should help alleviate some of these concerns. However, active feedback, as opposed to inherent feedback via the chassis of the prosthesis, is in all practical senses missing from deployed systems.

An additional concern with the majority of modern upper limb robotic prostheses is the requirement for a user to maintain visual and cognitive attention on the robotic prosthesis during operation (noted by Atkins, Heard, and Donovan 1996; Bongers et al. 2012). Prosthetic hands lack meaningful sensory feedback and must be carefully watched at all times to perform even simple tasks. Visual attention demands are an area where improved sensory feedback may play an important role, and feedback systems are thus a major area of development (Antfolk et al. 2013; Schofield et al. 2014). Other remaining concerns include prostheses being generally too large or heavy for most of their users due to the engineering requirements for actuation and robustness (Atkins, Heard, and Donovan 1996; Sensinger, Lock, and Kuiken 2014), and that users cannot always reliably use their devices in protracted or vigorous ADL (Atkins, Heard, and Donovan 1996). As described in the next section, these difficulties are being addressed by a significant body of ongoing industrial, clinical, and fundamental research.

In the lower limb, barriers to use mainly relate to socket comfort (Dillingham et al. 2001; Pezzin et al. 2004), although dissatisfaction with cosmesis may also play a role to a greater degree than previously appreciated, based on recent surveys in which patients listed concerns with respect to shape of the prosthesis matching the cosmesis to the sound limb, free prosthetic joint movement underneath the cosmesis, and natural fit of clothing over the cosmesis (Cairns et al. 2014). Interestingly, gait deviation has been reported as unimportant to the amputee, with self-reported functional ability and attitudes toward the prosthesis having the strongest correlation to satisfaction following lower limb amputation (Kark and Simmons 2011).

Future Directions

The intent of this section is to briefly introduce a range of frontier directions for improving the outcomes of patients with amputations. A focus is placed on breadth as opposed to depth, such that a wide range of topics can be covered, ranging from the conceptual (TRL 1–5) to those nearing practical use (TRL 5–8). Specifically, this section addresses ongoing work that aims to further close the loop between a person and the person's robotic prosthesis, the deployment of implantable technologies, the use of machine learning and intelligent systems for advanced control, and groundbreaking new robotic prostheses that significantly extend the function of currently available devices.

Bidirectional Control and Feedback

Targeted Motor and Sensory Reinnervation

Surgical reconstruction of the amputated limb plays an essential role in maximizing outcomes for prosthetic applications. In addition to advances in bone management, residual muscle management, and skin coverage, advanced nerve procedures have been developed to improve the ability to extract the rich control signals that are lost after upper limb amputation. **Targeted reinnervation (TR)** surgically redirects the amputated nerve endings that used to innervate the hand and wrist muscles to new muscle sites to provide physiologically natural motor command signals for myoelectric control (Kuiken, Schultz Feuser, and Barlow 2013). The surgically redirected nerves reinnervate purposely denervated remaining muscles, which then act as biological amplifiers for the neural signals that are still under voluntary (brain) control. These muscle responses, which are intuitively activated, are then linked to the action of the prosthesis. After reinnervation, patients are able to operate multiple degrees of freedom of advanced prosthetic devices with increased ease. Combining newer surface EMG recording techniques (such as pattern recognition) with TR may allow even more signals to be extracted for prosthetic control. Recently, in subjects with upper limb amputation having undergone TR, simultaneous pattern recognition control was found to be superior in preference and performance to both sequential pattern recognition and conventional myoelectric control (Young et al. 2013).

In addition to improved motor control, TR provides a potential avenue for sensory feedback. Redirection of the amputated sensory nerves to denervated skin restores the sensation of the hand and fingers on the new target area of skin (Hebert, Elzinga et al. 2014; Marasco, Schultz, and Kuiken 2009). This "transfer sensation" from reinnervation of the sensory afferents is a possible access point to provide physiologically natural and appropriate avenues of cutaneous touch and proprioceptive feedback through robotic devices (Hebert, Olson et al. 2014). Ongoing research in this area is linking haptic feedback to tactor devices that stimulate the skin and muscle in proportion to sensors on the prosthesis, thereby providing real-time bidirectional feedback in a noninvasive socket system.

Noninvasive Recording Alternatives

While sEMG from a small number of recording sites has become the dominant approach to controlling robotic prostheses, a number of alternatives have been proposed to help increase the view of the prosthesis into the intent of its user. As reviewed by Castellini et al. (2014) and Founger et al. (2012), there have been promising demonstrations of prosthesis control using ultrasound, high-density EMG arrays, topographic force mapping within the socket, acceleration measurement, mechanomyography (the measurement at the skin of muscle-contraction-related mechanical disturbances), and others. Each method has its own benefits in terms of the features of a user's upstream control intent that it provides. Each method also has specific implementation challenges that potentially limit deployment in take-home settings. Considered as a whole, the move to more diverse and more detailed recording of user intent—novel noninvasive recording modalities coupled with conventional sEMG technology—promises to alleviate significant failure modes of sEMG and increase the robustness of next-generation systems (Castellini et al. 2014).

Implantable Technology

Osseointegration

Osseointegration refers to the direct structural and functional connection between living bone and the surface of an artificial metal implant. Worldwide, osseointegration is used in joint replacement, dental implants, craniofacial deficiencies, maxillofacial reconstruction, orbital prostheses, and bone-anchored hearing aids. The technique for prosthetic attachment using a transdermal implant for limb amputation has been an accepted clinical treatment technique in Europe since the 1990s (Hagberg 2009) and in Australia since 2009 (Al Muderis, Tetsworth et al. 2016), and recently has been approved for investigational device exemption in the United States. The primary advantage of osseointegration is that the weight and functional leverage of the prosthetic limb is transferred directly to the skeleton, eliminating the need for a prosthetic socket. A titanium fixture is placed in the center of the amputated limb bone, with a replaceable titanium abutment extending through a skin opening. The end of the abutment serves as the mounting point for the prosthetic limb. The skin adheres to the bone at the junction where the percutaneous abutment traverses the skin to minimize communication with the underlying structures. The main persisting complication is that of intermittent skin infections that can occur at the percutaneous junction (reported in 34–55% of patients, with implant survival rates from 92% to 96%) (Al Muderis, Khemka et al. 2016; Brånemark 2014). Techniques of management of the skin–implant interface continue to evolve in attempts to reduce this relatively high rate of infection. Reports on the function and quality of life benefits of osseo-integration in general indicate improved prosthetic use, mobility, physical function, and global improvement in quality of life (Al Muderis, Tetsworth et al. 2016; Branemark 2014; Jönsson 2011; Lundberg 2011; van de Meent 2013). In addition to benefits of greater range of motion and control due to lack of requirement for a socket, there is a phenomenon of "osseopercep-tion" described, whereby the individual feels tactile and proprioceptive feedback through vibrations transmitted directly to the skeleton.

New techniques of osseointegration have shortened the rehabilita-tion time and in some cases combined osseointegrated limb attachments with joint replacement, in order to address the most challenging cases of prosthetic application (Khemka 2015). Recent exciting advances combine neural machine interfaces with osseointegration for proximal upper limb loss, which promises a "plug-and-play" system where the individual is functionally and structurally connected to his or her robotic prosthesis through a single abutment attachment (Ortiz-Catalan 2014).

Implantable Muscle Recording
Surface recording of EMG signals for prosthetic control is limited by the variability of the interface between the electrode and the skin and imprecision of the recorded signal due to cross talk and other artifacts. To address these limitations and improve the precision of myoelectric recording for prosthesis control, the Alfred Mann Foundation developed and deployed implantable and fully wireless EMG electrodes (Merrill et al. 2011; Pasquina et al. 2015). These Implantable Myoelectric Sensors (IMES®) are cylindrical devices with a very small footprint (2.5 by 16 mm) that, when implanted inside muscle tissue, can accurately sample multi-ple channels of EMG and report the resulting values over a wireless link to receivers outside the body (Pasquina et al. 2015). Epimysial electrodes are another type of muscle-sensing electrode implanted on the surface of the muscle belly (sewn to the muscle casing), and they have been widely

used in humans, commonly for functional electrical stimulation and more recently for neuroprosthetic control (Ortiz-Catalan et al. 2012; Ortiz-Catalan, Hakansson, and Branemark 2014).

The IMES system has seen active development and recently a first-in-human demonstration, wherein eight IMES units were implanted in eight different muscles of the residual forearm of a subject with transradial amputation. The subject reported satisfaction with the system and a number of qualitative gains over his previous myoelectric control; he further reported the ability to effectively and intuitively use IMES to perform a number of functional tasks with his robotic prosthesis (Pasquina et al. 2015). This demonstration shows great promise and, while preliminary, suggests a number of fruitful combinations with other innovations, such as TR (described previously) and advanced pattern recognition approaches (described in the material that follows). The estimated life span of IMES units is suggested to be upward of 80 years (Merrill et al. 2011). If successful in long-term deployment, IMES paves the way for significant gains in both the usability and the functionality of robotic prostheses, including easy donning and doffing of prostheses, simultaneous control of multiple joints, and greater dexterity in the control of individual actuators.

Peripheral Nerve Recording and Stimulation
Direct communication with the peripheral nervous system has been investigated through the use of implanted intraneural electrodes and nerve cuff approaches. Studies in amputee subjects using longitudinal intrafascicular electrodes (LIFEs) (Rossini et al. 2010), transverse intrafascicular multichannel electrodes (TIMEs) (Raspopovic et al. 2014), the Utah Slant Array (which penetrates the nerve fiber bundles), and the flat interface nerve electrode (FINE) have all shown the ability to use sensory input feedback with simultaneous motor control in amputee subjects. Research is ongoing to demonstrate long-term viability of the implants, but some have been in place as long as 2 years. These investigations are exciting advances that will likely lead to significant changes in the approach to sensory motor restoration in the future through the ability to directly tap into neural control and feedback signals.

Advanced Control Paradigms

Pattern Recognition
Pattern recognition, an approach to classifying a user's intended motions based on learned patterns of myoelectric activity, has seen recent

commercial availability. However, there is significant ongoing work under way to improve the interpretation of myoelectric patterns from users (Castellini et al. 2014; Micera, Carpaneto, and Raspopovic 2010). Recent work includes approaches to the simultaneous pattern recognition control of multiple functions and to increase the robustness of pattern recognition to the rigors of daily life—for example, decreasing the sensitivity of classifiers to the position of the residual limb, to other simultaneous bodily activities, or to ongoing fatigue (Hargrove, Lock, and Simon 2013; Hargrove, Simon et al. 2013; Scheme and Englehart 2011; Scheme, Hudgins, and Englehart 2013). Another active area of ongoing research is supervised adaptation (by way of prespecified or intermittent retraining of a pattern recognition system) and unsupervised adaptation (automatic retraining or updating of a pattern recognition system, without the need for specific training periods) to allow a device to modify its operation to new users or new situations (Sensinger, Lock, and Kuiken 2009; Tommassi 2013). Continual, real-time adaptation of pattern recognition is considered to be a major area of clinical interest (Scheme and Englehart 2011), as are ways to better structure the training of pattern recognition systems. For the interested reader, Castellini et al. (2014) provided a comprehensive review of ways in which pattern recognition is being enhanced to better leverage sEMG for more precise and user-friendly pattern recognition.

Machine Learning, Intelligent Systems, and Shared Control

Pattern recognition represents one form of autonomy and machine learning on the part of a robotic prosthesis (Oskoei and Hu 2007). The prosthetic control system is observing complex patterns from the user and making moment-by-moment decisions regarding which of the many functions on the device the user will control. In this case, the control system's choices are based on learned predictions of a user's motor intent. Pattern recognition and other forms of autonomy have been demonstrated to be desirable for the users of robotic prostheses (Castellini et al. 2014). One simple example of autonomy now deployed in commercial systems is slip detection for grasping, such that a system will hold on to an object even when a user is not attending to his or her grasp. These examples suggest how even modest intelligence on the part of an assistive technology can help support the user of that technology. More advanced examples include research into ways that a prosthetic hand could automatically preshape its grip to accommodate specific objects in an environment (as reviewed by Castellini et al. 2014) or how a robotic system may in fact build up knowledge about the user in the form of predictions and control policies to better inform the simultaneous control of multiple movements or functions (Edwards et al. 2016; Pilarski, Dawson et al. 2013; Pilarski, Dick, and Sutton 2013; Pulliam, Lambrecht, and Kirsch 2011).

Taken as a whole, there is a growing body of evidence to suggest that intelligence and agency on the part of a robotic prosthesis will extend the potential abilities of a prosthetic user (e.g., the idea of a prosthesis-human partnership developing shared *communicative capital* through ongoing interactions, as proposed by Pilarski, Sutton, and Mathewson 2015). More specifically, increased and more general machine intelligence in the control systems of robotic prostheses is expected to greatly increase the robustness, adaptability, and situational awareness of current systems to better meet the needs of users (Castellini et al. 2014). This hypothesis remains to be rigorously proved or disproved.

Next-Generation Robotic Prostheses

New physical and computational interfaces will form a keystone for improving the life of the next generation of prosthetic users. One principal reason to expect improvement is a corresponding surge in advanced robotic prostheses that vastly exceed the functionality of their predecessors but are not yet at the point of commercial readiness (TRL 7 and below). The intent of this section is to briefly describe the capabilities and highlights of some of the most notable advanced bionic limbs. While the summary is by no means complete, the reader will gain an understanding of the potential for future improvements in form, function, control, and feedback that evolve from game-changing new technology.

As one recent example, researchers from the University of New Brunswick and the Rehabilitation Institute of Chicago (RIC) have demonstrated the RIC Arm: a small, lightweight, modular prosthetic arm-and-hand solution with multiple actuators (TRL 7–8) (Sensinger, Lock, and Kuiken 2014). By incorporating custom motors tuned to the requirements of daily life, the RIC Arm is designed to be suitable for use by a 25th-percentile female, as opposed to the 75th-percentile male population that is the target of most prostheses. This provides the first multifunction prosthesis of many alternatives, it is hoped, to further increase the opportunities for prostheses that are personalized in all aspects to their different users—a major change from one-size-fits-all solutions of previous decades.

A representative example of one of the most advanced engineered limbs is the Modular Prosthetic Limb (MPL) developed by the Applied Physics Laboratory of Johns Hopkins University as part of the Defense Advanced Research Projects Agency (DARPA) Revolutionizing Prosthetics Program

(Bridges, Para, and Mashner 2011; Johannes et al. 2011; Ravitz et al. 2013). Now in its third generation, the MPL is arguably the most dexterous upper limb prosthesis developed to date. The hand of the MPL is actuated using small motors placed within the palm and fingers and involves multiple contact sensors; thermal, capacitive sensors; and other sensors (>100 sensors in total) located throughout the fingers, hand, and arm. The hand of the MPL also features computing hardware and embedded control electronics for the entire arm (Johannes et al. 2011; Ravitz et al. 2013). This configuration enables independent finger flexion and extension, finger deviations from their midline, thumb flexion and rotation. A third-generation MPL is shown in Figure 4.1d and Figure 4.5. In addition, the MPL features three degrees of freedom for wrist actuation, elbow flexion and extension, humeral rotation, and two axes of shoulder motion. As such, it provides a first approximation to the degrees of actuation in a biological limb and a viable recording source for a diverse set of sensory feedback modalities.

Another powerful new DARPA limb technology is the DEKA Arm (Resnik 2014). This system provides a number of actuators that greatly

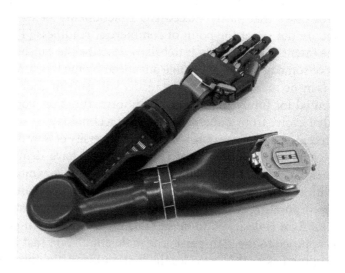

Figure 4.5   Third-generation modular prosthetic limb (HDT Global), with battery compartment in the forearm and showing the following actuators: shoulder (two actuators), humeral rotator in the middle of the upper arm, elbow, wrist (three actuators), and dexterous hand (independent finger and thumb actuation). This system, as shown, would be connected to the harness technology for someone with a shoulder disarticulation but can also be broken down into modules for other levels of amputation and socket integration.

exceeds those of commercially deployed prostheses, and, while featuring less actuation than the MPL, it is an example of a robust system that is suitable for use in deployed end-user environments; it has been through aggressive testing in military and civilian applications (TRL 8–9). The DEKA Arm recently received Food and Drug Administration (FDA) approval in the United States. As such, it is one example of an advanced upper limb device that is nearing the point of clinical translation to widespread use, although testing is still needed to determine the most effective control modalities for all settings and other factors affecting user acceptance.

With respect to the lower limb, recent work has demonstrated powered knee and ankle robots with and without pattern recognition control that promise to greatly extend locomotion abilities (Hargrove, Simon et al. 2013; Ingraham et al. 2016; Schultz, Lawson, and Goldfarb 2015), and in a high-profile example allowed one subject to climb more than 100 flights of stairs to summit the Chicago Willis Tower. Significant work on powered lower limb robots is also being conducted by the team led by Hugh Herr at the Massachusetts Institute of Technology, giving subjects with lower limb amputations the power to run, to climb, and even to return to precise and graceful activities such as ballroom dancing (e.g., Eilenberg, Geyer, and Herr 2010; Rouse et al. 2015).

Advanced robotic prostheses currently in development represent the future of limb replacement—a future in which the function, strength, speed, and dexterity of a replaced limb equals or even exceeds that of a lost biological limb. With the advent of nonphysiological prostheses (artificial limbs that do not mirror the look or operation of a biological limb) and supernumerary limbs for users without amputations (Llorens-Bonilla and Asada 2014; Parietti and Asada 2014), the potential for prosthetic technology to improve lives is vast. As a remaining challenge to unlocking the power of these systems, it will be important to continue to accelerate the state of the art in control and interface technology to keep pace with the potential power of available robotic hardware and rigorously develop robotic prostheses such that they can be brought to effective function in the daily life of users (TRL 9).

STUDY QUESTIONS

1. How do robotic prostheses differ from other assistive rehabilitation robots?
2. What are four main principles or components for creating effective robotic prostheses?
3. What are the main limitations in the control of an upper limb robotic prosthesis?

4. List four common reasons why prosthetic users may reject their prosthetic robotic device.

5. What would be an acceptable time delay for a prosthetic user to see the motion of the prosthetic device compared to when they activate their control signal?

6. How does appearance or cosmesis typically relate to function in prosthetic applications?

7. How does feedback influence control and usability of an upper limb prosthesis?

8. What types of feedback are provided to users in current prosthetic systems?

9. What are the core principles of providing feedback to a user from the user's robotic limb?

10. Why is the phenomenon of embodiment potentially relevant for prosthetic applications?

11. Describe the technological readiness of current robotic prostheses.

12. What are the main components of a robotic prosthesis?

13. How are the main components of a robotic prosthesis integrated?

14. What is the main difference in the control approaches being used for upper and lower limb robotic prostheses?

15. Why is modularity of robotic components important to prosthetic prescription?

16. What barriers are cited as reasons for users to reject robotic prostheses?

17. What advances are being made in interfacing of control signals and feedback?

18. Describe in detail one advanced prosthetic device.

19. What are machine intelligence and advanced pattern recognition, and why are they important for improving the control of robotic prostheses?

20. Describe the technological readiness of major research robotic prostheses for the upper and lower limbs.

References

Al Muderis, M., Khemka, A., Lord, S.J., Van de Meent, H., and Frölke, J.P.M. 2016. Safety of osseointegrated implants for transfemoral amputees: A two-center prospective cohort study. *J Bone Joint Surg Am.* 98, no. 11: 900–909.

Al Muderis, M., Tetsworth, K., Khemka, A., Wilmot, S., Bosley, B., Lord, S.J., and Glat, V. 2016. The Osseointegrated Group of Australia Accelerated Protocol (OGAAP-1) for two-stage osseointegrated reconstruction of amputated limbs. *Bone Joint J* 98-B: 952–60.

Alley, R.D., Williams, T.W., Albuquerque, M.J., and Altobelli, D.E. 2011. Prosthetic sockets stabilized by alternating areas of tissue compression and release. *J Rehab Res Dev* 48, no. 6: 679–696.

Antfolk, C., D'Alonzo, M.D., Rosen, B., Lundborg, G., Sebelius, F., and Cipriani, C. 2013. Sensory feedback in upper limb prosthetics. *Expert Rev Med Devices* 10, no. 1: 45–54.

Armel, K.C., and Ramachandran, V.S. 2003. Projecting sensations to external objects: Evidence from skin conductance response. *Proc R Soc London B Biol Sci* 270, no. 1523: 1499–1506.

Atkins, J.D., Heard, D.C., and Donovan, W.H. 1996. Epidemiologic overview of individuals with upper limb loss and their reported research priorities. *J Prosthet Orthot* 8, no. 1: 2–11.

Belter, J.T., Segil, J.L., Dollar, A.M., and Weir, R.F. 2013. Mechanical design and performance specifications of anthropomorphic prosthetic hands: A review. *J Rehabil Res Dev* 50, no. 5: 599–618.

Biddiss, E., and Chau, T. 2007a. Upper-limb prosthetics: Critical factors in device abandonment. *Am J Phys Med Rehabil* 86, no. 12: 977–987.

Biddiss, E.A., and Chau, T.T. 2007b. Upper limb prosthesis use and abandonment: A survey of the last 25 years. *Prosthet Orthot Int* 31, no. 3: 236–257.

Bongers, R.M., Kyberd, P.J., Bouwsema, H., Kenney, L., Plettenburg, D.H., and Van Der Sluis, C.K. 2012. Bernstein's levels of construction of movements applied to upper limb prosthetics. *J Prosthet Orthot* 24: 67–76.

Botvinick, M. 2004. Probing the neural basis of body ownership. *Science* 305: 782–783.

Botvinick, M., and Cohen, J. 1998. Rubber hands "feel" touch that eyes see. *Nature* 391: 756.

Brånemark, R., Berlin, O., Hagerg, K., Bergh, P., Gunterberg, B., and Rydevik, B. 2014. A novel osseointegrated percutaneous prosthetic system for the treatment of patients with transfemoral amputation: A prospective study of 51 patients. *Bone Joint J* 96-B, no. 1: 106–113.

Bridges, M.M., Para, M.P., and Mashner, M.J. 2011. Control system architecture for the Modular Prosthetic Limb. *Johns Hopkins APL Tech Dig* 30, no. 3: 217–222.

Cairns, N., Murray, K., Corney, J., and McFadyen, A. 2014. Satisfaction with cosmesis and priorities for cosmesis design reported by lower limb amputees in the United Kingdom: Instrument development and results. *Prosthet Orthot Int* 38, no. 6: 467–473.

Castellini, C., Artemiadis, P., Wininger, M., Ajoudani, A., Alimusaj, M., Bicchi, A., Caputo, B. et al. 2014. Proceedings of the First Workshop on Peripheral Machine Interfaces: Going beyond traditional surface electromyography. *Front Neurorobotics* 8: Article 22. doi:10.3389/fnbot.2014.00022.

Childress, D. 1985. Historical aspects of powered limb prostheses. *O&P Library* 9, no. 1: 2–13. http://www.oandplibrary.org/cpo/1985_01_002.asp.

Childress, D.S. 1992. Control of limb prostheses. In *Atlas of Limb Prosthetics: Surgical, Prosthetic, and Rehabilitation Principles*. 2nd ed., AAOS. J.H. Bowker and J.W. Michael, eds. St. Louis, MO: Mosby-Year Book; 1992, pp. 175–198.

Condie, E., Scott, H., and Treweek, S. 2006. Lower limb prosthetic outcome measures: A review of the literature 1995 to 2005. *J Prosthet Orthot* 18, no. 1S: 13–45.

Daley, H., Englehart, K., Hargrove, L., and Kuruganti, U. 2012. High density electromyography data of normally limbed and transradial amputee subjects for multifunction prosthetic control. *J Electromyogr Kines* 22, no. 3: 478–484.

D'Alonzo, M., Clemente, F., and Cipriani, C. 2015. Vibrotactile stimulation promotes embodiment of an alien hand in amputees with phantom sensations. *IEEE Trans Neural Syst Rehabil Eng* 23, no. 3: 450–457.

Dawson, M.R., Carey, J.P., and Fahimi, F. 2011. Myoelectric training systems. *Expert Rev Med Device* 8, no. 5: 581–589.

Deathe, A.B., Wolfe, D.L., Devlin, M., Hebert, J.S., Miller, W.C., and Pallaveshi, L. 2009. Selection of outcome measures in lower extremity amputation rehabilitation: ICF activities. *Disabil Rehabil* 31, no. 18: 1455–1473.

Dillingham, T.R., Pezzin, L.E., MacKenzie, E.J., and Burgess, A.R. 2001. Use and satisfaction with prosthetic devices among persons with trauma-related amputations: A long-term outcome study. *Am J Phys Med Rehabil* 80, no. 8: 563–571.

Edwards, A.L., Dawson, M.R., Hebert, J.S., Sherstan, C., Sutton, R.S., Chan, K.M., and Pilarski, P.M. 2016. Application of real-time machine learning to myoelectric prosthesis control: A case series in adaptive switching. *Prosthet Orthot Int*, 40, no. 5: 573–581.

Ehrsson, H.H., Rosen, B., Stockselius, A., Ragno, C., Kohler, P., and Lundborg, G. 2008. Upper limb amputees can be induced to experience a rubber hand as their own. *Brain* 131: 3443–3452.

Eilenberg, M.F., Geyer, H., and Herr, H. 2010. Control of a powered ankle-foot prosthesis based on a neuromuscular model. *IEEE Trans Neural Syst Rehabil Eng* 18, no. 2: 164–173.

Fougner, A., Stavdahl, O., Kyberd, P.J., Losier, Y.G., and Parker, P.A. 2012. Control of upper limb prostheses: Terminology and proportional myoelectric control—A review. *IEEE Trans Neural Syst Rehabil Eng* 20, no. 5: 663–677.

Gailey, R.S., Gaunaurd, I.A., Raya, M.A., Roach, K.E., Linberg, A.A., Campbell, S.M., Jayne, D.M. et al. 2013. Development and reliability testing of the Comprehensive High-Level Activity Mobility Predictor (CHAMP) in male service members with traumatic lower-limb loss. *J Rehabil Res Dev* 50, no. 7: 905–918.

Gallagher, S. 1986. Body image and body schema: A conceptual clarification. *J Mind Behav* 7: 541–554.

Goldfarb, M., Lawson, B.E., and Shultz, A. 2013. Realizing the promise of robotic leg prostheses. *Sci Transl Med* 5, no. 210: 210ps15.

Hagberg, K., and Brånemark, R. 2009. One hundred patients treated with osseo-integrated transfemoral amputation prostheses—Rehabilitation perspective. *J Rehabil Res Dev* 46, no. 3: 331–344.

Hargrove, L.J., Lock, B.A., and Simon, A.M. 2013. Pattern recognition control out-performs conventional myoelectric control in upper limb patients with tar-geted muscle reinnervation. *Proc IEEE Conf Eng Med Biol Soc* 2013: 1599–1602.

Hargrove, L.J., Simon, A.M., Young, A.J., Lipschutz, R.B., Finucane, S.B., Smith, D.G., and Kuiken, T.A. 2013. Robotic leg control with EMG decoding in an amputee with nerve transfers. *N Engl J Med* 369: 1237–1242. doi:10.1056 /NEJMoa1300126.

Hebert, J.S., Elzinga, K., Chan, K.M., Olson, J.L., and Morhart, M.J. 2014. Updates in targeted sensory reinnervation for upper limb amputation. *Curr Surg Rep* 2, no. 3: 45–53. doi:10.1007/s40137-013-0045-7.

Hebert, J.S., Olson, J.L., Morhart, M.J., Dawson, M.R., Marasco, P.D., Kuiken, T.A., and Chan, K.M. 2014. Novel targeted sensory reinnervation tech-nique to restore functional hand sensation after transhumeral amputation. *IEEE Trans Neural Syst Rehabil Eng* 22, no. 4: 765–773. doi:10.1109/TNSRE .2013.2294907.

Hebert, J.S., Wolfe, D.L., Miller, W.C., Deathe, A.B., Devlin, M., and Pallaveshi, L. 2009. Outcome measures in amputation rehabilitation: ICF body functions. *Disabil Rehabil* 31, no. 19: 1541–1554.

Heinemann, A.W., Connelly, L., Ehrlich-Jones, L., and Fatone, S. 2014. Outcome instruments for prosthetics: Clinical applications. *Phys Med Rehabil Clin N Am* 25: 179–198.

Hill, W., Kyberd, P., Hermansson, L.N., Hubbard, S., Stavdahl, Ø., and Swanson, S. 2009. Upper limb prosthetic outcome measures (UPLOM): A working group and their findings. *J Prosthet Orthot* 21, no. 9: 69–82. doi:10.1097/JPO .0b013e3181ae970b.

Ingraham, K.A., Fey, N.P., Simon, A.M., and Hargrove, L.J. 2016. Assessing the relative contributions of active ankle and knee assistance to the walking mechanics of transfemoral amputees using a powered prosthesis. *PLoS One* 11, no. 1: e0147661. doi:10.1371/journal.pone.0147661.

Johannes, M.S., Bigelow, J.D., Burck, J.M., Harshbarger, S.D., Kozlowski, M.V., and Van Doren, T. 2011. An overview of the developmental process for the mod-ular prosthetic limb. *Johns Hopkins APL Tech Dig* 30, no. 3: 207–216.

Jönsson, S., Caine Winterberger, K., and Brånemark, R. 2011. Osseointegration amputation prostheses on the upper limbs: Methods, prosthetics and reha-bilitation. *Prosthet Orthot Int* 35, no. 2: 190–200.

Kark, L., and Simmons, A. 2011. Patient satisfaction following lower limb ampu-tation: The role of gait deviation. *Prosthet Orthot Int* 35, no. 2: 225–233. doi:10.1177/0309364611406169.

Kaufman, K.R., Levine, J.A., Brey, R.H., Iverson, B.K., McCrady, S.K., Padgett, D.J., and Joyner, M.J. 2007. Gait and balance of transfermoral amputees using passive mechanical and microprocessor controlled prosthetic knees. *Gait Posture* 26, no. 4: 489–493.

Khemka, A., Frossard, L., Lord, S.J., Bosley, B., and Al Muderis, M. 2015. Osseointegrated total knee replacement connected to a lower limb prosthesis: 4 cases. *Acta Orthop* 86, no. 6: 740–744.

Kuiken, T.A., Schultz Feuser, A.E., and Barlow, A.K., eds. 2013. *Targeted Muscle Reinnervation: A Neural Interface for Artificial Limbs.* Boca Raton, FL: Taylor & Francis.

Lawson, B.E., Varol, H., Huff, A., Erdemir, E., and Goldfarb, M. 2013. Control of stair ascent and descent with a powered transfemoral prosthesis. *IEEE Trans Neural Syst Rehabil Eng* 21, no. 3: 466–473.

Longo, M.R., Schüür, F., Kammers, M.P.M., Tsakiris, M., and Haggard, P. 2008. What is embodiment? A psychometric approach. *Cognition* 107: 978–998.

Llorens-Bonilla, B., and Asada, H.H. 2014. A robot on the shoulder: Coordinated human-wearable robot control using coloured petri nets and partial least squares predictions. *Proc 2014 IEEE Int Conf Robotics Automation* May 31–June 7: 119–125.

Lundberg, M., Hagberg, K., and Bullington, J. 2011. My prosthesis as a part of me: A qualitative analysis of living with an osseointegrated prosthetic limb. *Prosthet Orthot Int* 35, no. 2: 207–214.

Lundborg, G., and Rosen, B. 2001. Sensory substitution in prosthetics. *Hand Clin* 17, no. 3: 481–488.

Marasco, P.D., Kim, K., Colgate, J.E., Peshkin, M.A., and Kuiken, T.A. 2011. Robotic touch shifts perception of embodiment to a prosthesis in targeted reinnervation amputees. *Brain* 134: 747–758.

Marasco, P.D., Schultz, A.E., and Kuiken, T.A. 2009. Sensory capacity of reinnervated skin after redirection of amputated upper limb nerves to the chest. *Brain* 132: 1441–1448.

Merrill, D.R., Lockhart, J., Troyk, P.R., Weir, R.F., and Hankin, D.L. 2011. Development of an implantable myoelectric sensor for advanced prosthesis control. *Artif Organs* 35, no. 3: 249–52. doi:10.1111/j.1525-1594.2011.01219.x.

Micera, S., Carpaneto, J., and Raspopovic, S. 2010. Control of hand prostheses using peripheral information. *IEEE Rev Biomed Eng* 3: 48–68.

Millstein, S.G., Heger, H., and Hunter, G.A. 1986. Prosthetic use in adult upper limb amputees: A comparison of the body powered and electrically powered prostheses. *Prosthet Orthot Int* 10, no. 1: 27–34.

Orendurff, M.S. 2013. Literature review of published research investigating microprocessor-controlled prosthetic knees: 2010–2012. *J Prosthet Orthot* 25, no. 4S: P41.

Ortiz-Catalan, M., Brånemark, R., Håkansson, B., and Delbeke, J. 2012. On the viability of implantable electrodes for the natural control of artificial limbs: Review and discussion. *Biomed Eng Online* 11: 33.

Ortiz-Catalan, M., Hakansson, B., and Branemark, R. 2014. An osseointegrated human-machine gateway for long-term sensory feedback and motor control of artificial limbs. *Sci Transl Med* 6, no. 257: 257.

Oskoei, M.A., and Hu, H. 2007. Myoelectric control systems—A survey. *Biomed Signal Proc Control* 2, no. 4: 275–294.

Parietti, F., and Asada, H.H. 2014. Supernumerary robotic limbs for aircraft fuselage assembly: Body stabilization and guidance by bracing. *2014 IEEE Int Conf Robotics Automation (ICRA)* 1176–1183. doi:10.1109/ICRA .2014.6907002.

Parker, P., Englehart, K.B., and Hudgins, B. 2006. Myoelectric signal processing for control of powered limb prostheses. *J Electromyogr Kines* 16, no. 6: 541–548.

Pasquina, P.F., Evangelista, M., Carvalho, A.J., Lockhart, J., Griffin, S., Nanos, G., McKay, P. et al. 2015. First-in-man demonstration of a fully implanted myoelectric sensors system to control an advanced electromechanical prosthetic hand. *J Neurosci Methods* 15, no. 244: 85–93.

Peerdeman, B., Boere, D., Witteveen, H., Huis In Tveld, R., Hermens, H., Stramigioli, S., Rietman, H., Veltink, P., and Misra, S. 2011. Myoelectric forearm prostheses: State of the art from a user-centered perspective. *J Rehabil Res Dev* 48, no. 6: 719–737.

Pezzin, L.E., Dillingham, T.R., Mackenzie, E.J., Ephraim, P., and Rossbach, P. 2004. Use and satisfaction with prosthetic limb devices and related services. *Arch Phys Med Rehabil* 85, no. 5: 723–729.

Pilarski, P.M., Dawson, M.R., Degris, T., Carey, J.P., Chan, K.M., Hebert, J.S., and Sutton, R.S. 2013. Adaptive artificial limbs: A real-time approach to prediction and anticipation. *IEEE Robotics Automation Magazine* 20, no. 1: 53–64.

Pilarski, P.M., Dick, T.B., and Sutton, R.S. 2013. Real-time prediction learning for the simultaneous actuation of multiple prosthetic joints. Proceedings of the 2013 IEEE International Conference on Rehabilitation Robotics (ICORR), Seattle, June 24–26.

Pilarski, P.M., Sutton, R.S., and Mathewson, K.W. 2015. Prosthetic devices as goal-seeking agents. Presented at the Second Workshop on Present and Future of Non-Invasive Peripheral-Nervous-System Machine Interfaces: Progress in Restoring the Human Functions (PNS-MI), Singapore, August 11.

Pulliam, C.L., Lambrecht, J.M., and Kirsch, R.F. 2011. Electromyogram-based neural network control of transhumeral prostheses. *J Rehabil Res Dev* 48, no. 6: 739–754.

Raspopovic, S., Capogrosso, M., Petrini, F.M., Bonizzato, M., Rigosa, J., Di Pino, G., Carpaneto, J. et al. 2014. Restoring natural sensory feedback in real-time bidirectional hand prostheses. *Sci Transl Med* 6, no. 222: 222ra19. doi:10.1126/scitranslmed.3006820.

Ravitz, A.D., McLoughlin, M.P., Beaty, J.D., Tenore, F.V., Johannes, M.S., Swetz, S.A., Helder, J.B. et al. 2013. Revolutionizing prosthetics—Phase 3. *Johns Hopkins APL Tech Dig* 31, no. 4: 366–376.

Resnik, L. 2011. Development and testing of new upper-limb prosthetic devices: Research designs for usability testing. *J Rehabil Res Dev* 48, no. 6: 697–706.

Resnik, L., Klinger, S.L., and Etter, K. 2014. The DEKA Arm: Its features, functionality, and evolution during the Veterans Affairs Study to optimize the DEKA Arm. *Prosthet Orthot Int* 38, no. 6: 492–504.

Resnik, L., Meucci, M.R., Lieberman-Klinger, S., Fantini, C., Kelty, D.L., Disla, R., and Sasson, N. 2012. Advanced upper limb prosthetic devices: Implications for upper limb prosthetic rehabilitation. *Arch Phys Med Rehabil* 93, no. 4: 710–717.

Rossini, P.M., Micera, S., Benvenuto, A., Carpaneto, J., Cavallo, G., Citi, L., Cipriani, C. et al. 2010. Double nerve intraneural interface implant on a human amputee for robotic hand control. *Clin Neurophysiol* 121: 777–783.

Rouse, E.J., Villagaray-Carski, N.C., Emerson, R.W., and Herr, H.M. 2015. Design and testing of a bionic dance prosthesis. *PLoS One* 10, no. 8: e0135148.

Scheme, E., and Englehart, K. 2011. Electromyogram pattern recognition for control of powered upper-limb prostheses: State of the art and challenges for clinical use. *J Rehabil Res Dev* 48, no. 6: 643–659.

Scheme, E., Hudgins, B., and Englehart, K. 2013. Confidence based rejection for improved pattern recognition myoelectric control. *IEEE Trans Biomed Eng* 60: 1563–1570. doi:10.1109/TBME.2013.2238939.

Schofield, J.S., Evans, K.R., Carey, J.P., and Hebert, J.S. 2014. Applications of sensory feedback in motorized upper extremity prostheses: A review. *Expert Rev Med Devices* 11, no. 5: 499–511. doi:10.1586/17434440.2014.929496.

Schultz, A.H., Lawson, B.E., and Goldfarb, M. 2015. Running with a powered knee and ankle prosthesis. *IEEE Trans Neural Syst Rehabil Eng* 23, no. 3: 403–412. doi:10.1109/TNSRE.2014.2336597.

Sensinger, J.W., Lock, B.A., and Kuiken, T.A. 2009. Adaptive pattern recognition of myoelectric signals: Exploration of conceptual framework and practical algorithms. *IEEE Trans Neural Sys Rehab* 17, no. 3: 270–278.

Shannon, C.E. 1948. A mathematical theory of communication. *Bell Syst Tech J* 27: 379–423, 623–656.

Silcox, D.H., Rooks, M.D., Vogel, R.R., and Fleming, L.L. 1993. Myoelectric prostheses. A long-term follow-up and a study of the use of alternate prostheses. *J Bone Joint Surg Am* 75: 1781–1789.

Sup, F., Varol, H.A., and Goldfarb, M. 2011. Upslope walking with a powered knee and ankle prosthesis: Initial results with an amputee subject. *IEEE Trans Neural Syst Rehabil Eng* 19, no. 1: 71–78.

Sutton, L.G., Clawson, A., Williams, T.W., Lipsey, J.H., and Sensinger, J.W. 2011. Towards a universal coupler design for modern powered prostheses. *Proc MEC '11 Raising the Standard* August: 271–275.

Tikandylakis, G., Berlin, Ö., and Brånemark, R. 2014. Implant survival, adverse events, and bone remodeling of osseointegrated percutaneous implants for transhumeral amputees. *Clin Orthop Relat Res* 472, no. 10: 2947–2956.

Tkach, D.C., Young, A.J., Smith, L.H., and Hargrove, L.J. 2012. Performance of pattern recognition myoelectric control using a generic electrode grid with targeted muscle reinnervation patients. *Proc IEEE Eng Med Biol Soc* 4319–4323. doi:10.1109/EMBC.2012.6346922.

Tsakiris, M., and Haggard, P. 2005. The rubber hand illusion revisited: Visuotactile integration and self-attribution. *J Exp Psychol Hum Percept Perform* 31, no. 1: 80–91.

Van de Meent, H., Hopman, M.T., and Frolke, J.P. 2013. Walking ability and quality of life in subjects with transfemoral amputation: A comparison of osseointegration with socket prostheses. *Arch Phys Med Rehabil* 94, no. 11: 2174–2178.

Weir, R.F.F. 2004. Design of artificial arms and hands for prosthetic applications. In *Standard Handbook of Biomedical Engineering and Design*. M. Kutz, ed. New York: McGraw-Hill; pp. 32.1–32.61.

Williams, R.M., Turner, A.P., Orendurff, M., Segal, A.D., Klute, G.K., Pecoraro, R.N., and Czerniecki, J. 2006. Does having a computerized prosthetic knee influence cognitive performance during amputee walking? *Arch Phys Med Rehab* 87, no. 7: 989–994.

Williams, T.W. 2011. Guest editorial: Progress on stabilizing and controlling powered upper-limb prostheses. *J Rehabil Res Dev* 48, no. 6: ix–xix.

World Health Organization. 2001. *International Classification of Functioning, Disability and Health*. Geneva: World Health Organization.

Wright, T.W., Hagan, A.D., and Wood, M.B. 1995. Prosthetic usage in major upper extremity amputations. *J Hand Surg Am* 20, no. 44: 619–622.

Young, A.J., Smith, L.H., Rouse, E.J., and Hargrove, L.J. 2014. A comparison of the real-time controllability of pattern recognition to conventional myoelectric control for discrete and simultaneous movements. *J Neuroeng Rehabil.* 11, no. 1: 5. doi:10.1186/1743-0003-11-5.

Zuo, K.J., and Olson, J.L. 2014. The evolution of functional hand replacement: From iron prostheses to hand transplantation. *Can J Plast Surg* 22, no. 1: 44–51.

5

Smart Wheelchairs for Assessment and Mobility

Pooja Viswanathan, Richard C. Simpson,
Geneviève Foley, Andrew Sutcliffe, and Julianne Bell

Contents

> **Learning Objectives**
> After completing this chapter, readers will be able to
>
> 1. Describe how smart wheelchairs may be used to improve the assessment process for powered wheelchairs.
> 2. Describe how smart wheelchairs may be used to increase independent mobility.
> 3. Compare the advantages and disadvantages of sensors, feedback mechanisms, and input modalities used by smart wheelchairs.

Principles

Several researchers, mainly in computer science and engineering, have been developing "smart wheelchairs" with the goal of increasing safe and effective navigation of powered wheelchairs (PWCs). These wheelchairs

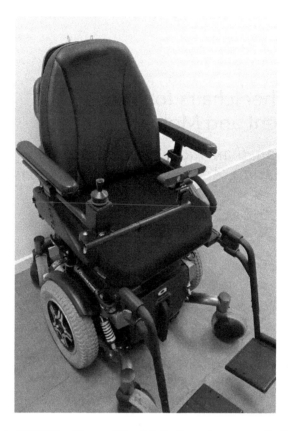

Figure 5.1   A CANWheel Smart Wheelchair (http://www.canwheel.ca/) research prototype, not yet commercially available.

are intended to provide a range of functions, including collision avoidance, autonomous navigation to locations, wall following, and virtual path following and have been implemented using various sensors and user interfaces. Although smart wheelchairs have been described in the literature since at least the mid-1980s (Madarasz et al. 1986), few smart wheelchairs have ever been used by a person with a disability, and no smart wheelchair has achieved more than a modest degree of commercial success. An example of a smart wheelchair is shown in Figure 5.1.

Independent Mobility

Independent mobility has been identified as a key component of physical well-being and happiness, enabling people to interact with their surroundings (Bourret et al. 2002). Unfortunately, the mobility and independence of many individuals are often reduced due to physical disabilities. Reduced mobility often results in decreased opportunities to explore and socialize, leading to social isolation and depression. For example, one study has reported that, among noninstitutionalized U.S. adults, 31% of people with major mobility difficulties were frequently depressed or anxious, versus only 4% of those without mobility difficulties (Iezzoni et al. 2001). Loss of mobility also results in increased dependence on caregivers to fulfill daily tasks. A National Population Health Survey was conducted by Statistics Canada in 1995 with more than 2,000 residents from 232 long-term care facilities. According to survey results, "Half the residents spent most of the day in a bed or chair" (Tully and Mohl 1995, 29). Wheelchairs have been found to positively enhance the mobility of several long-term care residents (Pawlson, Goodwin, and Keith 1986). However, independent propulsion of manual wheelchairs within a facility is often an unmet goal for wheelchair users (Fuchs and Gromak 2003). Despite this evidence for inadequate wheelchair self-mobility, there is often minimal recognition of these issues by caregiving staff (Pawlson, Goodwin, and Keith 1986).

Power wheelchairs can enable independent mobility and are typically prescribed by clinicians for individuals who lack the strength to propel themselves in manual wheelchairs. However, safe operation of a PWC requires a significant level of cognitive function, including decision-making, memory, judgment, and self-awareness (Brighton 2003). In fact, it was estimated in 2008 that over one million individuals in the United States who needed a PWC experienced symptoms such as loss of attention and impulse control, agitation, spasticity, tremor, and visual field neglect, which are linked to Alzheimer's disease, cerebral palsy, amyotrophic lateral sclerosis, multiple sclerosis, stroke, and other pathologies (Simpson, LoPresti, and Cooper 2008). These symptoms can pose safety risks and often lead to exclusion from PWC use (Mortenson et al. 2006).

Components of a Smart Wheelchair

An information flow diagram for a smart wheelchair is shown in Figure 5.2. Critical components of a smart wheelchair include sensors for identifying features in the environment, input methods for the user to provide commands to the system, methods for the system to provide feedback to the user, and a control algorithm that coordinates input from the user, the sensors, and the PWC to determine the system's behavior.

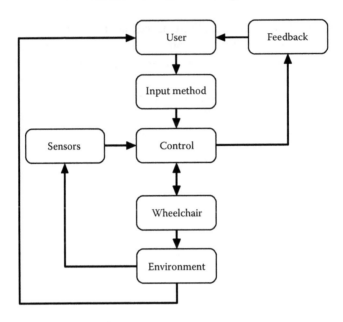

Figure 5.2 Information flow diagram for a smart wheelchair.

Sensors

To avoid obstacles, smart wheelchairs need sensors to perceive their surroundings. A variety of sensors have been used in smart wheelchairs (LoPresti et al. 2002), but no sensor (or combination of sensors) has been identified that is sufficiently accurate, inexpensive, small, lightweight, and impervious to environmental conditions (e.g., lighting, precipitation, temperature) and requires little power. A comparison of sensors used in smart wheelchairs described in the literature is provided in Table 5.1.

Input Methods

Smart wheelchairs have been used to explore a variety of alternatives to the more "traditional" input methods associated with power wheelchairs (e.g., joystick, pneumatic switches). More recent smart wheelchairs have used brain-computer interfaces (Carlson and del R. Millan 2013; Mandel et al. 2009), eye gaze (Rofer, Mandel, and Laue 2009), and voice recognition (Pineau et al. 2011; Simpson and Levine 2002). A summary of alternative input methods can be found in Table 5.2.

Feedback Modalities

Smart wheelchairs can provide feedback to the driver through various modalities and interfaces (Viswanathan, Zambalde et al. 2016; Wang,

TABLE 5.1 Summary of Sensors Used by Smart Wheelchairs

Sensor	Capability	Advantages	Disadvantages
Ultrasonic (sonar)	Measures distance to obstacles by emitting sound waves	• Small • Low power • Low cost	• Sensitive to obstacle properties (such as sound-absorbing material) • Cannot detect very small/thin or concave obstacles • Cross-talk issues with other sounds or multiple ultrasonic sensors • Cannot detect drop-offs unless sensor is pointed to the floor • Limited coverage
Infrared (IR)	Measures distance to obstacles by emitting light; can also detect transitions from light to dark lines	• Small • Low power • Low cost	• False positives in natural light (due to IR interference) • Sensitive to flooring materials (issues with dark, light-absorbent, transparent, and refractive surfaces) • Limited coverage
Laser range finder	Provides 180° scan of obstacles (distances) in the environment	• High precision • Good for longer ranges	• High cost • High power • Possible eye safety issues • Only detects objects at the height of the laser range finder
Stereovision camera	Captures color or black-and-white image and depth images of the environment	• Low power • Medium cost • Can be used for high-level scene understanding (e.g., object and location recognition) and head/eye tracking of users	• Cannot detect textureless objects • Cannot perform in poorly lit conditions • Challenges posed by reflective and transparent surfaces

(Continued)

TABLE 5.1 (CONTINUED)   Summary of Sensors Used by Smart Wheelchairs

Sensor	Capability	Advantages	Disadvantages
Structured light (e.g., Microsoft Kinect)	Captures color or black-and-white image and depth images (using projected IR) of the environment	• Low power • Low cost • Can be used for high-level scene understanding (e.g., object and location recognition) and head/eye tracking of users	• Challenges posed by outdoor environments (due to IR interference) • Sees through transparent surfaces (i.e., cannot be used to avoid collisions with glass doors) • Can demand a lot of processing power
Bump (tactile sensor)	Can detect if contact is made (force is exerted) by an object	• Low cost • Low power	• Requires contact (safety issues) • Increasing coverage (e.g., by using bumper skirt-like sensors) can lead to increased form factor and bulkiness
Wheelchair encoders	Measures number and speed of wheel rotations	• Can be used to easily gather information on distances traveled and speed	• Can be expensive to retrofit on wheelchairs • Wheel slippage can lead to errors
Inertial measurement units (IMUs)	Contain accelerometers, gyroscopes, and optional magnetometers that can be used to determine velocity, orientation, and position, respectively	• Low cost • Low power	• Prone to accumulated errors when used for longer distances • Higher-accuracy IMUs can be expensive
Global positioning system (GPS)	Provides location and time information	• Can give accurate location when GPS satellites are in an unobstructed line of sight • Low cost	• Does not work well indoors

TABLE 5.2 Alternative Input Methods Used in Smart Wheelchairs

Input	Capability	Advantages	Disadvantages
Brain-computer interface	Sensors may be worn on the head (e.g., electroencephalography, EEG) or implanted in the skull (e.g., electrocorticography, ECOG).	• Requires no physical movement	• Requires significant computational power • Expensive • Limited signals available for control • Sensors must be placed on or inside the skull
Eye gaze	Cameras pointed at the user's face track where the user is looking to determine where the PWC should steer.	• Requires limited physical movement • No sensors touch the user's body	• Requires significant computational power • Distinguishing between "looking to drive" and "looking to see" is challenging • Expensive
Voice recognition	Speech recognition software interprets steering commands from user.	• Low cost • No sensors touch the user's body	• Requires ability to speak clearly and consistently • Voice has limited bandwidth

Mihailidis et al. 2011). For example, speakers can be used to provide audio feedback, while small light-emitting diodes (LEDs) can be used to offer visual feedback (such as a flashing red light if the driver gets too close to an object). Haptic feedback can be provided by using small vibrations to warn the driver about obstacles. Touch screen displays can be used both to gather information from the driver (e.g., desired destination) and to display information (e.g., scheduled activities, way-finding assistance, virtual environments, etc.). Feedback modalities that have been described in the literature are summarized in Table 5.3.

Control Algorithm

Investigators have taken a variety of approaches to implement control software for smart wheelchairs, based on the functions supported by the smart wheelchair and the sensors it uses. Many smart wheelchairs implement semiautonomous behaviors (combining or switching between input from the driver and the intelligent system) rather than autonomous driving behaviors (where the driver's input is ignored) to offer the driver higher levels of control while ensuring safety. However, the exact mechanism of semiautonomous control that is both effective and acceptable to users is still under investigation (Viswanathan, Zambalde et al. 2016).

Critical Review of the Technology Available

Smart wheelchairs are at level 4 of NASA's progression of technology readiness levels (Mankins 1995); low-fidelity systems have been used to demonstrate basic functionality in controlled environments. Although a large number of prototypes have been described in the research literature, no smart wheelchairs are widely used today. The CALL Center smart wheelchair is sold in the United Kingdom and Europe by Smile Rehab Limited (Berkshire, U.K.) as the "Smart Wheelchair" (http://smilesmart-tech.com /assistive-technology-products/smile-smart-wheelchair.php), but this is intended to be a training tool rather than a permanent mobility aid. An overview of smart wheelchair designs described in the research literature can be found in Table 5.4.

A significant technical obstacle to commercialization is the cost/accuracy trade-off that must be made with existing sensors. There is reason for optimism, however, that the significant research in self-driving automobiles (Guizzo 2011) will lead to affordable technology that can also be used in smart wheelchairs. In 2014, the technology used in one of Google's self-driving cars cost approximately $320,000 (Tannert 2014),

TABLE 5.3   Summary of Feedback Modalities Used by Smart Wheelchairs

Modality	Implementation	Advantages	Disadvantages
Auditory	Feedback can be provided through intermittent sound (e.g., warning sirens), continuous sound (e.g., tone indicating distance to the nearest obstacle), or spoken words.	• Does not distract visual attention • Low cost	• May be washed out by ambient noise • Nonspoken feedback may be misinterpreted • Only available for a short period of time
Visual	Feedback can be provided through something as simple as individual lights or as complex as a "dashboard" implemented on a computer screen.	• Not affected by ambient noise • Remains available to user • Low cost	• Can distract visual attention
Haptic	Feedback can be provided through pressure applied to a joystick.	• Possible to give very precise feedback about the environment around the PWC • Does not distract visual attention	• Only works if the driver uses a joystick to operate the PWC • Expensive

TABLE 5.4 Overview of Semiautonomous Smart Wheelchairs

System	Functions	Control Method	Feedback	Sensors	Navigation
Feedback simulation (Wang, Gorski et al. 2011; Wang, Mihailidis et al. 2011)	Collision avoidance	Teleoperator	Audio (direction) Haptic (joystick blocked in obstacle direction) Visual (LEDs around joystick)	N/A	N/A
Wizard-of-Oz simulation (Mitchell et al. 2014; Rushton et al. 2014; Viswanathan, Zambalde et al. 2016)	Collision avoidance	Teleoperator Three modes: 1. Basic safety (stop to avoid collision, blocks direction of obstacle) 2. Steering correction (turns away from obstacle) 3. Autonomous	Audio (chair actions, directions) Haptic (direction or speed)	N/A	N/A
Anticollision contact sensor skirt (Wang, Gorski et al. 2011)	Collision avoidance	Stops when bumper hits obstacle	Indicator lights (directions)	Microswitches	Lights indicate possible directions following stop through sensor skirt contact

(*Continued*)

TABLE 5.4 (CONTINUED) Overview of Semiautonomous Smart Wheelchairs

System	Functions	Control Method	Feedback	Sensors	Navigation
Collaborative Assistive Robot for Mobility Enhancement (CARMEN) (Urdiales et al. 2010)	Collision avoidance	Continuously shared control weighted based on local evaluation of human and robot efficiency	None	Laser range finder Encoders	Three layers: safeguard; reactive (potential fields approach [PFA]: user and wheelchair goals are attractors); deliberative (reach intermediate goals) Efficiency based on smoothness (angle between current direction and upcoming motion vector); directness (angle between vector and destination); and safety
Collaborative controller (Carlson and Demiris 2012)	Obstacle avoidance Navigation assistance	Shared dynamically	None	Camera (two-dimensional [2-D] markers on ceiling)	Known indoor mapped environment; computer vision-based localization system using markers Determine user intent, verify action is safe with dynamic local obstacle avoidance (DLOA) algorithm If user deviates from safe minitrajectory, user is guided toward the minitrajectory with speed proportional to joystick deflection in that direction

(Continued)

TABLE 5.4 (CONTINUED)   Overview of Semiautonomous Smart Wheelchairs

System	Functions	Control Method	Feedback	Sensors	Navigation
Collaborative Wheelchair Assistant (CWA) (Zeng, Burdet, and Teo 2008; Zeng, Teo et al. 2008)	Navigation assistance	User controls speed; wheelchair mostly controls heading to reach user-defined destination Two options for user to deviate from path (collision avoidance): elastic path controller and graphical user interface	None	Encoders Scanner (bar code on floor)	Virtual path learned with walk-through programming (WTP) Path acts as tracks Elastic path controller: user can deviate but feels attraction to path
IATSL Intelligent Wheelchair System (IWS) (How 2010)	Obstacle avoidance Navigation assistance	Stops if user too close to obstacle	Audio (provides navigation prompts after chair has stopped)	Stereovision camera	Occupancy grid with blob detection for obstacle avoidance Direction of greatest freedom computed from occupancy grid for prompting

(Continued)

TABLE 5.4 (CONTINUED) Overview of Semiautonomous Smart Wheelchairs

System	Functions	Control Method	Feedback	Sensors	Navigation
JiaoLong wheelchair (Chen and Agrawal 2013)	Collision avoidance	Three modes: 1. Manual 2. Minimum vector field histogram (MVFH) aided (obstacle avoidance) 3. Dynamic shared control (DSC) algorithm: weighted control between user and wheelchair	None	Laser range finder Camera Encoders	Evaluation of performance in real time to determine user control weight with minimax multiobjective optimization algorithm based on 1. Safety 2. Comfort 3. Obedience
Levels-of-automation (LOA) wheelchair (Jipp 2013)	Collision avoidance navigation assistance	Three modes (LOAs): 1. Manual 2. Collision avoidance with eye tracking to determine intended direction; manual navigation and path planning 3. Autonomous driving based on user gaze to determine target; user-confirmed destination	Touch screen (mode 3)	Eye tracker Ultrasonic sensors	Autonomous navigation with A* algorithm: shortest path between position and goal Added button: pressed continually to move (mode 2) and emergency stop (mode 3)

(Continued)

TABLE 5.4 (CONTINUED) Overview of Semiautonomous Smart Wheelchairs

System	Functions	Control Method	Feedback	Sensors	Navigation
NavChair (Levine et al. 1999) behavior replicated in Hephaestus Smart Wheelchair System (Simpson, Poirot, and Baxter 2002)	Obstacle avoidance Navigation assistance	Three modes: 1. General obstacle avoidance (GOA) 2. Door passage (DP) 3. Automatic wall following (AWF)	None	Array of 12 ultrasonic sensors Encoders	Certainty grid to map obstacle locations and find direction with minimal obstacles closest to user input using MVFH Combined with vector force field (VFF) to avoid obstacles in chosen direction
Navigation and Obstacle Avoidance Help (NOAH) (Viswanathan 2012)	Obstacle avoidance Navigation assistance	Stops if user too close to obstacle	Audio prompts	Stereovision camera	Occupancy grid (obstacle detection) from camera Directional Control Logic Module (DCLM) to interrupt joystick message (stop) Internal map with Simultaneous Localization And Mapping (SLAM) Partially Observable Markov Decision Process (POMDP) to estimate user's cognitive state and issue adaptive prompts

(Continued)

TABLE 5.4 (CONTINUED) Overview of Semiautonomous Smart Wheelchairs

System	Functions	Control Method	Feedback	Sensors	Navigation
Smart Chair (Parikh et al. 2007)	Obstacle avoidance Navigation assistance	Three modes: 1. Shared (chair drives until user takes control of the joystick—checks consistency with goal) 2. Autonomous 3. Manual	None	Cameras: omnidirectional, human interaction Laser range finder IR sensors (back) Encoders	Three types of actions: 1. Deliberative path planning 2. Reactive obstacle avoidance 3. User initiated Visual interface to choose destination (video projection) Dead reckoning (encoders) + visual feedback (camera and markers on ceiling); triangulation with recognized landmarks Adaptable to user: level of autonomy, sensitivity

but industry reports predicted that the additional price a consumer will pay for self-driving car technology will be approximately $5,000 by 2030 (IHS Automotive 2014; Mosquet et al. 2015). Because approximately two-thirds of the cost of the technology underlying self-driving cars is actually devoted to geographic positioning system (GPS) technology (Davies 2015), the additional price of technology for a smart wheelchair might be as low as $2,000.

Critical Review of the Available Utilization Protocols

As stated, smart wheelchairs have not made the transition from research to clinical practice due to issues of cost and reliability. The first "real-world" use of smart wheelchair technology may be as training and assessment tools under controlled clinical environments, rather than as mobility aids in unconstrained real-world environments. To explore the use of smart wheelchairs as training and assessment tools, a multidisciplinary workshop, "Smart Wheelchairs in Assessment and Training" (SWAT), was recently conducted with 31 participants with experience in PWC interventions (Viswanathan et al. 2016a,b). Participants indicated that a variety of data may be collected while a client is using a smart wheelchair (e.g., during driving trials or long-term use), and these data (and the developed tools) may serve multiple purposes to augment clinical practices, including the following (Viswanathan et al. 2016a,b):

1. Identifying individuals who can learn to become safe drivers with additional training;
2. Bringing attention to specific aspects of driving that require further training and recommending training strategies to enhance driving performance;
3. Providing objective measures of driving performance using clinically relevant information (extracted from the data);
4. Verifying intervention outcomes through performance assessment and analysis of system/**tool use**; and
5. Long-term and real-world monitoring of drivers to assess safety risks, detect changes in driving ability, and prevent accidents.

Table 5.5 describes technological interventions in development during the last decade for the purposes of assessment and training of PWC users. Note that the goal of training systems is not simply to correct or prevent all driver errors (which several collision avoidance systems do), but rather

TABLE 5.5 Smart Wheelchair Technologies for Assessment and Training

Reference	Description of Technology	Target Population	Data Collected/Generated
Chen and Agrawal 2013	This system uses a mobile robot with a force-feedback joystick that provides a corrective bias during a line-following task if the driver deviates. It aims to train drivers in following a desired path with turns.	Special needs infants	• It collects joystick inputs and computes the robot's position and trajectory using the sensors.
Archambault et al. 2010	The data logger was developed for assessing performance of PWC driving tasks.	Any PWC user	• The data logger includes accelerometers, gyroscopes, wheel encoder, GPS, seat pressure sensors. • The data collected could be used to compute completion time, mean and variability of joystick direction, as well as maximal forward and backward velocity.
Jipp et al. 2009	A system for psychomotor profiling that can be used in assessment and in identifying areas for further training. It is suggested that this system could be used to automatically and dynamically determine the appropriate level of autonomy implemented by a smart wheelchair.	Any PWC user who might experience spasticity while driving	• The system consists of an ultrasonic sensor to detect distances to objects. • In addition, task completion times, velocities, distances traveled, number of input commands, number of changes in movement direction, mean translational and rotational joystick inputs, and corrective behaviors are recorded by the system. • The system produces an estimated quantitative measure of driving precision.

(Continued)

TABLE 5.5 (CONTINUED) Smart Wheelchair Technologies for Assessment and Training

Reference	Description of Technology	Target Population	Data Collected/Generated
Moghaddam et al. 2011	The system automatically recognizes specific events and driving activities during PWC use. The aim of the system is to characterize driving behavior to improve driving skills and PWC design with respect to safety and performance. The events consist of three types of impacts and two driving activities (rolling down slopes at different speeds).	Any PWC user	• The system uses GPS, ultrasonic sensors, and wheel encoders. • The system currently recognizes specific events only based on accelerometer data.
Manrique et al. 2007	An obstacle-sensing system that emits an intermittent beep when the wheelchair approaches an object. The beeping frequency gradually increases and becomes a continuous tone as the wheelchair gets closer to the object.	PWC users who experience mobility challenges due to cognitive or perceptual impairment	• The system computes distances to objects and produces audio feedback (a commercial obstacle-sensing system was used).
Marchal-Crespo, Furumasu, and Reinkensmeyer 2010	RObot-assisted Learning for Young drivers (ROLY) is a trainer that uses a force-feedback joystick to guide the driver in following a line on the floor. A mixed-reality environment was recently developed to semiautonomously train PWC driving skills. The PWC is used as the gaming input device to maneuver through floor-projected games. The mixed-reality environment is created using a multiprojector and multicamera tracking system.	Children with severe mobility impairment (for example, due to cerebral palsy)	• The system uses infrared sensors to detect obstacles and safely stop the wheelchair, as well as a webcam to track the line on the floor. • It offers force feedback through the joystick based on the driver error and duration of training (i.e., the feedback is proportional to the amount of assistance required). • The mixed-reality environment also provides force feedback through the joystick.

(Continued)

TABLE 5.5 (CONTINUED) Smart Wheelchair Technologies for Assessment and Training

Reference	Description of Technology	Target Population	Data Collected/Generated
Miro et al. 2011	A stand-alone sensor package, consisting of a laser range finder, camera, and inertial measurement unit. This system was created to aid clinicians in PWC competency assessment.	Target users of this system would be clinicians assessing PWC users, including older adults	• 2-D maps of the environment are generated. Visualizations of the driver's motion in the environment are captured and can be replayed later. • Examples of quantitative data that can be computed with the system include alignment with beds, proximity to doors, and linear and angular velocity profiles.
Nisbet et al. 1996	The CALL Smart Wheelchair (now manufactured by Smile Rehab) is a training tool that has the following features: different types of switches and controls, collision avoidance, line following, and feedback to the user.	Training tool originally developed for children with complex and severe disabilities	• Bump and ultrasonic sensors installed on the wheelchair provide information on obstacles in the environment. • A speech synthesizer provides feedback to the driver regarding system actions and confirms driving commands received from the driver.

to provide feedback to the driver that helps the driver learn how to drive safely and independently (eventually without any assistance).

Review of User Studies, Outcomes, and Clinical Evidence

Even if the technical barriers to developing a smart wheelchair are overcome, there remain issues of clinical acceptance and reimbursement that must be addressed before smart wheelchairs can be widely used. Third-party payers are unlikely to reimburse clients for the expense of smart wheelchairs until they have been proven to be efficacious, if not cost-effective. Unfortunately, enough data to demonstrate safety will be extremely difficult to accumulate. A recent analysis determined that autonomous vehicles would have to be driven hundreds of millions of miles to demonstrate reliability (Kalra and Paddock 2016). Even if smart wheelchairs need to be driven a fraction of this distance, there are significant obstacles to obtaining this amount of data.

The target user population for smart wheelchairs is small to begin with and, almost by definition, has difficulty traveling to a lab. Another significant obstacle to accurately evaluating smart wheelchairs is the need for extensive amounts of training. Smart wheelchair technologies are inherently difficult to master, especially when using a different technology outside the lab in between training sessions can interfere with retention of skills taught during training. A final obstacle to evaluating smart wheelchairs in the lab is the decision of what to measure. Investigators often emphasize speed at the expense of other valid measures such as accuracy, comfort, or workload. Smart wheelchairs, however, are likely to cause participants to take longer to complete navigation tasks because the technology slows the wheelchair in the presence of obstacles. A participant completing a navigation task without a smart wheelchair may drive straight from the start point to the goal if he or she chooses completing the navigation task in the shortest time possible at the expense of incurring multiple collisions.

An alternative to evaluating smart wheelchairs in the lab is to evaluate assistive technology (AT) "in the field" or "in the real world." Testing smart wheelchairs in unconstrained environments is appealing because that is how we ultimately hope they will be used, but there are challenges as well. For example, there may be only one existing prototype of the device being tested, which makes field trials much less efficient than laboratory trials. In addition, real-world environments are (by definition) less controlled than laboratories, making it difficult to replicate conditions across subjects. Field trials can also take much longer to generate data. For example, an entire day in a wheelchair user's life may feature much less driving than a single hour in a laboratory.

Thus, the usability, reliability, validity, and clinical utility of independent use of smart wheelchairs by users with disabilities, especially in uncontrolled environments, are yet to be established. In addition, there has been limited research that explores the use of smart wheelchairs in assessment and training by clinicians (Smith et al. 2014), possibly due to the lack of significant clinical involvement during the development of these systems. Table 5.6 provides details on user studies conducted with smart wheelchairs.

Future Directions

Smart wheelchairs have remained at technology readiness level 4 for decades because no smart wheelchair has been subjected to a rigorous, controlled evaluation that involves extended use in real-world settings. The primary obstacle to conducting long-term studies is the prohibitive hardware cost associated with constructing enough smart wheelchairs for such a study. Long-term studies are necessary, however, because the actual effects of using a smart wheelchair for an extended period of time are unknown. Some investigators (e.g., the CALL Center) have intended their smart wheelchair to be used as a means of developing the skills necessary to use standard wheelchairs safely and independently. Most investigators, however, have intended their smart wheelchair to be a person's permanent mobility solution or have not addressed the issue at all. It is possible that using a smart wheelchair could actually *diminish* an individual's ability to use a standard wheelchair, as that individual comes to rely on the navigation assistance provided by the smart wheelchair. Ultimately, it is likely that, for some users (particularly children), smart wheelchair technology will be effective "training wheels" that can be used to teach the most basic mobility skills (e.g., cause and effect, starting and stopping on command), and for other users, smart wheelchairs will be permanent solutions.

The distinction between using a smart wheelchair as a *mobility aid*, a *training tool*, or an *evaluation instrument* is also worthy of study. Each of these functions is unique and requires very different behavior on the part of the smart wheelchair. As a mobility aid, the smart wheelchair's goal is to help the user reach a destination as quickly and comfortably as possible. Feedback to the user is kept to a minimum to avoid distractions, and collisions are to be avoided.

TABLE 5.6 User Studies with Semiautonomous Smart Wheelchairs

System	Participants	Test/Task	Outcome Measures	Limitations
Feedback simulation (Wang, Gorski et al. 2011; Wang, Mihailidis et al. 2011)	5 adults with cognitive impairment	Power-Mobility Indoor Driving Assessment (PIDA) (Dawson, Chan, and Kaiserman, 1994)	Ability to perform self-identified goals and PIDA tasks Ability to perform 6 × 1 h of driving NASA Task Load Index (NASA-TLX) (Hart and Staveland, 1988) Quebec User Evaluation of Satisfaction with Assistive Technology (QUEST 2.0) (Demers, Weiss-Lambrou, and Ska 2002) Psychosocial Impact of Assistive Devices Scale (PIADS) (Jutai and Day, 2002)	Small sample size Not current PWC users (unable to contrast with standard PWC) Simulated smart wheelchair through teleoperation Audio feedback errors
Wizard-of-Oz simulation (Mitchell et al. 2014; Rushton et al. 2014; Viswanathan, Zambalde et al. 2016)	10 adults with cognitive impairment	PIDA: elevator, table docking, back-in parking, maneuverability, hallway	Pre–post semistructured interviews NASA-TLX QUEST 2.0 Sensor data	Small sample size Used under supervision for specific tasks, not independent in daily life Self-reported demographic data Simulated smart wheelchair through teleoperation Participants' cognitive impairment limited their ability to provide feedback in some cases

(Continued)

TABLE 5.6 (CONTINUED) User Studies with Semiautonomous Smart Wheelchairs

System	Participants	Test/Task	Outcome Measures	Limitations
Anticollision contact sensor skirt (Wang, Gorski et al. 2011)	5 adults with cognitive impairment	PIDA Manual wheelchair vs. smart wheelchair	Interviews and observation	Small sample size Slow speed required for safe stop on collision Response bias
Collaborative Assistive Robot for Mobility Enhancement (CARMEN) (Urdiales et al. 2010)	30 adults with physical or cognitive impairments	Two tasks: 1. Door passage (shared control only) 2. Hallway (shared control and manual)	Safety Directness Smoothness Trajectory curvature Time to destination Traveled distance Intervention level (number of times joystick used) Disagreement (difference between human output and robot output) Inconsistency (difference in user behavior for some situations) Joystick variation (>10% of joystick deflection) PIADS Amount of help provided at each point Stand-alone efficiency Subjective degree of satisfaction	In shared control, performance can't be compared to user or machine only since both inputs are continuously blended Joystick variation is not a good measurement of workload (lack of sensitivity)

(Continued)

TABLE 5.6 (CONTINUED) User Studies with Semiautonomous Smart Wheelchairs

System	Participants	Test/Task	Outcome Measures	Limitations
Collaborative controller (Carlson and Demiris 2012)	21 able-bodied adults; 1 adult wheelchair user	Manual vs. shared control Task of driving around an office (hallway, door passages, cluttered office space) Secondary task: press the right quadrant of a joypad corresponding to the lit quadrant on a screen	Number of collisions (head on or clipping) Task completion time Jerkiness (3rd derivative of position) Secondary task: reaction time and hit rates	User not used to dynamics of that particular wheelchair Chair does not detect overhanging tabletops
Collaborative Wheelchair Assistant (CWA) (Zeng, Burdet, and Teo 2008; Zeng, Teo et al. 2008)	5 able-bodied adults; 5 adults with cerebral palsy or traumatic brain injury	Two modes: free (FM) vs. guided (GM) Navigation through realistic office environment (obstacles, doorways)	Mean speed Joystick movement (variation of joystick position) and intervention level (intervention time) Safety (number of collisions) Task completion time	Little user input required (speed only) but still requires reactive action from user Relies on predetermined path Small sample sizes
IATSL Intelligent Wheelchair System (IWS) (How 2010)	3 adults with cognitive impairment	Obstacle course PWC vs. IWS	Number of collisions Location of collision on wheelchair Subtask success Task completion time NASA-TLX QUEST 2.0 Adherence to audio prompting False collision detections	Missed obstacles Incorrect prompts and limited adherence Small sample size Limited time to accustom to system

(Continued)

TABLE 5.6 (CONTINUED)   User Studies with Semiautonomous Smart Wheelchairs

System	Participants	Test/Task	Outcome Measures	Limitations
JiaoLong wheelchair (Li, Chen, and Wang 2011)	5 mobility-impaired adults	Three tasks: 1. hall tour 2. door passage 3. obstacle avoidance	Task completion time Collision times Trajectory smoothness (curvature), fluency (speed variation, length) User control weight Three evaluation indices Posttest questionnaire: self-reported task difficulty, operating difficulty, satisfaction	No high-level user control No report on qualitative results
Levels-of-automation (LOA) wheelchair (Jipp 2013)	21 able-bodied adults	Standardized course in office environment	Number of collisions, times driving backward, times turning > 90° User acceptance questionnaire (5-point Likert scale) 1. Usefulness: perceived safety and dependability 2. Ease of use: perceived operability, straightforwardness, comfort Motor performance test	Danger due to not detecting tabletop but only legs Limitations with eye tracking (quick head movements) Limited directability: choice to follow printed path or stop Controlled lab study: limited external validity Occasional failure of system in higher levels of automation Sample not consisting of potential users

(Continued)

TABLE 5.6 (CONTINUED)   User Studies with Semiautonomous Smart Wheelchairs

System	Participants	Test/Task	Outcome Measures	Limitations
Navigation and Obstacle Avoidance Help (NOAH) (Viswanathan 2012)	6 adults with cognitive impairment	Navigate through a maze to a target destination while minimizing collisions Eight repetitions/participant for baseline and intervention	Number of collisions Length of route Task completion time NASA-TLX QUEST 2.0 Self-reported confidence Custom questionnaire User comments and investigator observations	Static environment Positive responses to please investigator Participants' impaired memory could affect responses to posttask questionnaire Short duration of task and trial Small sample size
Smart Chair (Parikh et al. 2007)	50 able-bodied adults	Navigation in two rooms for each mode Secondary tasks: arithmetic operation, pick up object	Wheelchair and robotic experience NASA-TLX Task completion time Number of human–robot interactions (number of times user interacts with joystick) Secondary-task effectiveness Distance traveled Number of collisions Odometry Subjective rating of safety, control, rigidity of system, frustration and effort, overall assessment	Not tested on target users

Open clinical research questions associated with using a smart wheelchair as a mobility aid identified by SWAT participants include the following (Viswanathan et al. 2016a):

- How can smart wheelchairs be used for remediation?
- How can they be used for compensation?
- What kind of feedback is acceptable to users and appropriate to meet clinical goals?
- What type and level of shared control is acceptable to users and appropriate to meet clinical goals?

Open engineering/technology research questions associated with using a smart wheelchair as a mobility aid identified by SWAT participants include the following (Viswanathan et al. 2016a):

- How should feedback regarding control be implemented?
- How is a reliable, safe, and adaptive collision avoidance and navigation system developed?
- How and when should the type and level of shared control be modified?

As a training tool, the goal of using a smart wheelchair is to develop the skills needed for independent mobility. In this role, feedback is likely to be significantly increased, and the extent to which the smart wheelchair complies with the user's input will be a function of the actual training activity. As an evaluation instrument, the smart wheelchair's goal is to record activity without intervention. In this case, there would likely be no feedback or active navigation assistance to the user. Open clinical research questions associated with using a smart wheelchair as a training or an evaluation instrument identified by SWAT participants include the following (Viswanathan et al. 2016a):

- How can sensor data (e.g., proximity to obstacles, driving patterns, navigated routes, weight distribution) be presented to provide meaningful information to clinicians regarding, for example, safety, activity, participation, or pressure sores, at a given point in time?
- How can these data be integrated into current clinical practice and be used to track changes over time?
- What are the **security** concerns and ethics with regard to collecting user data for training and evaluation purposes?
- What attitudes do the client, caregiver, and trainer have toward these kinds of systems?

Open engineering/technology research questions associated with using a smart wheelchair as a training or assessment tool identified by SWAT participants include the following (Viswanathan et al. 2016a):

- How can rich environmental data be synthesized in semantically meaningful ways?
- How can video and sensor data be collected and analyzed while respecting the privacy of the user and the people with whom the user interacts?

STUDY QUESTIONS

1. Name three different types of sensors used in smart wheelchairs and explain the strengths and weaknesses of each.
2. John F. Kennedy said, "We choose to go to the moon," in 1962, and the first manned moon landing occurred seven years later, in 1969. By comparison, one of the earliest peer-reviewed journal articles describing a smart wheelchair (Madarasz et al. 1986) was published in 1986, and smart wheelchairs are still not in general use. Does this mean it is harder to make a wheelchair that does not hit things than it is to send humans to the moon and back safely?
3. Describe how smart wheelchairs may be used to increase independent mobility.
4. Name three different types of input methods that have been explored with smart wheelchairs.
5. Name three different types of feedback modalities that have been used by smart wheelchairs.
6. If you could have a smart wheelchair or an exoskeleton (which provided independent mobility, the ability to traverse stairs, and the ability to manipulate objects), which would you choose? Why?

References

Archambault, P. S., Sorrento, G., Routhier, F., and Boissy, P. (2010). Assessing improvement of powered wheelchair driving skills using a data logging system. Presented at RESNA annual conference, June, Las Vegas, NV. http://www.resna.org/sites/default/files/legacy/conference/proceedings /2010/WheeledMobility/ArchambaultP.html.

Bourret, E. M., Bernick, L. G., Cott, C. A., and Kontos, P. C. (2002). The meaning of mobility for residents and staff in long-term care facilities. *Journal of Advanced Nursing*, *37*(4), 338–345. http://doi.org/10.1046/j.1365-2648.2002.02104.x.

Brighton, C. (2003). Rules of the road. *Rehab Management*, *16*(3), 18–21. http:// www.ncbi.nlm.nih.gov/pubmed/12741254.

Carlson, T., and del R. Millan, J. (2013). Brain-controlled wheelchairs: A robotic architecture. *IEEE Robotics and Automation Magazine, 20*(1), 65–73. http://doi.org/10.1109/MRA.2012.2229936.

Carlson, T., and Demiris, Y. (2012). Collaborative control for a robotic wheelchair: Evaluation of performance, attention, and workload. *IEEE Transactions on Systems, Man, and Cybernetics. Part B, Cybernetics, 42*(3), 876–888. http://doi.org/10.1109/TSMCB.2011.2181833.

Chen, X., and Agrawal, S. K. (2013). Assisting versus repelling force-feedback for learning of a line following task in a wheelchair. *IEEE Transactions on Neural Systems and Rehabilitation Engineering, 21*(6), 959–968. http://doi.org/10.1109/TNSRE.2013.2245917.

Davies, A. (2015). Turns out the hardware in self-driving cars is pretty cheap. http://www.wired.com/2015/04/cost-of-sensors-autonomous-cars/.

Dawson, D., Chan, R., and Kaiserman, E. (1994). Development of the power-mobility indoor driving assessment for residents of long-term care facilities: A preliminary report. *Canadian Journal of Occupational Therapy, 61*(5), 269–276. http://doi.org/10.1177/000841749406100507.

Demers, L., Weiss-Lambrou, R., and Ska, B. (2002). The Quebec User Evaluation of Satisfaction with Assistive Technology (QUEST 2.0): An overview and recent progress. *Technology and Disability, 14*, 101–105. http://content.iospress.com/articles/technology-and-disability/tad00095.

Fuchs, R. H., and Gromak, P. A. (2003). Wheelchair use by residents of nursing homes: Effectiveness in meeting positioning and mobility needs. *Assistive Technology, 15*(2), 151–163. http://doi.org/10.1080/10400435.2003.10131899.

Guizzo, E. (2011). How Google's self-driving car works. http://spectrum.ieee.org/automaton/robotics/artificial-intelligence/how-google-self-driving-car-works.

Hart, S. G., and Staveland, L. E. (1988). Development of NASA-TLX (Task Load Index): Results of empirical and theoretical research. *Advances in Psychology, 52*(1), 139–183.

How, T.-V. (2010). *Development of an Anti-collision and Navigation System for Powered Wheelchairs.* Toronto, Canada: University of Toronto. http://hdl.handle.net/1807/25621.

Iezzoni, L. I., McCarthy, E. P., Davis, R. B., and Siebens, H. (2001). Mobility difficulties are not only a problem of old age. *Journal of General Internal Medicine, 16*(4), 235–243. http://www.pubmedcentral.nih.gov/articlerender.fcgi?artid=1495195&tool=pmcentrez&rendertype=abstract.

IHS Automotive. (2014). *Emerging Technologies: Autonomous Cars—Not If, But When.* Englewood, CO: IHS.

Jipp, M. (2013). Levels of automation: Effects of individual differences on wheelchair control performance and user acceptance. *Theoretical Issues in Ergonomics Science, 15*(5), 479–504. http://doi.org/10.1080/1463922X.2013.815829.

Jipp, M., Bartolein, C., Badreddin, E., Abkai, C., and Hesser, J. (2009). Psychomotor profiling with Bayesian neworks. In C.L. Philip Chen (ed.), *2009 IEEE International Conference on Systems, Man and Cybernetics* (pp. 1680–1685). Piscataway, NJ: IEEE. http://doi.org/10.1109/ICSMC.2009.5346795.

Jutai, J., and Day, H. (2002). Psychosocial Impact of Assistive Devices Scale (PIADS). *Technology and Disability, 14*, 107–111. Amsterdam: IOS Press. http://content.iospress.com/articles/technology-and-disability/tad00094.

Kalra, N., and Paddock, S. M. (2016). *Driving to Safety: How Many Miles of Driving Would It Take to Demonstrate Autonomous Vehicle Reliability?* Santa Monica, CA: RAND. http://www.rand.org/pubs/research_reports/RR1478..html.

Levine, S. P., Bell, D. A., Jaros, L. A., Simpson, R. C., Koren, Y., and Borenstein, J. (1999). The NavChair assistive wheelchair navigation system. *IEEE Transactions on Rehabilitation Engineering, 7*(4), 443–451. http://www.ncbi.nlm.nih.gov/pubmed/10609632.

Li, Q., Chen, W., and Wang, J. (2011). Dynamic shared control for human-wheelchair cooperation. In LI Zexiang (ed.), *2011 IEEE International Conference on Robotics and Automation* (pp. 4278–4283). Piscataway, NJ: IEEE. http://doi.org/10.1109/ICRA.2011.5980055.

LoPresti, E. F., Simpson, R. C., Miller, D., and Nourbakhsh, I. (2002). Evaluation of sensors for a smart wheelchair. In J. Smith (ed.), *Proceedings of the RESNA 2002 Annual Conference* (pp. 166–168). Arlington, CA: Resna.

Madarasz, R., Heiny, L., Cromp, R., and Mazur, N. (1986). The design of an autonomous vehicle for the disabled. *IEEE Journal on Robotics and Automation, 2*(3), 117–126. http://doi.org/10.1109/JRA.1986.1087052.

Mandel, C., Luth, T., Laue, T., Rofer, T., Graser, A., and Krieg-Bruckner, B. (2009). Navigating a smart wheelchair with a brain-computer interface interpreting steady-state visual evoked potentials. In Ning Xi (ed.), *2009 IEEE/RSJ International Conference on Intelligent Robots and Systems* (pp. 1118–1125). Piscataway, NJ: IEEE. http://doi.org/10.1109/IROS.2009.5354534.

Mankins, J. C. (1995). Technology readiness levels: A white paper. http://www.hq.nasa.gov/office/codeq/trl/trl.pdf.

Manrique, L., Radideau, G., Reinhold, G., and Hoffman, A. (2007). Using an obstacle sensing system in power wheelchair training of children: A pilot study. In Ray Grott (ed.), *RESNA Annual Conference*. Phoenix, AZ: RESNA Press.

Marchal-Crespo, L., Furumasu, J., and Reinkensmeyer, D. J. (2010). A robotic wheelchair trainer: Design overview and a feasibility study. *Journal of Neuroengineering and Rehabilitation, 7*:40. http://doi.org/10.1186/1743-0003-7-40.

Miro, J. V., Black, R., De Bruijn, F., and Dissanayake, D. (2011). Semi-autonomous competency assessment of powered mobility device users. In Robert Riener (ed.), *IEEE International Conference on Rehabilitation Robotics, 2011*, 5975364. Piscataway, NJ: IEEE. http://doi.org/10.1109/ICORR.2011.5975364.

Mitchell, I. M., Viswanathan, P., Adhikari, B., Rothfels, E., and Mackworth, A. K. (2014). Shared control policies for safe wheelchair navigation of elderly adults with cognitive and mobility impairments: Designing a Wizard of Oz study. In Dawn Tilbury (ed.), *2014 American Control Conference* (pp. 4087–4094). Piscataway, NY: IEEE. http://doi.org/10.1109/ACC.2014.6859446.

Moghaddam, A. K., Pineau, J., Frank, J., Archambault, P., Routhier, F., Audet, T., Polgar, J. et al. (2011). Mobility profile and wheelchair driving skills of powered wheelchair users: Sensor-based event recognition using a support vector machine classifier. In *Annual International Conference of the IEEE Engineering in Medicine and Biology Society. 2011*, 7336–7339. http://doi.org/10.1109/IEMBS.2011.6091711.

Mortenson, W. B., Miller, W. C., Boily, J., Steele, B., Crawford, E. M., and Desharnais, G. (2006). Overarching principles and salient findings for inclusion in guidelines for power mobility use within residential care facilities. *Journal of Rehabilitation Research and Development*, 43(2), 199–208. http://www.pubmedcentral.nih.gov/articlerender.fcgi?artid=3614519&tool=pmcentrez&rendertype=abstract.

Mosquet, X., Agrawal, R., Dauner, T., Lang, N., Rubmann, M., Mei-Pochtler, A., and Schmieg, F. (2015). *Revolution in the Driver's Seat: The Road to Autonomous Vehicles*. Boston: bcg.perspectives. https://www.bcgperspectives.com/content/articles/automotive-consumer-insight-revolution-drivers-seat-road-autonomous-vehicles/.

Nisbet, P., Craig, J., Odor, P., and Aitken, S. (1996, January 1). "Smart" wheelchairs for mobility training. *Technology and Disability*, 5(1):49–62. http://doi.org/10.3233/TAD-1996-5107.

Parikh, S. P., Grassi, V., Jr., Kumar, V., and Okamoto, J., Jr. (2007). Integrating human inputs with autonomous behaviors on an intelligent wheelchair platform. *IEEE Intelligent Systems*, 22(2), 33–41. http://doi.org/10.1109/MIS.2007.36.

Pawlson, L. G., Goodwin, M., and Keith, K. (1986). Wheelchair use by ambulatory nursing home residents. *Journal of the American Geriatrics Society*, 34(12), 860–964. http://www.ncbi.nlm.nih.gov/pubmed/3782699.

Pineau, J., West, R., Atrash, A., Villemure, J., and Routhier, F. (2011). On the feasibility of using a standardized test for evaluating a speech-controlled smart wheelchair. *International Journal of Intelligent Control and Systems*, 16(2), 124–131.

Rofer, T., Mandel, C., and Laue, T. (2009). Controlling an automated wheelchair via joystick/head-joystick supported by smart driving assistance. In Kiyoshi Nagai (ed.), *2009 IEEE International Conference on Rehabilitation Robotics* (pp. 743–748). Piscataway, NJ: IEEE. http://doi.org/10.1109/ICORR.2009.5209506.

Rushton, P. W., Mortenson, B., Viswanathan, P., Wang, R. H. L., and Clarke, L. H. (2014). Intelligent power wheelchairs for residents in long-term care facilities: Potential users' experiences and perceptions. In Alisa Brownlee (ed.), *RESNA Annual Conference*. Indianapolis, IN: RESNA Press. http://www.resna.org/sites/default/files/conference/2014/WheeledMobility/Rushton.html.

Simpson, R. C., and Levine, S. P. (2002). Voice control of a powered wheelchair. *IEEE Transactions on Neural Systems and Rehabilitation Engineering, 10*(2), 122–125. http://doi.org/10.1109/TNSRE.2002.1031981.

Simpson, R. C., LoPresti, E. F., and Cooper, R. A. (2008). How many people would benefit from a smart wheelchair? *Journal of Rehabilitation Research and Development, 45*(1), 53–71. http://www.ncbi.nlm.nih.gov/pubmed/18566926.

Simpson, R. C., Poirot, D., and Baxter, F. (2002). The Hephaestus smart wheelchair system. *IEEE Transactions on Neural Systems and Rehabilitation Engineering, 10*(2), 118–122. http://doi.org/10.1109/TNSRE.2002.1031980.

Smith, E., Miller, W. C., Mortenson, W. B., Mihailidis, A., Viswanathan, P., Lo, J., and Pham, P. (2014). Interface design for shared control tele-operated power wheelchair technology. Presented at the 8th International Convention on Rehabilitation Engineering and Assistive Technology, June, Singapore.

Tannert, C. (2014). Will you ever be able to afford a self-driving car? FastCompany.com. http://www.fastcompany.com/3025722/will-you-ever-be-able-to-afford-a-self-driving-car.

Tully, P., and Mohl, C. (1995). Older Residents of Health Care Institutions. *Health Reports, 27*(3), 27–30. http://www.statcan.gc.ca/pub/82-003-x/1995003/article/2452-eng.pdf.

Urdiales, C., Peula, J. M., Fdez-Carmona, M., Barrué, C., Pérez, E. J., Sánchez-Tato, I., del Toro, J. C. et al. (2010). A new multi-criteria optimization strategy for shared control in wheelchair assisted navigation. *Autonomous Robots, 30*(2), 179–197. http://doi.org/10.1007/s10514-010-9211-2.

Viswanathan, P. (2012). *Navigation and Obstacle Avoidance Help (NOAH) for Elderly Wheelchair Users with Cognitive Impairment in Long-Term Care.* Vancouver: University of British Columbia. https://open.library.ubc.ca/cIRcle/collections/ubctheses/24/items/1.0052150.

Viswanathan, P., Zambalde, E. P., Foley, G., Bell, J. L., Wang, R. H., Adhikari, B., Mackworth, A. K. et al. (2016). Intelligent wheelchair control strategies for older adults with cognitive impairment: User attitudes, needs, and preferences. *Autonomous Robots: Special Issue on Assistive and Rehabilitation Robotics.* 1–16. Springer, USA. doi:10.1007/s10514-016-9568-y

Viswanathan, P., Wang, R. H., Sutcliffe, A., Kenyon, L., Foley, G., Miller, W. C., and the SWAT participants. (2016a). Smart Wheelchairs in Assessment and Training (SWAT): State of the Field (submitted).

Viswanathan, P., Wang, R. H., Sutcliffe, A., Kenyon, L., Foley, G., Miller, W. C., and the SWAT participants. (2016b). State of the field: Findings from the 2014 Smart Wheelchairs in Assessment and Training (SWAT) workshop. Proceedings of the 5th European Seating Symposium, June, Dublin, Ireland.

Wang, R .H., Gorski, S. M., Holliday, P. J., and Fernie, G. R. (2011). Evaluation of a contact sensor skirt for an anti-collision power wheelchair for older adult nursing home residents with dementia: Safety and mobility. *Assistive Technology, 23*(3): 117–134.

Wang, R. H., Mihailidis, A., Dutta, T., and Fernie, G. R. (2011). Usability testing of multimodal feedback interface and simulated collision-avoidance power wheelchair for long-term-care home residents with cognitive impairments. *Journal of Rehabilitation Research and Development, 48*(7), 801–822. http://www.ncbi.nlm.nih.gov/pubmed/21938666.

Zeng, Q., Burdet, E., and Teo, C. L. (2008). User evaluation of a collaborative wheelchair system. *Annual International Conference of the IEEE Engineering in Medicine and Biology Society.* August 20–25, 1956–1960. http://doi.org/10.1109/IEMBS.2008.4649571.

Zeng, Q., Teo, C. L., Rebsamen, B., and Burdet, E. (2008). A collaborative wheelchair system. *IEEE Transactions on Neural Systems and Rehabilitation Engineering, 16*(2), 161–170. http://doi.org/10.1109/TNSRE.2008.917288.

6

Exoskeletons as an Assistive Technology for Mobility and Manipulation

Jaimie Borisoff, Mahsa Khalili, W. Ben Mortenson, and H. F. Machiel Van der Loos

Contents

Learning Objectives

After completing this chapter, readers will be able to

1. Describe the principles that underlie the performance criteria for a particular exoskeleton technology when it is implemented as an assistive technology for mobility or manipulation.
2. List the walking exoskeletons (lower limb exoskeletons, LLEs) that are either commercially available or nearing production.
3. List the **upper limb exoskeletons (ULEs)** for manipulation that are either commercially available or nearing production.
4. Describe and list the client populations, and their associated disabilities, that are candidate users for exoskeleton technologies.
5. Discuss the current limitations of exoskeletons for use in the community.
6. Describe the activities, applications, and environments suitable for exoskeleton use as a mobility device, both currently and in the future.

Principles

In 2013, it was estimated that over 41 million people in the United States (approximately 13% of the population) had a mobility disability, the most prevalent type of disability (Courtney-Long et al. 2015). In 2009, it was estimated that over 24 million people in the United States used assistive technology (AT) (Ilunga Tshiswaka et al. 2016), and in 2010, over 3.6 million used a wheelchair (Brault 2010). Wheelchairs, in particular, have progressed to the point that, regardless of their notoriety as a limiting factor, they are, in fact, empowering and paramount to many people in terms of achieving a high quality of life, independence, and participation in the community. Wheelchairs do present some problems when used chronically, however. Two problems are: (1) health (conventional, seated wheelchair use is associated with a variety of potential health concerns, such as skin breakdown and overuse injuries); and (2) access (the built and natural environments in which we live invariably impose barriers to full access and participation by wheelchair users). In addition, wheelchairs are simply not *transformative*; that is, they do not allow persons with a disability a level of mobility performance that approaches that of their nondisabled peers (Cowan et al. 2012).

As well as gait or mobility disabilities, some conditions affect *manipulation*. Manipulation, in this context, involves the use of arms, hands, and fingers to manipulate objects in the environment for a variety of reasons, but usually related to performing activities of daily living (ADLs), such as eating and interacting with computers, tasks that require a minimum level of upper limb functionality, including reaching and grasping. Upper extremity disorders can significantly reduce the independence of individuals and consequently decrease their quality of life. Some upper limb impairments can be reversed after undergoing intensive rehabilitation, whereas other disorders are progressive and may leave individuals with permanent impairment. Some of the latter disorders include brachial plexus injury (BPI), high-level spinal cord injury (SCI), stroke, multiple sclerosis (MS), amyotrophic lateral sclerosis (ALS), among other upper limb impairments affecting disabled and elderly populations. Just considering stroke, there are more than 6 million survivors in the United States alone, and stroke is the leading cause of serious long-term disability (Mozaffarian et al. 2016). It is well known that poor outcomes for upper limb function after stroke are common (Gowland 1982). Despite research that has been conducted in the area of upper limb functional improvement, there seems to be a substantial gap between commercially available solutions and the need in the community for viable devices.

To improve function for people with mobility and manipulation-related disabilities, *exoskeletons* have been developed and now represent an emerging AT sector. An exoskeleton, as defined in this chapter, is a powered robotic orthosis for people with disabilities. They are designed for mobility or manipulation and are wearable and autonomously operated; ideally, if used as AT, exoskeletons could be deployed in daily life scenarios (Van der Loos, Reinkensmeyer, and Guglielmelli 2015). More specifically, with regard to lower limb exoskeletons (LLEs), we use the definition of Louie et al. (2015, 1): "a multi-joint orthosis that uses an external power source to move at least two joints on each leg, which is portable, and can be used independent of a treadmill or body-weight support." It is important to note that these are *active* devices; thus, we are not considering any *passive* exoskeletons or other types of orthoses.

While the focus of discussions on exoskeletons is usually on standing and walking, upper limb exoskeletons (ULEs) are being developed to improve manipulation and are also reviewed here. Manipulation is simply mobility of the upper extremities to perform a task, although, certainly with regard to medical applications, one significant distinguishing difference between ULE and LLE designs is that ULE designs are focused on precise control while LLEs are focused more on the power necessary for standing and walking. Consistent with the LLE definition cited, a definition for a ULE designed for manipulation would be that it is a wearable, portable, and autonomously operated multijoint orthosis that uses an external power source to move at least two joints on the upper limb for use in daily life scenarios.

In this chapter, we do not consider ULEs that need external attachment to a base of support (other than to a wheelchair), hence preserving their portability and assistive functionality. Exoskeletons with nonportable stable supports are considered to be robotic manipulators. Other robotic manipulators are portable (e.g., attached, like the JACO [Maheu et al. 2011], to a wheelchair). Robotic manipulators (Chapter 3) are meant to substitute movements for disabled upper extremities (Maciejasz et al. 2014), rather than assisting functionally natural movements of the limbs themselves. Robotic prostheses are addressed in Chapter 4. We also do not consider single-joint exoskeletons, such as ankle-only or knee-only powered orthoses (Lajeunesse et al. 2015).

Young and Ferris (2016) have categorized exoskeletons based on their intended use into three classes:

1. Augmentation of able-bodied people for increases in strength, speed, or endurance. This is usually associated with military applications, but industrial uses are proposed as well, including use by factory workers or health care professionals (e.g., for assisting patient transfers).

2. Rehabilitation or therapy devices, a class of exoskeletons that is outside the scope of this book.
3. Exoskeletons as an AT, as we consider in this chapter.

There is possible overlap in these three classes of technology; for example, a design with variable assistive control and seamless user-intentional control may be usable in the future by a person with a disability for rehabilitation and AT purposes, as well as used as an augmentation exoskeleton for military-industrial uses by an able-bodied person. There has been some effort in the literature to distinguish exoskeletons that were developed to expressly augment the physical capabilities of able-bodied individuals from powered orthoses. For instance, Herr has stated: "In general, the term 'exoskeleton' is used to describe a device that augments the performance of an able-bodied wearer, whereas the term 'orthosis' is typically used to describe a device that is used to assist a person with a limb pathology" (Herr 2009, 1). On the other hand, we propose to use the terminology adopted by the U.S. Food and Drug Administration (FDA), which recently approved the ReWalk exoskeleton, the first LLE to be approved, for supervised therapeutic use at home: "The device is assigned the generic name powered lower extremity exoskeleton, and it is identified as a prescription device that is composed of an external, powered, motorized orthosis that is placed over a person's paralyzed or weakened limbs for medical purposes" (U.S. Food and Drug Administration, HHS 2015, 25227).

Almost exclusively, exoskeletons are being used today for rehabilitation purposes under supervision by a therapist. However, exoskeletons could actually become a replacement or adjunct for wheelchairs or other ATs. As of this writing (March 2016), there was little evidence to suggest this is likely in the short term. Nevertheless, this chapter discusses the potential for exoskeletons to become true mobility or manipulation assistive devices, reviews the products available today, and describes known efforts under way in research laboratories.

To develop a better understanding of the potential for exoskeletons to be used as mobility devices, it is important to understand how AT is defined. The Technology Related Assistance to Individuals with Disabilities Act of 1988 (U.S. Code Chapter 31 2011) described AT devices as "any item, piece of equipment, or product system, whether acquired commercially off the shelf, modified, or customized, that is used to increase, maintain, or improve functional capabilities of individuals with disabilities." Similarly, the International Organization for Standardization (ISO) defined assistive products, in part, as any product (including devices, instruments, and equipment) used by persons with disability for participation, and to support or substitute for body functions, or to prevent activity limitations (ISO 2011). Although these definitions suggest that AT devices can be used for either compensation (environmentally focused interventions) or rehabilitation (interventions focused on changing/restoring the abilities of the individual), AT is usually conceived as a compensatory strategy (Russell et al. 1997). From this perspective, Cowan et al. (2012) described how some technologies, such as robotic exercise devices, may have an indirect effect on mobility by improving the capabilities of the user, whereas ATs have a direct effect on mobility without changing the body of the person. It is only when a device is used in the real world for purposeful activities that it becomes AT. That said, the relationship between compensation and rehabilitation is somewhat ambiguous, as devices such as manual wheelchairs may compensate for problems with ambulating, but at the same time provide a form of exercise, which may reduce the risk of more general deconditioning.

According to the Human Activity Assistive Technology (HAAT) model (Cook and Polgar 2015), successful AT prescription requires careful consideration of the person, the targeted activity, the AT that can be used, and the context in which it will be used. With the HAAT model, activity is a broad term that includes both the execution of a task and social participation as defined in the World Health Organization's (WHO's) International Classification of Functioning, Disability and Health (Svestkova 2008). For example, the provision of mobility AT requires a thorough understanding of the abilities of the individuals, activities that they want to perform (in terms of both mobility-related activities they want to take part in and activities they want to take part in using their mobility devices), the features of each device being considered, the accessibility of the environment, and availability of assistance.

The AT choices invariably involve compromises (Jutai et al. 2005). For example, someone may have difficulty self-propelling a manual wheelchair but might not want to use a power wheelchair because of the difficulty in transporting it in his or her current vehicle and would be unable to go places that did not have curb cuts (manual wheelchairs can be lifted up onto curbs). There may also be a temporal component to these deliberations in terms of seasonal climatic conditions (e.g., snow and ice) (Ripat, Brown, and Ethans 2015; Ripat and Colatruglio 2016); funding availability (e.g., one device every five years); condition trajectory (progressive vs. stable); or functional variability (e.g., diurnal variation in fatigue with MS).

Six principles were identified by WHO that need to be considered to meet the obligations for AT provision described in the Convention on the Rights of Persons with Disabilities. These are acceptability (e.g., efficiency, reliability, simplicity, safety, and aesthetics); accessibility; adaptability (i.e., can the AT be customized to meet individual needs?); affordability; availability; and quality. All six are certainly applicable to the use of exoskeletons as an AT for ambulation or manipulation. In terms of acceptability, safety is perhaps the key concern (Wolff et al. 2014). Although concerns about the potential for injury with exoskeletons frequently focus on the user, it is also important to consider the potential for injury to those around them. Reliability is also related to safety. If people begin to depend on exoskeletons as assistive devices, equipment breakdowns could become potentially dangerous (e.g., being stuck outside and unable to move in subzero temperatures). Speed is also likely factored into acceptability. Slow gait speeds might be a source of frustration for users or potentially a safety concern for activities such as street crossing. Effort is also a consideration, so that fatigue from ambulation using an exoskeleton does not limit capacity to perform other activities. Training requirements are critical; if the use of an AT is not second nature, it cannot be fully integrated into a person's daily routines (i.e., habituation) (Mortenson et al. 2012).

Some people may only be willing to use an AT if they can do so independently. Ease of use is an important aspect for users, as they would prefer devices that are easy to doff and don and do not interfere with other activities, such as transfers. Similarly, exoskeletons should be easy to control (i.e., not difficult to program) and not be cognitively taxing.

Although exoskeletons might be considered a means of improving accessibility, there may be limitations in terms of the kinds of surfaces they can operate on, inclines they can go up and down, height of curbs and stairs they can negotiate, and transportation requirements (e.g., Could the user get in and out of a standard passenger vehicle? Would the user need to sit down when using public transportation?).

Any technology device will be poorly regarded if it can only be used during specific "windows of control" when the system is capable of being controlled. This is called "synchronous control" and plagues other advanced experimental technology, such as brain-computer interfaces (BCIs; Borisoff, Mason, and Birch 2006). Thus, the ability for exoskeletons to be operated under asynchronous control, a more natural and preferred control scheme, will be important. This would allow users to be able to operate an exoskeleton whenever they would like. This also likely affects a rarely considered characteristic of AT: spontaneity. Spontaneity represents the integration of many of the elements listed previously (e.g., ease of use, donning and doffing, and asynchronous control) and gets at the concept of transformative technology, which is at the heart of future innovations.

When considering these characteristics of effective AT devices, it quickly becomes apparent that exoskeletons are lacking at this time. A more instructive approach may be to question the short-term feasibility of exoskeletons as mobility or manipulation devices and provide some guidance about the necessary features needed to be considered for a successful design to be realized.

Critical Review of the Available Technology

We described the difference between exoskeletons as an AT device or as a rehabilitation tool. Young and Ferris (2016) recently reviewed their three categories of exoskeletons. Although relatively little is known about the current state of the art of military-industrial exoskeletons, their history and known capabilities have been documented (Herr 2009; Young and Ferris 2016). None has made a commercial impact, to our knowledge, in any military or industrial application to date. Young and Ferris also described exoskeletons for therapy, which generally include stationary devices coupled to a treadmill such as the Lokomat. They classify the portable LLEs, which we describe further in this chapter, as AT devices for people with mobility impairments. We consider these devices, with the Rex as one exception, as LLEs for over-ground therapy or more simply as portable versions of stationary exoskeletons for therapeutic purposes. No study is known that documents the feasibility of LLEs as an AT community use device for ambulation or general mobility. The capability of a technology to ambulate an individual, under supervision of a trained therapist, is not enough evidence to recommend it as a potential AT device when one considers the definition and background described in the first section. Nevertheless, a review of these devices illuminates the current state of technology readiness of exoskeletons as AT. It is hoped this will also assist the community in further technology development efforts and increase our understanding and ability to incorporate the requirements that wheelchair users need in their daily mobility needs (Table 6.1).

Each listed technology described in Table 6.2 is categorized using its technology readiness level (TRL) considering its use as an AT device. TRL scoring was done by considering the current state of each technology in terms identified by the TRL scale, as well as considering how each technology currently aligns with the six WHO principles of AT: acceptability, accessibility, adaptability, affordability, availability, and quality. For instance, the minimum speed reported necessary to safely cross a street is 0.5–0.6 m/s (Andrews et al. 2010; Bryce, Dijkers, and Kozlowski 2015);

TABLE 6.1　LLE Device Characteristics

Device Name, Company	Joint Type	Supported Movements	Target Users	Type of Control	Device Weight; Modular Design	Reported Walking Speed
ReWalk™ by ReWalk Robotics	Actuated hip and knee Spring-assisted ankle	Sit to stand Stand to sit Walking Ascending and descending stairs	Personal use: SCI at levels T7 to L5 Rehabilitation settings: SCI at levels T4 to L5	Forward COG shift detection, lateral COG shift to clear swing foot Wireless wrist-worn controller	20.9 kg; No	Maximum speed: 0.6 m/s
Ekso™ GT by Ekso Bionics	Actuated hip and knee Variable stiffness ankle	Sit to stand Stand to sit Walking	Complete SCI at level C7 or lower Any level of incomplete SCI Stroke	Forward and lateral COG shift detection; crutch-attached controller	20.4 kg; No	Maximum speed: 0.89 m/s
HAL® for Medical Use (Lower Limb Type) by CYBERDYNE	Actuated hip and knee Spring-assisted ankle	Sit to stand Stand to sit Walking Ascending and descending stairs	SCI Stroke	Forward and lateral COG shift detection to one leg EMG detection of intentional walking	15.0 kg; No	Minimum speed (reported for one subject): 0.11 m/s

(Continued)

TABLE 6.1 (CONTINUED) LLE Device Characteristics

Device Name, Company	Joint Type	Supported Movements	Target Users	Type of Control	Device Weight; Modular Design	Reported Walking Speed
Indego® by Parker Hannifin	Actuated hip and knee Fixed orthotic ankle	Sit to stand Stand to sit Walking	Personal use: SCI at levels T7 to L5 Rehabilitation settings: SCI at levels T4 to L5	Forward COG shift detection	12.3 kg; Yes	Mean speed: 0.22 m/s
Rex® P by Rex Bionics	Hip flexion/extension Hip abduction/adduction Knee flexion/extension Ankle dorsiflexion/plantar flexion Ankle inversion/eversion	Sit to stand Stand to sit Walking Ascending and descending stairs	SCI up to C4/5 level Muscular dystrophy Multiple sclerosis Postpolio syndrome	Hand-directed joystick control	38.0 kg; No	Speed: 0.08 m/s

Note: COG, center of gravity; EMG, electromyographic.

walking exoskeleton speeds are generally below this threshold. In addition, most LLEs require supervision for safety reasons. Almost all current LLEs need to be used with other mobility aids, such as a walker or forearm crutches. This limits their use to people with relatively good upper extremity function. In addition, the use of mobility aids restricts the functional activities that someone could do with a device (e.g., shopping or holding a drink), although future generations will likely include self-balancing features that would obviate this need. Poor speed, safety, and functional limitations certainly do not meet the acceptability quotient of the WHO principles and thus contribute to a low TRL score. All are prohibitively expensive, most are not widely available, and most rank poorly in accessibility, in terms of both use of the LLE to access the environment and the ease with which a user can transfer into or don the device. On the other hand, adaptability is generally well implemented. Quality is generally unknown, as there are simply not enough long-term data for any LLE products in the marketplace.

A final and critical criterion used in determining the TRL of LLEs as AT devices is the notion of independent use, although the WHO principles do not refer to independence as one of their six key principles of effective AT. There are many examples where dependent use can still be effective use of AT, given the HAAT model ensures both the disability and the context are considered. For instance, a "sip-and-puff" power wheelchair cannot be used independently (from start to stop) by the user (e.g., a high-level tetraplegic), as it entails an assisted transfer and device setup each time first use is initiated early in a day. After that, the device enables a high degree of independent mobility and is rightly considered an effective AT. In comparison, the ReWalk and Indego LLEs were recently approved by the FDA for home use for sit to stand and walking, but under *constant* supervision and assistance from a trained companion (U.S. Food and Drug Administration, HHS 2015). Furthermore, only people with spinal cord injuries of thoracic level 7 and below are approved to use the device. This population typically uses an ultralight wheelchair, which is used fully independently in most circumstances to support a high level of participation in the community. Using an exoskeleton necessitates dependence on a caregiver, far worse basic mobility outcomes, negligible secondary mobility outcomes, and potential safety issues. In contrast to the power wheelchair example, almost no one would consider this an effective form of AT. Hence, for the potential target population for LLE use, independence (and concomitant safety designs and procedures) must be considered as a core principle. Thus, all but one LLE have a TRL of only 1 (Table 6.2) because none of these has any research evidence of safe and

TABLE 6.2   LLE Device Characteristics and Technology Readiness Level Score

Name of Device	Variable Assistance	Upper Extremity Strength Required	Battery Life (Hours) (Continuous Operation)	Regulatory Approval Institutional Use	Regulatory Approval Personal Use	Approximate Cost (U.S.$)	TRL
ReWalk™	No	Yes	8	FDA CE Mark	FDA CE Mark	$70,000–85,000	1
Ekso™ GT	Yes	Yes	4	FDA CE Mark	None	$100,000	1
HAL®	Yes	Yes	2.5	CE Mark	None	$14,000–$19,000	1
Indego®	Yes	Yes	4	FDA CE Mark	FDA CE Mark	$80,000	1
Rex®	No	No	2	FDA CE Mark	CE Mark	$150,000	8

independent use without close supervision. Higher scores are found with the ULEs (Table 6.3). A caveat to our use of TRL scores here is that these are our best estimates given the incomplete nature of data from manufacturers and uncertainty of current technology status because the available research and documentation might only be representative of the product's status some time ago.

Lower Limb Exoskeletons

Lajeunesse et al. (2015) conducted a systematic review of LLEs for use by people with SCI; Lajeuness et al. identified five LLE systems. We used similar methodology and updated the results to reflect publications available up to February 2016. Several other recent reviews of LLEs have also been conducted with similar results (Arazpour et al. 2016; Federici et al. 2015; Louie et al. 2015; Young and Ferris 2016). Our general search strategy identified systems that adhere to the definition of LLE used in this chapter and that were studied during use by people with a disability. This section describes systems ready or nearly ready for commercialization, that is, the developers have demonstrated the technology and have a commercial partner. Research-only systems are also briefly mentioned if they have been the subject of a clinical trial or case study with a target population. In the following, we briefly describe each of the identified exoskeleton systems. These are shown in Figure 6.1. Refer to Tables 6.1 and 6.2 for specific details of each system.

The first commercially available exoskeleton for home use in the United States was the **ReWalk** exoskeleton by ReWalk Robotics (http://rewalk.com/) (Asselin et al. 2015; Benson et al. 2015; Esquenazi et al. 2012; Fineberg et al. 2013; Sale et al. 2012; Spungen 2012; Spungen et al. 2013; Yang et al. 2015; Zeilig et al. 2012), formerly Argo Medical Technologies in Israel. The ReWalk consists of a full lower limb orthosis with knee and hip actuators and has supported orthotic ankle joints. The four actuators, two each at the knees and hips, are a common design template for all but one of the LLEs described here. A shoulder-slung backpack contains the battery. The latest ReWalk Personal 6.0 device dispenses the backpack with installation of the battery in the pelvis portion of the device, a similar architecture to that of the Indego. Straps at the knee, thigh, torso, and shoulders connect the user to the device. Foot orthoses are placed inside shoes; this potentially makes donning the device difficult for some users. Control of the ReWalk is through a wrist-worn controller and a tilt sensor in the pelvis area for detection of shifts in center of gravity (COG). The

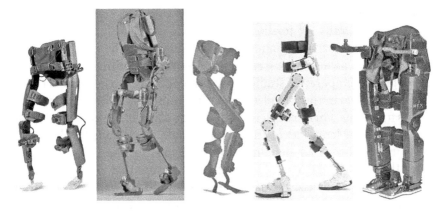

Figure 6.1 The lower limb exoskeletons. From left to right: ReWalk™ 6.0; Ekso™ GT; Indego®; HAL® for Medical Use (Lower Limb Model); and Rex®. (Photographs courtesy of ReWalk Robotics; Ekso Bionics; Parker Hannifin Corporation; Prof. Sankai, University of Tsukuba/Cyberdyne, Incorporated; and Rex Bionics, respectively.)

controller is used to select the operation mode (e.g., sit to stand or stair climbing). The device detects a user's forward lean to initiate a step. The ReWalk has demonstrated modes to enable sit to stand, stand to sit, walking, turning, and ascending and descending stairs. It is typically used with a walker or forearm crutches for stability. The ReWalk is available in several jurisdictions, including the European Union. The U.S. FDA cleared the ReWalk for home use in 2015, albeit with several conditions, including no approval for its use on stairs (U.S. Food and Drug Administration, HHS 2015). The FDA stated its approval for use "with assistance from a trained companion, such as a spouse or home health aide," a notable difference from the company's marketing materials, which include testimonials, such as allowing one "to regain independence, to use the system to walk and stand on my own."

The **Ekso GT** (Kozlowski, Bryce, and Dijkers 2015; Sale et al. 2016) is made by Ekso Bionics, Berkeley, California (http://www.eksobionics .com/). This is the latest generation of the eLEGS system of Berkeley Bionics, a company founded to commercialize the military/industrial exoskeleton technology developed by Kazerooni and colleagues. The Ekso GT consists of a full foot-shank-thigh-torso orthotic frame in which the user is attached to the device with straps at each section. Shoulder straps are further used to position the device tightly to the torso, rather than as a support for a backpack. Two other structural elements are worth noting. First, the user's shoes are placed on top of footplates, instead of having orthotics within shoes. Second, the thigh section incorporates a hinge that swings laterally 90° to allow the wearer to more easily transfer from a wheelchair to an armless stationary chair supporting the LLE. These two features may enable easier transfers and donning/doffing of the device, although no comparative studies have been published. The Ekso GT uses pressure sensors in the foot plates and tilt sensors in the torso area to control its functions. Forward-lateral shifts by the user initiate each step by the leg opposite the lateral lean. Thus, a user would alternate left-right lateral leans for synchronized stepping, similar to most of the LLEs described here. The Ekso GT also has a variable assist feature that enables configurable variable power assist to each or either leg and allows this to be tuned prior to each session to suit therapeutic improvements in strength.

The Hybrid Assistive Limb (**HAL**) exoskeleton (Kawamoto et al. 2013; Kubota et al. 2013; Nilsson et al. 2014) was developed in Japan at the University of Tsukuba and commercialized by CYBERDYNE, Incorporated, of Tsukuba, Japan (http://www.cyberdyne.jp/english/). It has recently been studied for use by people with brain, spinal cord, and neuromuscular diseases and has received the CE (Conformité Européene [European Conformity]) Marking for Medical Devices in the European Union for distribution to hospitals. It has also been approved as a medical device by the Japanese regulatory authorities and is covered under public medical insurance based on medical evidence. HAL looks like a mechanically conventional LLE, with laterally placed hip and knee actuators. The foot-ankle component comprises a built-in shoe the user has to don and a passive sprung ankle joint. Joint angles, device tilt, and floor reaction forces are sensed for control strategies. Notably, HAL for Medical Use (Lower Limb Type) is the only commercial LLE system that can use brain-derived bioelectrical signals for control (Cruciger et al. 2014). Surface electrodes placed on the users' legs detect bioelectrical signals at the skin from attempted movements. This enables voluntary and intuitive control of the device by simply attempting to walk; even if the bioelectrical signals are too faint to generate muscle movement, the signals can be detected, amplified, filtered, and fed into a cooperative control system whereby the onboard actuators support the user's own power generation throughout the gait cycle. A second control system for users with complete paralysis uses reference trajectories and COG shifts in a manner similar to the other LLE systems (Sankai 2011).

The **Indego** exoskeleton by Parker Hannifin, Cleveland, Ohio (http://indego.com/indego/en/home), evolved from a prototype developed at Vanderbilt University (Farris, Quintero, and Goldfarb 2011; Ha, Murray, and Goldfarb 2016). The Indego is available for sale in the European

Union; it was also the second LLE granted FDA approval for personal use in the United States. The Indego is compatible for use with functional electrical stimulation (FES), whereby additional power is harnessed from the user to cooperatively augment the onboard actuators of the device. The published reports of Indego used in the clinic involved the actuator-only version of the device. However, one study has shown cooperative FES control of the original Vanderbilt device when used by one person with SCI (Ha, Murray, and Goldfarb 2016). The Indego is perhaps the lightest and slimmest of the commercially available exoskeletons, weighing 26 lb (12 kg). The company claims it is compatible with normal wheelchairs use due to its slim design. However, users may find that, to accommodate the exoskeleton, they would have to migrate to a wider wheelchair than the one they would regularly use, as any additional mechanical components at the hips and pelvis would require a larger-than-ideal wheelchair. The Indego is unique in terms of its modularity, as the system breaks down into five pieces: two foot-and-shank components; two thigh sections, each housing two motors; and the pelvis/torso section containing the battery. This modularity supports the claim of the Indego to be easily and independently donned and doffed by the user. Video evidence of this is shown on the company website (http://indego.com/indego/en/Product). While it appears independence is indeed possible, the process is slow for some people; mean times for donning the Indego were reported to be 8.5 minutes (Hartigan et al. 2015). It is encouraging that researchers are addressing the usability of these devices (in this example, the ease of donning and doffing). However, it is feared that time-consuming transitions to actually being able to stand up and walk away from one's wheelchair will limit LLE adoption or contribute to product abandonment. A related factor is portability, which is the ability to transport the device to any desired location. The Indego modularity should be beneficial in this regard. Portability and donning/doffing ease are components of spontaneity of use, one of the AT principles described. It should be emphasized that all manufacturers need to address these issues moving forward to the realization of an LLE as a personal AT product. The Indego is not alone in this regard, and today it is one of the better designs for this aspect of achieving use as an AT for mobility.

Unique among the exoskeletons reviewed here, **Rex** is a self-balancing device (Barbareschi et al. 2015; Tamez-Duque et al. 2015). Rex Bionics, Auckland, New Zealand (http://www.rexbionics.com/), claims that Rex is "completely self-supporting," which enables stability, dynamic balancing, and full hands-free use when standing. When walking, a user's hands are mostly free, only needing to operate an armrest-mounted joystick to direct the walking movement. Thus, controlling Rex is akin to controlling a power wheelchair. Rex allows for standing up or sitting down, walking and turning on level surfaces, and walking up and down stairs. However, there are questions about how well the Rex can be used on stairs: No research has documented stair use, and it has been reported that only specific atypical stair geometries are traversable, with tread depth greater than 30.7 cm (12.1 in.) and tread rise less than 18 cm (7 in.) (Lajeunesse et al. 2015). Significant slopes up to 7° in inclination are also claimed to be walkable. In contrast to the other exoskeletons that are designed to be as light and sleek as possible, Rex is large and heavy, utilizing its inherent bulk and wide footprint (including large footpads), to enable its self-balancing function.

Although no published report is available, Rex is generally thought to be the slowest of the exoskeletons, perhaps due to its mass and self-balancing primary function. This size may also affect the ability to transfer into and out of the device, but no published evidence is available in this regard. Regarding size, it should be noted that while Rex claims to be usable by a wide range of user heights (from 142 to 193 cm), it is limited to a hip width of 38 cm or less; this would be rather limiting for general use by disabled populations and raises concerns about whether larger users could be accommodated in the future.

Unlike the other exoskeletons described previously, Rex uses 10 actuators to power its movement. Although little information on specifications is available, it appears that these actuators power hip extension/flexion, hip abduction/adduction, knee extension/flexion, ankle dorsiflexion/plantar flexion, and ankle eversion/inversion on both legs. The company claims that two hours of walking are possible, while also noting that standing alone does not consume power.

Although not available in the United States for home use at this time, Rex is perhaps the one exoskeleton closest to being classified as an AT device for mobility. The company actually states its personal use is as a "robotic mobility device designed for use at work or home" and that "REX® is designed to allow hands-free standing and walking." It certainly appears to achieve the latter claim through video presentations and demonstrations at trade shows, although no supporting published research was found. There are several testimonials that speak to Rex's ability to enable many activities while standing, such as benchtop work or socializing. One study, after testing REX in an able-bodied subject, summarized the differences between REX's static balancing gait patterns and the dynamic balancing of human walking: "In terms of usage as an assistive technology, the ability to safely support the wearer through the whole cycle, while leaving the upper limbs free for additional tasks, can represent a great advantage" (Barbareschi et al. 2015, 6731). As such, we score the Rex for its stated use with a TRL of 8. It is also interesting to note that the company is endeavoring to position Rex as capable of facilitating "robotic assisted physiotherapy." This is not neurorehabilitation for improving walking (as performed by the other LLEs); rather, it is stand-assisted upper limb exercise. No evidence is available at this time concerning this.

A few research-only systems have been developed and studied for different purposes. The MINA, or X1 Robotic Exoskeleton LLE, was developed with knee and hip actuators similar to the others discussed and has been tested with two subjects with SCI (Neuhaus et al. 2011). Future work includes the development of **compliant control** strategies in hopes of realizing more versatile walking capabilities on different terrains and by users with different residual function. The MINDWALKER was developed to eventually integrate BCI control to exoskeleton walking, as well as to investigate electromyographic (EMG) control and self-balancing capabilities. It uses hip adduction/abduction as well as the common hip and knee flexion/extension actuators. It has been tested with four people with SCI (Sylos-Labini et al. 2014; Wang et al. 2015). The ATLAS LLE was developed by adding hip and knee actuation to an existing torso-hip-knee-ankle-foot orthosis. Designed for children with mobility impairments, it has been validated with a single quadriplegic subject using a walking frame for balance (Garcia, Cestari, and Sanz-Merodio 2014; Sanz-Merodio et al. 2012).

Upper Limb Exoskeletons

A similar approach to identifying LLEs was used to identify ULE systems. We adhered to our definition of ULE for manipulation with potential for use as an AT and included only systems that have been studied during use by people with a disability. A similar search strategy was employed as a recent systematic review (Maciejasz et al. 2014) to compile this list of ULE systems; the notable difference was the necessity for systems to be demonstrated for use with ADLs rather than for rehabilitation. The search revealed only one commercially available ULE, but also found were some research-only systems that were developed around the world. All these required multiple actuated joints to be included, consistent with our exoskeleton definition as a "multi-joint orthosis that uses an external power source to move at least two joints" for use in daily life scenarios. Thus, several systems with only a single actuator were not included; also not included were systems incorporating an upper limb orthosis with movements initiated by FES alone rather than incorporating external actuators. Several systems with demonstrated use only by able-bodied study participants were also not included. Table 6.3 lists specific details of each system. Maciejasz et al. (2014) included a list of systems that did not meet our criteria for inclusion here.

The **MyoPro Motion-G**, a portable elbow-wrist-hand orthosis, was recently launched by the medical device company Myomo, Incorporated, of Cambridge, Massachusetts (http://www.myomo.com/). The MyoPro Motion-G is the third generation of a previously developed arm (elbow) orthosis called Myomo e100 (Stein 2009). Myomo e100 was developed and FDA approved in 2007 as a class II medical device, with class II devices subject to special controls with a higher level of assurance of user safety than class I devices. The MyoPro Motion-G (Table 6.2) provides flexion/extension actuation at the elbow joint and grasping capabilities to perform ADL, including feeding, reaching, and lifting. User intention is detected by the use of EMG signals recorded from biceps, triceps, forearm flexor, and forearm extensor muscle group activations. Because the device uses residual muscle activity, it cannot be used by those with complete paralysis. For any individual user, the level of assistance provided by the orthosis is set based on the user's individual muscle signals as measured by a certified orthotist. Several training sessions are necessary to acquire a base level of proficiency. The target population for this orthosis is people with upper limb disorders, including neuromuscular conditions such as BPI, traumatic brain injury, SCI, MS, ALS, and stroke. The company claims that the MyoPro Motion-G can improve a person's independence in performing ADLs and also emphasizes that, unlike most of the LLEs, this device is not intended as a rehabilitation device. Rather, its objective design use is as an AT (Figure 6.2).

MUNDUS (Multimodal Neuroprosthesis for Daily Upper limb Support) was a focused ULE research project that ended in 2013 and was funded by the European Commission. MUNDUS was developed as an AT research platform to perform reaching and grasping of objects and positioning the arm in space (Pedrocchi et al. 2013). The exoskeleton is a lightweight, antigravity orthosis that provides 2 degrees of freedom (DOF) at the shoulder joint (shoulder elevation in the sagittal plane and shoulder rotation in the horizontal elevation plane) and 1 DOF at the elbow joint. If there is no residual hand function, an actuated hand orthosis is included. Electromagnetic brakes are implemented in the mechanical design of the exoskeleton to provide weight support during use. Neuromuscular electrical stimulation (NMES) is applied to the upper arm muscles to control the motion of the upper extremity; thus, it is debatable whether this

TABLE 6.3   ULE Device Characteristics and Technology Readiness Level Score

Device Name	Joint Type	Supported Movements	Target Users	Type of Control	Commercially Available	TRL
MyoPro® Motion-G	Elbow flexion/extension Hand grasping function	Reaching Grasping	Brachial plexus injury Traumatic brain injury SCI, ALS, stroke Multiple sclerosis	Intention detection through residual EMG activity	Yes	8
MUNDUS	Shoulder elevation/rotation Elbow flexion/extension Actuated hand grasp (optional)	Reaching Grasping	SCI, ALS Friedreich ataxia Multiple sclerosis	Joystick control by opposite hand	No	6
WOTAS	Elbow flexion/extension Forearm pronation/supination Wrist flexion/extension	Tremor suppression	Any neurological disorders that cause tremor	Real-time tremor suppression algorithm	No	6

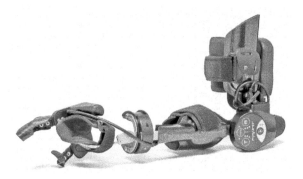

Figure 6.2 The MyoPro® Motion-G upper limb exoskeleton, intended for use as an assistive technology. (Photograph courtesy of Myomo, Incorporated.)

device should be included in this chapter because only the hand module has externally actuated control (i.e., a single joint of external actuation and another 2 DOF controlled by NMES).

According to the severity of the impairment, three different control strategies were implemented in the first MUNDUS prototype. The first mode used EMG sensors and residual activation of the user's muscles to execute a certain task. The second mode was designed for those with lack of arm and hand muscle activity and detects user intention with an eye-tracking system. In the ultimate progression of some diseases, the user may have no gaze control; in this case, the third control mode utilizes an EEG-based BCI. Functionality of the device is restricted to a set of pre-defined tasks when the second or third control strategy is deployed. The MUNDUS system was a research prototype, but was stated to be currently under commercial development (Pedrocchi et al. 2013).

WOTAS (Wearable Orthosis for Tremor Assessment and Suppression) is a portable, powered ULE that aims to suppress tremors. Three DOF are considered in the mechanical structure of the device, corresponding to elbow flexion/extension, forearm pronation/supination, and wrist flexion/extension. Both kinematic and kinetic sensors are used to measure the state of the joint angles, angular velocities, as well as interaction forces between limb and orthosis. Signals are then used to develop a control strategy to be delivered to the onboard motors. This results in the application of an equal and opposite force that cancels out tremulous movement (Rocon et al. 2007).

A brief introduction of other ULE devices that were designed and tested, but did not meet our inclusion criteria with published testing results when used by a person with a disability, follows. MULOS

(Motorized Upper-Limb Orthotic System) is a 5-DOF, electrically powered, wheelchair-mounted device (Johnson et al. 2001). The design provides 3 DOF at the shoulder, 1 DOF at the elbow, and 1 DOF at the forearm to perform pronation/supination. The device can be directly worn by the user and is controlled by a 5-DOF joystick that is operated by the intact side of the user's body. The target population for the use of this device is considered to be the elderly and people in general with upper limb disabilities.

The upper limb–type HAL (HAL-UL) is a wearable robotic suit that provides meal assistance, developed by the same Japanese group who developed the LLE HAL. The design has 3 DOF in the shoulder joint, 1 DOF in the elbow joint, and 3 DOF in the wrist joint. Although the mechanical structure of the system seems to have the potential to provide different manipulation tasks, the only published study regarding the use of this exoskeleton suit addressed performing a meal assistance task (Kawamoto et al. 2011).

The 7 degrees of freedom upper limb motion assist exoskeleton robot (SUEFUL-7) is an upper limb exoskeleton robot that is controlled by residual EMG signals. The SUEFUL-7 assists the motions of shoulder vertical and horizontal flexion/extension, shoulder internal/external rotation, elbow flexion/extension, forearm supination/pronation, wrist flexion/extension, and wrist radial/ulnar deviation. Several kinematic and kinetic sensors are used to evaluate the real-time postural configuration of the user as well as forces and torques that are generated between the arm and the orthosis. An experimental study showed that the EMG levels were reduced when the device was used, thus indicating that the device provided external assistance during movements (Gopura, Kiguchi, and Yi 2009).

Critical Review of the Available Utilization Protocols: How Can Exoskeletons Be Used?

As stated throughout this chapter, exoskeletons designed for people with disabilities are currently used for rehabilitation and health purposes only and typically only used in clinical settings. However, we review the target populations for the existing devices, their requirements for use, and exclusion criteria that may limit their use by specific people. We also look forward and address exoskeleton use as AT devices, discussing how exoskeletons may be used and which applications and functional tasks may be possible.

Lower Limb Exoskeletons

Most LLE exoskeleton companies list persons with a SCI as their target population for use. The identified populations for each technology are listed in Table 6.1. Of the LLEs, the FDA-approved systems are only intended for use by users with paraplegia and only specific levels of SCI at that: "ReWalk is for people with paraplegia due to spinal cord injuries at levels T7 (seventh thoracic vertebra) to L5 (fifth lumbar vertebra) when accompanied by a specially trained caregiver. It is also for people with spinal cord injuries at levels T4 (fourth thoracic vertebra) to T6 (sixth thoracic vertebra) where the device is limited to use in rehabilitation institutions" (U.S. Food and Drug Administration 2014, fifth paragraph). Persons with other levels of injury, including incomplete tetraplegia with significant remaining arm function, are also using LLEs in clinical and research studies. Uniquely, the Rex LLE can be used by persons with SCI up to C4/5, similar to those who can use a joystick-driven power wheelchair. SCI is the largest documented etiology of mobility impairment studied during LLE use, as well described in the Federici et al. 2015 review.

Individuals with stroke make up the second-most-targeted disease population for LLE studies (Federici et al. 2015). In particular, the variable assist feature in the Ekso GT, and similar control methods, are claimed useful for stroke rehabilitation, as well as for incomplete SCI. In the broadest sense, Ekso claims that any person with paralysis or hemiparesis due to neurological disease or injury may be appropriate for use of the Ekso GT. This statement mirrors the literature as well, as after SCI and stroke, "gait disorders of unspecified etiology" were the only other category of disability identified by Federici et al. (2015). In terms of potential use as an AT, and ignoring the technical limitations of current exoskeletons, it is reasonable to assume that any mobility-impaired population currently part of investigational studies would be an appropriate candidate for using exoskeletons as AT mobility devices.

Regardless of the target population for exoskeleton use, there are several general inclusion and exclusion criteria for use of LLEs. Federici et al. (2015) provided some information about these criteria, with more found on inspection of companies' websites. Users must be medically cleared by a physician, with consideration of bone density, contractures, spasticity, orthostatic hypotension, cognitive function, and arm function sufficient for walker or crutch use.

Exoskeleton technologies can be controlled in several different ways. Yan et al. (2015), in an in-depth review about control strategies of broadly defined LLEs, characterized seven different strategies. For our purposes, only two strategies are employed by the devices reviewed here: predefined joint trajectories and cooperative or model-based control. The predefined joint trajectory strategy incorporates well-known patterns of healthy gait, scaled appropriately to a user's size and the desired gait parameters (e.g., walking speed and stride length). This strategy is common, forming the basis of at least one mode of control on all identified LLEs described previously. It is appropriate for users with complete paralysis and thus dependent on full assistance from the exoskeleton.

The cooperative or model-based control strategy uses an integrated human-device model and typically combines joint trajectory control with a human-based control signal, which is a signal somehow derived from or applied to the user directly. The Indego LLE combines actuator-controlled joint trajectories with an FES controller to effect cooperative control of external and human power (Ha, Murray, and Goldfarb 2016). The HAL LLE has been demonstrated with cooperative control using residual EMG signals of the user (Cruciger et al. 2014). The Ekso GT LLE has its variable-assist operation modes, whereby in "Adaptive Assist" mode the users' own muscle activity participates in the joint trajectory control strategy, with the external actuators compensating as needed.

What are the limitations currently on use of exoskeletons in the community? Most LLEs are not approved for use in the United States (with the exception of ReWalk and very recently Indego in March 2016), but most do have approval in Europe for use at home. In these cases, the described operation modes of the previous sections apply. For LLEs in the United States, it is interesting to note that the FDA classified these as class II medical devices and placed "special controls" on the use of the device. This not only includes their use only with a companion, but also specifies the training necessary for the user and companion and restricted environments of use (e.g., small slopes and no stairs).

Adapting (Cowan et al. 2012), we can consider a reduced scope of mobility-based functions when considering new technologies, including postural control; balance; transfers (or donning and doffing the exoskeleton); walking on level ground and turning; stair climbing; walking on slopes (both up and down and across slopes) and uneven terrain; transitions between sitting, standing, and walking; and using transportation. Little information about any of these functions, besides basic walking distance and speed, is provided in the literature.

Bryce, Dijkers, and Kozlowski (2015) have recently presented a framework for assessing LLE usability. This was not done solely with AT use in mind; rather, it considered a wide array of uses for LLEs, including early and late rehabilitation, exercise, and as a wheelchair replacement. The proposed framework documented six components to consider when assessing LLE use: functional applications, personal factors, device factors, external factors, activities, and health outcomes (Bryce, Dijkers, and Kozlowski 2015). This framework may prove useful when considering future LLE use for mobility, both at home and in the community. Measuring and documenting exoskeleton features and predicted functional impact may guide device prescription, as well as provide insight to guide future device development.

Depending on the environment of use and activities performed, there would be different requirements to allow an LLE exoskeleton to function effectively as an AT. Some of these are summarized here. Because many activities require the use of the upper extremities (e.g., cleaning, cooking, shopping), it would be important to be able to have the users' hands free while standing for short periods of time. Battery life and charging would also be important considerations. Most users would likely require a minimum battery life to make donning and doffing the device worthwhile. Potentially, inductive charging pads might be one option so that the device would not need to be plugged in for charging. Currently, many devices have restrictions about the minimum seat dimensions and height from which they can rise. If used in a specific setting, chairs that met these criteria could be used. If used in other settings, then a way to appraise the appropriateness of different seating surfaces or more flexibility in types of seating that can be used would be beneficial. Ease of doffing and donning is also an important consideration, especially in terms of toileting and dressing. Currently, level changes (e.g., curbs, slopes, and stairs) are challenging with most devices. This is an area for development. For outdoor mobility, walking speed would need to be sufficient for street crossing within timed light cycles. In the future, it may be possible to design exoskeletons to enable people to perform complex lower limb activities, such as car driving (including transfers in and out and use of pedals) or sports. Finally, safety is perhaps the most significant requirement moving forward, a topic more fully addressed in the section on future directions.

Upper Limb Exoskeletons

An effective ULE for AT able to perform all of the functions of the upper limb of someone who is able-bodied requires considerable development, especially given that each upper extremity has 30 DOF (7 from the shoulder to the wrist and 23 for the hand), whereas each lower extremity only has 12 DOF (Apkarian, Naumann, and Cairns 1989). This may account for only one ULE currently commercially available for use as AT. During future development of ULEs, it is likely that the DOF provided will be curtailed initially, and the devices will only be suitable for performing a limited number of tasks in fairly controlled environments. Also, many ADLs can be performed effectively using a reduced number of DOF (e.g., only using two fingers). As with AT exoskeletons for the lower extremity, it will be important to consider a variety of factors, including control function, safety, comfort, cost, ease of use (including donning and doffing), and portability or capability of being mounted on a wheelchair.

There are several important challenges with ULEs. First, conditions like SCI and some neurodegenerative diseases have a distal-to-proximal presentation; that is, impairments first affect distal functions such as grasp, while higher or more severe injuries also affect proximal functions such as shoulder movements. Unfortunately, although movements of the hand are smaller and require less force, they are also far more complex, which would require very refined control strategies. Second, although there are fewer DOF from the shoulder to the wrist, having full range of the shoulder would likely require a bulky and unaesthetic design. Third, the market for ULEs may likely be smaller than the market for LLEs because problems such as stroke typically only affect one extremity, and many people are able to compensate using the other extremity to perform upper limb tasks. Nevertheless, given the body of research that has been conducted in the area of ULEs for rehabilitation and the existing gap between commercially available ATs and actual need for devices in the community, it seems only a matter of time before more devices become available commercially.

Review of User Studies, Outcomes, and Clinical Evidence

Lower Limb Exoskeletons

A recent systematic review of the evidence for rehabilitation outcomes, especially neurorehabilitation benefits, due to exoskeleton use was written by Federici and colleagues (2015). It concluded that rehabilitation using LLEs has been effective in improving gait function and is safe during supervised use. However, they concluded that this evidence is limited due to little, if any, comparisons between exoskeleton rehabilitation and traditional therapy.

Some LLE research related to mobility functions, such as gait speed, has been performed. A recent systematic review of 15 studies documented the gait speed of people using powered robotic exoskeletons after SCI (Louie et al. 2015). The mean gait speed attained by nonambulatory participants with SCI (n = 84) while wearing an LLE was 0.26 m/s. This modest speed was positively correlated with older participants, lower levels of injury, and number of training sessions. Age of subjects was thought to exert its effects due to older people presenting with less-traumatic SCI and thus retaining greater motor function. This speed is far below one reported mean speed in able-bodied community ambulators of 1.32 m/s and below the minimum necessary speed of 0.49 m/s to safely cross streets (Andrews et al. 2010). In summary, individuals with more residual function and training time in the LLE walked faster, although rarely at speeds necessary for community ambulation.

The evidence of an expanded list of mobility outcomes and putative use of exoskeletons as AT was recently reviewed by Lajeunesse and colleagues (2015). They presented the evidence from seven papers, including outcomes of walking speed, distance, and duration (10-m walk test and 6-minute walk test). Some studies also reported the timed duration of sit to stand as an outcome. Their final conclusion was that "the applicability and effectiveness of lower limb exoskeletons as assistive devices in the community have not been demonstrated" (Lajeunesse et al. 2015, 1).

A review by Arazpour and colleagues (2016) included a large number of other less-sophisticated ankle-knee-hip orthoses that incorporate actuation of a single joint. Many of the systems considered in this review share functional similarities with the exoskeletons described previously. Arazpour and colleagues also compared those orthoses to the full LLEs described in this chapter. Their findings support others that LLEs can improve walking ability after SCI. However, they also found poor evidence for LLE usefulness in providing gait *function* for persons with paraplegia, concluding that, "These types of orthosis, even the hybrid one with reciprocating and FES, are not enough to provide a functional, efficient gait for the paraplegic patient" (Arazpour et al. 2016, 9). This evidence certainly does not support their more general use as an AT for mobility.

Although many studies confound the definitions of mobility device, AT, and restoration of walking function, two studies involving LLEs have reported outcomes associated with LLE use as an AT. The first studied seven participants using the ReWalk and measured their ability to do different tasks that may be appropriate at home and in the community (Spungen et al. 2013). All subjects were able to transfer into and out of the device and independently manage the chest, thigh, and calf straps. Six needed assistance to put their feet into shoes. Five of seven were able to use the wrist-worn controller to input operation modes. Only four subjects were able to retrieve an object from a shelf above their head while standing in the device. Regarding secondary mobility skills, five subjects could stop walking on command or operate an automatic push-button door. Four of seven could use a wall to support themselves for resting or use an elevator independently. Only three subjects could walk without assistance on concrete or uneven ground or use a revolving door. And only two could walk on carpet or a slight slope. No subjects could navigate a curb without assistance. The second study reported on another AT outcome during use of the Indego LLE: the time taken to don and doff the device. The mean times for donning and doffing the Indego by 16 subjects with SCI were reported to be 8.5 minutes and 4.0 minutes, respectively (Hartigan et al. 2015). No comparative data for other LLEs were included in this study.

The physical effort required by people to use a LLE for walking has been studied recently (Asselin et al. 2015; Evans et al. 2015; Kressler et al. 2014). This work has two different implications. The first is whether it is physically difficult to use an exoskeleton, thus potentially limiting its applicability as a mobility device for daily use. If a person becomes physically exhausted simply undertaking basic mobility needs, then mobility, participation, and quality of life will surely suffer. The second is less important to LLE use as an AT: whether a user can actually receive cardiovascular exercise benefits from walking with LLE assistance. This is of interest to researchers due to the profound increase of cardiovascular disease risk seen in people with SCI (Cragg et al. 2013) and the difficulty for this population to access appropriate and regular cardiovascular exercise. It may be that passive leg movements, with appropriate upper limb exercise, may improve cardiovascular exercise outcomes over conventional arm-only exercise modalities (West et al. 2015). One study of five people with SCI found that walking in the Indego LLE resulted in an acute cardiorespiratory outcome response akin to moderate intensity exercise, and that metabolic responses increased with speed of walking (Evans et al. 2015). This study indicated that LLE use may benefit cardiovascular fitness depending on how it is used. A ReWalk study about SCI similarly found potential for improved fitness with use (Asselin et al. 2015). Conversely, a study about the Ekso GT LLE and SCI found that its use resulted in exercise effects that were small or nonexistent (Kressler et al. 2014); that is, LLE use did not impose unwieldy physical demands during use. This contrast may have been due to different study parameters, as in this last study participants walked slowly for about an hour with many rest breaks; in the former studies, participants walked at self-selected speeds for 2 to 6 minutes at a time. Taken together, it may be possible to adjust the metabolic demand of using an LLE depending on its motivation for use and style of walking: lower demand for AT-like activities and higher demand for exercise benefits.

Some research has documented the time and effort required to *learn to use* an exoskeleton, that is, the training period necessary for use proficiency. This is somewhat difficult to compare, as training time will be affected by many factors, including trainer proficiency, user skill and learning capacity, user function (i.e., level of injury), device characteristics, manufacturer protocols, training goal, level of supervision required, and institutional or study constraints. Nevertheless, it has been reported that users took an average of 5–15 sessions to walk independently (i.e., with no assistance but with "close" supervision) on level ground and 15–25 sessions to ascend stairs in the ReWalk (Spungen et al. 2013) and 8–28 sessions to walk on level ground in the Ekso GT (Kozlowski, Bryce, and Dijkers 2015) with similar levels of supervision. The proficiency of Indego LLE use after only five training sessions was also recently studied (Hartigan et al. 2015). Sixteen subjects with SCI (injury levels ranging from T12, American Spinal Injury Association Impairment Scale [AIS] A to C5, AIS B) obtained a mean walking speed of 0.34 m/s. Of the 16 subjects, during the fifth day of training, two (both tetraplegic) required moderate assistance by a therapist, six required minimal assistance, and eight required only close supervision for safety reasons.

If we consider the potential secondary health outcomes that may result from exoskeleton use, several more studies are found. These are summarized here due to the difference between these outcomes and the more typical neuromuscular rehabilitation outcomes. It is also likely that changes in secondary health outcomes would occur if LLEs were used truly as AT devices at home and in the community. Using the Ekso GT for six weeks, Kressler et al. (2014) found a reduction in pain severity in three subjects with complete SCI. Cruciger et al. (2014) found similar pain benefits with two subjects using the HAL for Medical Use (Lower Limb Type), as well as improvements in a quality-of-life outcome measure. The ReWalk was studied with a variety of self-report outcome measures in 11 subjects with SCI following each LLE walking session: Pain reduction was consistently reported by five subjects; three reported decreased spasticity; and five subjects reported improvements in bowel routines (Esquenazi et al. 2012). Note that all these studies were anecdotal and should only be considered as feasibility experiments at this time as none had adequate sample size or controls to be considered strong evidence of any health benefits that may arise due to LLE use.

An online survey of therapists regarding potential LLE end uses was conducted to ascertain the therapists' perceptions about the reasons for using LLE technology as well as the perceived importance of a variety of device characteristics and functions (Wolff et al. 2014). Secondary health benefits and rehabilitation purposes were the highest-ranked reasons for use. Social uses and daily mobility tasks, both associated with AT functionality, were ranked lower. Seventeen LLE design features were scored on a Likert scale from 1 to 5 for their perceived importance. Four features had the highest median rank of 5 or "very important": minimization of falls risk, comfort, donning and doffing the device, and purchase cost. The two lowest scores of median 3 or "neither important nor unimportant" were appearance/aesthetics and length of training time needed for proficiency. When analyzing the data by considering the percentage of participants ranking each feature as important (either 4 or 5, i.e., "important" or "very important"), most features were deemed important by the vast majority of participants. Of note, the four lowest-scored features (i.e., ranked important by less than 65% of end users) were appearance/aesthetics, length of training time needed for proficiency, walking speed, and ability to use without arm supports (i.e., self-balancing capabilities). A qualitative analysis of open-ended questions about further reasons to use an exoskeleton was also performed. The three themes with the highest percentage of participants citing them were psychosocial benefits, which included items such as roles and relationships, psychological, quality of life, independence, and eye-level social interaction; health and physical benefits, which included items such as pressure management, pain management, walking, standing, exercise, and transfers; and uses in daily life, which included items such as leisure, employment, functional day-to-day tasks, access, and outdoor use. This type of user-directed input may prove useful for developers when considering where to direct research efforts into future LLE designs.

In summary, the research to date indicates that LLEs can be safely used under supervision to effect basic walking function, particularly by people with SCI. However, the evidence also shows that LLEs are not yet capable of being used as AT in the community. Finally, it is possible that a host of secondary health complications may be improved with LLE use by people with SCI, although more research is needed to confirm this.

Upper Limb Exoskeletons

Relatively little research has been done regarding ULE studies with people with disabilities when using the devices as AT for manipulation, reflective of the very few systems described in the previous sections.

The only commercially available device, the myoelectrically controlled MyoPro, has seen some study, although little work has been published on the current design or specifically about AT activities, compared to evidence for rehabilitation purposes, such as increasing range of elbow motion. An experiment conducted on stroke survivors indicated that the earlier Myomo e100 could be successfully controlled (Stein et al. 2007), although this was a single-joint (elbow) powered orthosis only and did not have any AT-related outcome measures. The design and functionality of the more current MyoPro Motion-G originated from a single DOF grasping hand orthosis that was tested many years ago by C6 level SCI subjects and one with a BPI (Benjuya and Kenney 1990). Little current peer-reviewed research is available, although the company states that functional task studies, including home use, with the latest commercial design are under way.

The MUNDUS ULE was evaluated with five potential end users (three with SCI and two with MS) (Pedrocchi et al. 2013). The level of device assistance provided, as well as the control mode, was adapted for each subject. One subject used the full exoskeleton system, including the robotic hand module; the other four subjects only tested various forms of NMES control of the passive orthosis. Subjects performed two tasks, each of which was scored by expert evaluators: a drinking task and a general reaching task. The user's intention was detected with 100% success. The functionality of all modules was claimed to be successfully demonstrated. Donning time ranged from 6 to 65 minutes. The authors concluded that the MUNDUS platform can provide functional assistance to daily life activities, although it is clear that much more work is needed to validate this claim, especially as it pertains to the full ULE configuration, including the hand module with external actuators.

The WOTAS ULE for tremor suppression and manipulation assistance has been tested on 10 users with different pathologies, including different levels of essential tremor (ET), MS, post-traumatic tremor, and mixed tremor (Rocon et al. 2007). The device was tested during three tasks: to keep the arm outstretched, to point at the nose with a finger, and to keep the arm in a rest position. The results showed an overall 40% reduction in tremor power for all users, and that voluntary motion was not hindered.

The authors also mentioned that users anecdotally reported that the device would not be considered as a solution to their problem due to its bulk and weight, while also expressing their wish for the system to be slim enough to be worn under clothing. Finally, subjects were concerned that use of the device in its current form may cause social exclusion (see discussion of **stigma** in Chapter 10).

In summary, little research has been published about ULE use as an AT. Only one system is available for purchase. ULEs for use as AT appear to be an understudied area of research.

Future Directions

It is clear from the literature and anecdotal reports from users and therapists that exoskeletons are not yet effective AT devices for either mobility or manipulation. This is especially true for LLE mobility devices, which would essentially be replacing a wheelchair for some or all of one's daily mobility needs and activities. Of course, an LLE could be used in conjunction with a conventional daily use wheelchair, much like one would use a sports-specific wheelchair a few times per week. The issue becomes one of cost and usability then, although it is possible to foresee a large decrease in unit cost with these technologies given the innovations occurring in robotics and other mechatronic consumer products. Unfortunately, though, cost will always be an important factor and has been acknowledged by many, including the authors of the usability framework paper (Bryce, Dijkers, and Kozlowski 2015) and a survey of stakeholder perceptions on LLE technology (Wolff et al. 2014).

Regarding usability, it is known that many factors contribute to device abandonment (Biddiss and Chau 2007; Cowan et al. 2012; Kittel, Di, and Stewart 2002). Although walking speed was ranked as somewhat less important than other LLE design features (Wolff et al. 2014), when one is relying on the device for daily mobility needs, speed will surely affect how frequently the device is used. Donning, doffing and portability will also be considerations. Taken together, these issues support a concept under development that integrates an LLE with a wheelchair (Borisoff, Mattie, and Rafer 2013). In this design concept, a releasable LLE is attached to a wheelchair frame to create a device with the following features: (1) seating analogous to existing wheelchairs (i.e., that are easy to transfer into and capable of all-day use); (2) equivalent wheelchair mobility speeds; (3) a full range of adjustable seating positions, including recline, elevated seating, and standing; and (4) a detachable LLE for walking sojourns and rehabilitation. Such a concept attempts to merge the best features of an LLE with the effectiveness of wheeled mobility to create a mobility device that could provide benefits throughout the entire day of a wheelchair user.

Another concept merging powered orthoses with wheels is the ABLE project, described as a "biped-type leg-wheeled robot system" (Mori et al. 2011). With the ABLE prototype, a user is supported through sit to stand and passive standing with the powered orthosis. The feet of the orthosis are attached to small wheeled platforms that enable rolling mobility somewhat akin to a power standing wheelchair. Although walking function is not supported, the device can enable stair climbing by locking the wheeled platforms and using the powered orthosis to perform stepping up or down stairs. Perhaps other concepts that merge orthoses and wheels for improved mobility outcomes will emerge in the future.

Other types of powered orthoses have been developed, but did not meet the strict inclusion criteria we laid forth in the beginning of this chapter. These criteria may have to be revisited in future treatments of this topic, as developers continue to add actuation and sensors to more conventional passive orthoses. Exoskeletons are also evolving to be lighter, slimmer, less battery dependent, and more similar to conventional orthoses. Some LLE development is also under way exploring lower DOFs. One example, the Phoenix, is a design from the SuitX Company (http://www.suitx .com/phoenix). Phoenix was developed in part by Kazerooni, the original developer of the system that became the Ekso GT exoskeleton. Phoenix does not use a full knee actuator; rather, it uses only a brake for maintaining upright standing during the stance phase of gait. They claim this results in a lighter, more battery-efficient and cheaper exoskeleton; however, no studies have been published.

Some more advanced technology research experiments have been performed about direct brain control of exoskeletons (Kwak, Muller, and Lee 2015; Wang et al. 2015). Although any practical applications of BCI and exoskeletons must be considered far off at the moment, there is ample impetus to evolve control strategies to make exoskeleton use easy and more natural. One example is the HAL ULE, only tested on healthy subjects, which uses a vision system to track intentional positioning and grasp control for eating assistance (Kawamoto et al. 2011).

Finally, it is imperative to mention the elephant in the room when it comes to true LLE use as an AT device for daily mobility: *safety*. Although there are several studies documenting completely safe use of LLEs during research use, it must be pointed out that all LLE walking is performed with a trained therapist attending close behind the user to arrest any falls that may otherwise occur. Nevertheless, there are several anecdotal reports of falls, which may or may not have been mitigated by the attendant, as well as stories of attendant injuries due to the effort required to help arrest a person falling while wearing an LLE. Research is needed for fall prevention, mitigation, and recovery. Regarding fall mitigation, it is most important to protect the user's head. A possible method may be to detect a fall and have the LLE enter a mitigation program to utilize the onboard sensors and actuators to position the user to minimize any head impact. Unfortunately, a likely scenario, at least in backward falling, would be to invoke hip flexion and aim for the buttocks to take the brunt of the fall similarly to bipedal robots and normal human falling. This would be counterproductive due to the fragility of a user's pelvis, with the users most likely being people with SCI. Protecting the skin integrity of the buttocks is one of the most important requirements in wheelchair seating prescription. Obviously, a design strategy would have to take this protective requirement into account. As LLE designs begin to enter home and community use, people will use them in ways not intended by manufacturers or regulatory bodies. It is easy to envision that people will use them independently without an attendant, as well as use them in environments not fully vetted, such as stairs and rougher terrain. Falls will occur. It is beneficial to all stakeholders interested in LLEs to acknowledge this and begin to study methods to mitigate the effects.

Although far less research and development activity appears to be occurring around ULEs, the path to market for ULE use as AT in the community seems far less daunting. Safety, in particular, appears to be much less of an issue, with one example of a potential adverse event being injury from spilling hot coffee. Demonstrations of effective use of commercially available ULEs for ADLs and other activities in the community are needed to support their widespread adoption. Do these devices truly improve daily activities or are common compensatory strategies preferred long term? Of course, this question might be affected by the ease of donning and doffing the devices, either independently or with help of a caregiver. Improvements here would surely improve ULE use. Aesthetics of ULEs may be a greater concern than for LLEs, perhaps due to the more intimate and personal nature of upper limb tasks compared to locomotion.

Several of the ULEs described used electrically stimulated muscle function rather than external actuators; thus, systems for use by those with fully paralyzed upper limbs remains understudied, unfortunately neglecting a potential user population most in need of the purported function. The major outstanding issue for ULEs for completely paralyzed hands and arms may be the control method. LLEs can be controlled by the users' hands or upper body movements to direct walking intention (e.g., leaning forward). Effective control of ULEs, at least in the most extreme examples of impairments, remains elusive. Perhaps BCI progress is needed before these devices are truly effective and transformative for a broad population of people with upper limb disabilities.

STUDY QUESTIONS

1. What characteristics distinguish the use of exoskeletons as an AT from their use as therapeutic equipment?
2. What six principles, described by WHO, comprise a set of performance criteria for any particular technology when it is implemented as an AT for mobility or manipulation?
3. Which LLE has the highest TRL for its use as an AT?
4. What specific feature is responsible for this score and distinguishes it from the other LLEs?
5. Which is the only ULE commercially available for use as an AT for manipulation?
6. What level of scientific evidence exists to support ULE use as AT for manipulation?
7. Which disability group is the most prevalent potential target population for use of LLEs?
8. Name two disabilities prevalent in potential target populations who may benefit from use of an ULE.
9. What factors currently limit LLEs for use in the community?
10. What are some applications or uses of ULEs for manipulation?
11. To simulate human extremities, how many DOF would a ULE require as compared to a LLE?
12. What environments are suitable for LLE use as a mobility device, both currently and in the future?

References

Andrews, A. W., S. A. Chinworth, M. Bourassa, M. Garvin, D. Benton, and S. Tanner. 2010. "Update on Distance and Velocity Requirements for Community Ambulation." *Journal of Geriatric Physical Therapy* 33 (3): 128–134.

Apkarian, J., S. Naumann, and B. Cairns. 1989. "A Three-Dimensional Kinematic and Dynamic Model of the Lower Limb." *Journal of Biomechanics* 22 (2): 143–155.

Arazpour, M., M. Samadian, K. Ebrahimzadeh, M. Ahmadi Bani, and S. W. Hutchins. 2016. "The Influence of Orthosis Options on Walking Parameters in Spinal Cord-Injured Patients: A Literature Review." *Spinal Cord* 54 (6): 412–422.

Asselin, P., S. Knezevic, S. Kornfeld, C. Cirnigliaro, I. Agranova-Breyter, W. A. Bauman, and A. M. Spungen. 2015. "Heart Rate and Oxygen Demand of Powered Exoskeleton-Assisted Walking in Persons with Paraplegia." *Journal of Rehabilitation Research and Development* 52 (2): 147–158.

Barbareschi, G., R. Richards, M. Thornton, T. Carlson, and C. Holloway. 2015. "Statically versus Dynamically Balanced Gait: Analysis of a Robotic Exoskeleton Compared with a Human." *Conference Proceedings: Annual International Conference of the IEEE Engineering in Medicine and Biology Society* August 25–29: 6728–6731.

Benjuya, N., and S. B. Kenney. 1990. "Myoelectric Hand Orthosis." *Journal of Prosthetics and Orthotics* 2 (2): 149–154.

Benson, I., K. Hart, D. Tussler, and J. J. van Middendorp. 2015. "Lower-Limb Exoskeletons for Individuals with Chronic Spinal Cord Injury: Findings from a Feasibility Study." *Clinical Rehabilitation* 30 (1): 73–84.

Biddiss, E., and T. Chau. 2007. "Upper-Limb Prosthetics: Critical Factors in Device Abandonment." *American Journal of Physical Medicine & Rehabilitation* 86 (12): 977–987.

Borisoff, J. F., S. G. Mason, and G. E. Birch. 2006. "Brain Interface Research for Asynchronous Control Applications." *IEEE Transactions on Neural Systems and Rehabilitation Engineering* 14 (2): 160–164.

Borisoff, J. F., J. Mattie, and V. Rafer. 2013. "Concept Proposal for a Detachable Exoskeleton-Wheelchair to Improve Mobility and Health." *Conference Proceedings: IEEE International Conference on Rehabilitation Robotics.* doi:10.1109/ICORR.2013.6650396.

Brault, M. 2010. *Americans with Disabilities.* Washington, DC: U.S. Census Bureau.

Bryce, T. N., M. P. Dijkers, and A. J. Kozlowski. 2015. "Framework for Assessment of the Usability of Lower-Extremity Robotic Exoskeletal Orthoses." *American Journal of Physical Medicine & Rehabilitation* 94 (11): 1000–1014.

Cook, A. M., and J. M. Polgar. 2015. *Cook and Hussey's Assistive Technologies: Principles and Practice.* 4th ed. St. Louis, MO: Mosby.

Courtney-Long, E. A., D. D. Carroll, Q. C. Zhang, A. C. Stevens, S. Griffin-Blake, B. S. Armour, and V. A. Campbell. 2015. "Prevalence of Disability and Disability Type among Adults—United States, 2013." *MMWR. Morbidity and Mortality Weekly Report* 64 (29): 777–783.

Cowan, R. E., B. J. Fregly, M. L. Boninger, L. Chan, M. M. Rodgers, and D. J. Reinkensmeyer. 2012. "Recent Trends in Assistive Technology for Mobility." *Journal of Neuroengineering and Rehabilitation* 9: 20.

Cragg, J. J., V. K. Noonan, A. Krassioukov, and J. Borisoff. 2013. "Cardiovascular Disease and Spinal Cord Injury: Results from a National Population Health Survey." *Neurology* 81 (8): 723–728.

Cruciger, O., T. A. Schildhauer, R. C. Meindl, M. Tegenthoff, P. Schwenkreis, M. Citak, and M. Aach. 2014. "Impact of Locomotion Training with a Neurologic Controlled Hybrid Assistive Limb (HAL) Exoskeleton on

Neuropathic Pain and Health Related Quality of Life (HRQoL) in Chronic SCI: A Case Study." *Disability and Rehabilitation. Assistive Technology* 10: 1–6.

Esquenazi, A., M. Talaty, A. Packel, and M. Saulino. 2012. "The ReWalk Powered Exoskeleton to Restore Ambulatory Function to Individuals with Thoracic-Level Motor-Complete Spinal Cord Injury." *American Journal of Physical Medicine & Rehabilitation* 91 (11): 911–921.

Evans, N., C. Hartigan, C. Kandilakis, E. Pharo, and I. Clesson. 2015. "Acute Cardiorespiratory and Metabolic Responses during Exoskeleton-Assisted Walking Overground among Persons with Chronic Spinal Cord Injury." *Topics in Spinal Cord Injury Rehabilitation* 21 (2): 122–132.

Farris, R. J., H. A. Quintero, and M. Goldfarb. 2011. "Preliminary Evaluation of a Powered Lower Limb Orthosis to Aid Walking in Paraplegic Individuals." *IEEE Transactions on Neural Systems and Rehabilitation Engineering* 19 (6): 652–659.

Federici, S., F. Meloni, M. Bracalenti, and M. L. De Filippis. 2015. "The Effectiveness of Powered, Active Lower Limb Exoskeletons in Neurorehabilitation: A Systematic Review." *NeuroRehabilitation* 37 (3): 321–340.

Fineberg, D. B., P. Asselin, N. Y. Harel, I. Agranova-Breyter, S. D. Kornfeld, W. A. Bauman, and A. M. Spungen. 2013. "Vertical Ground Reaction Force-Based Analysis of Powered Exoskeleton-Assisted Walking in Persons with Motor-Complete Paraplegia." *The Journal of Spinal Cord Medicine* 36 (4): 313–321.

Garcia, E., M. Cestari, and D. Sanz-Merodio. 2014. "Wearable Exoskeletons for the Physical Treatment of Children with Quadriparesis." *Conference Proceedings: IEEE International Conference on Humanoid Robotics* November 18–20: 425–430.

Gopura, R. A. R. C., K. Kiguchi, and Y. Yi. 2009. "SUEFUL-7: A 7DOF Upper-Limb Exoskeleton Robot with Muscle-Model-Oriented EMG-Based Control." *2009 IEEE/RSJ International Conference on Intelligent Robots and Systems, IROS* October 10–15: 1126–1131.

Gowland, C. 1982. "Recovery of Motor Function Following Stroke: Profile and Predictors." *Physiotherapy* 34: 77–84.

Ha, K., S. Murray, and M. Goldfarb. 2016. "An Approach for the Cooperative Control of FES with a Powered Exoskeleton during Level Walking for Persons with Paraplegia." *IEEE Transactions on Neural Systems and Rehabilitation Engineering* 24 (4): 455–466.

Hartigan, C., C. Kandilakis, S. Dalley, M. Clausen, E. Wilson, S. Morrison, S. Etheridge et al. 2015. "Mobility Outcomes Following Five Training Sessions with a Powered Exoskeleton." *Topics in Spinal Cord Injury Rehabilitation* 21 (2): 93–99.

Herr, H. 2009. "Exoskeletons and Orthoses: Classification, Design Challenges and Future Directions." *Journal of NeuroEngineering and Rehabilitation* 6: 21.

Ilunga Tshiswaka, D., S. Loggins Clay, C.-Y. Chiu, R. Alston, and A. Lewis. 2016. "Assistive Technology Use by Disability Type and Race: Exploration of a Population-Based Health Survey." *Disability and Rehabilitation: Assistive Technology* 11 (2): 124–132.

International Organization for Standardization (ISO). 2011. ISO-9999. *Assistive Products for Persons with Disability—Classification and Terminology.* Geneva: International Organization for Standardization.

Johnson, G. R., D. A. Carus, G. Parrini, S. Scattareggia Marchese, and R. Valeggi. 2001. "The Design of a Five-Degree-of-Freedom Powered Orthosis for the Upper Limb." *Proceedings of the Institution of Mechanical Engineers. Part H, Journal of Engineering in Medicine* 215 (3): 275–284.

Jutai, J. W., M. J. Fuhrer, L. Demers, M. J. Scherer, and F. DeRuyter. 2005. "Toward a Taxonomy of Assistive Technology Device Outcomes." *American Journal of Physical Medicine & Rehabilitation/Association of Academic Physiatrists* 84 (4): 294–302.

Kawamoto, H., K. Kamibayashi, Y. Nakata, K. Yamawaki, R. Ariyasu, Y. Sankai, M. Sakane et al. 2013. "Pilot Study of Locomotion Improvement using Hybrid Assistive Limb in Chronic Stroke Patients." *BMC Neurology* 13: 141-2377-13-141.

Kawamoto, H., T. Shiraki, T. Otsuka, and Y. Sankai. 2011. "Meal-Assistance by Robot Suit HAL using Detection of Food Position with Camera." *2011 IEEE International Conference on Robotics and Biomimetics, (ROBIO)* December 7–11: 889–894.

Kittel, A., M. A. Di, and H. Stewart. 2002. "Factors Influencing the Decision to Abandon Manual Wheelchairs for Three Individuals with a Spinal Cord Injury." *Disability and Rehabilitation* 24 (1–3): 106–114.

Kozlowski, A. J., T. N. Bryce, and M. P. Dijkers. 2015. "Time and Effort Required by Persons with Spinal Cord Injury to Learn to Use a Powered Exoskeleton for Assisted Walking." *Topics in Spinal Cord Injury Rehabilitation* 21 (2): 110–121.

Kressler, J., C. K. Thomas, E. C. Field-Fote, J. Sanchez, E. Widerstrom-Noga, D. C. Cilien, K. Gant et al. 2014. "Understanding Therapeutic Benefits of Overground Bionic Ambulation: Exploratory Case Series in Persons with Chronic, Complete Spinal Cord Injury." *Archives of Physical Medicine and Rehabilitation* 95 (10): 1878–1887.e4.

Kubota, S., Y. Nakata, K. Eguchi, H. Kawamoto, K. Kamibayashi, M. Sakane, Y. Sankai et al. 2013. "Feasibility of Rehabilitation Training with a Newly Developed Wearable Robot for Patients with Limited Mobility." *Archives of Physical Medicine and Rehabilitation* 94 (6): 1080–1087.

Kwak, N. S., K. R. Muller, and S. W. Lee. 2015. "A Lower Limb Exoskeleton Control System Based on Steady State Visual Evoked Potentials." *Journal of Neural Engineering* 12 (5): 056009.

Lajeunesse, V., C. Vincent, F. Routhier, E. Careau, and F. Michaud. 2015. "Exoskeletons' Design and Usefulness Evidence According to a Systematic Review of Lower Limb Exoskeletons used for Functional Mobility by People with Spinal Cord Injury." *Disability and Rehabilitation: Assistive Technology* 4: 1–13.

Louie, D. R., J. J. Eng, T. Lam, and Spinal Cord Injury Research Evidence (SCIRE) Research Team. 2015. "Gait Speed Using Powered Robotic Exoskeletons After Spinal Cord Injury: A Systematic Review and Correlational Study." *Journal of Neuroengineering and Rehabilitation* 12: 82.

Maciejasz, P., J. Eschweiler, K. Gerlach-Hahn, A. Jansen-Troy, and S. Leonhardt. 2014. "A Survey on Robotic Devices for Upper Limb Rehabilitation." *Journal of Neuroengineering and Rehabilitation* 11: 3.

Maheu, V., J. Frappier, P. S. Archambault, and F. Routhier. 2011. "Evaluation of the JACO Robotic Arm: Clinico-Economic Study for Powered Wheelchair Users with Upper-Extremity Disabilities." *2011 IEEE International Conference on Rehabilitation Robotics (ICORR)* June 29–July 1: 5975397.

Mori, Y., K. Maejima, K. Inoue, N. Shiroma, and Y. Fukuoka. 2011. "ABLE: A Standing Style Transfer System for a Person with Disabled Lower Limbs (Improvement of Stability when Traveling)." *Industrial Robot: An International Journal* 38 (3): 234–245.

Mortenson, W. B., John L. Oliffe, William C. Miller, and Catherine L. Backman. 2012. "Grey Spaces: The Wheeled Fields of Residential Care." *Sociology of Health & Illness* 34 (3): 315–329.

Mozaffarian, D., E. J. Benjamin, A. S. Go, D. K. Arnett, M. J. Blaha, M. Cushman, S. R. Das et al. 2016. "Heart Disease and Stroke Statistics—2016 Update: A Report from the American Heart Association." *Circulation* 133 (4): e38-e360.

Neuhaus, P. D., J. H. Noorden, T. J. Craig, T. Torres, J. Kirschbaum, and J. E. Pratt. 2011. "Design and Evaluation of Mina: A Robotic Orthosis for Paraplegics." *Conference Proceedings: IEEE International Conference on Rehabilitation Robotics* June 29–July 1: 5975468.

Nilsson, A., K. S. Vreede, V. Haglund, H. Kawamoto, Y. Sankai, and J. Borg. 2014. "Gait Training Early After Stroke with a New Exoskeleton—The Hybrid Assistive Limb: A Study of Safety and Feasibility." *Journal of Neuroengineering and Rehabilitation* 11: 92.

Pedrocchi, A., S. Ferrante, E. Ambrosini, M. Gandolla, C. Casellato, T. Schauer, C. Klauer et al. 2013. "MUNDUS Project: MUltimodal Neuroprosthesis for Daily Upper Limb Support." *Journal of Neuroengineering and Rehabilitation* 10: 20.

Ripat, J., and A. Colatruglio. 2016. "Exploring Winter Community Participation among Wheelchair Users: An Online Focus Group." *Occupational Therapy in Health Care* 30 (1): 95–106.

Ripat, J. D., C. L. Brown, and K. D. Ethans. 2015. "Barriers to Wheelchair Use in the Winter." *Archives of Physical Medicine and Rehabilitation* 96 (6): 1117–1122.

Rocon, E., J. M. Belda-Lois, A. F. Ruiz, M. Manto, J. C. Moreno, and J. L. Pons. 2007. "Design and Validation of a Rehabilitation Robotic Exoskeleton for Tremor Assessment and Suppression." *IEEE Transactions on Neural Systems and Rehabilitation Engineering* 15 (3): 367–378.

Russell, J. N., G. E. Hendershot, F. LeClere, L. J. Howie, and M. Adler. 1997. "Trends and Differential Use of Assistive Technology Devices: United States, 1994." *Advance Data* (292): 1–9.

Sale, P., M. Franceschini, A. Waldner, and S. Hesse. 2012. "Use of the Robot Assisted Gait Therapy in Rehabilitation of Patients with Stroke and Spinal Cord Injury." *European Journal of Physical and Rehabilitation Medicine* 48 (1): 111–121.

Sale, P., E. F. Russo, M. Russo, S. Masiero, F. Piccione, R. S. Calabro, and S. Filoni. 2016. "Effects on Mobility Training and De-Adaptations in Subjects with Spinal Cord Injury due to a Wearable Robot: A Preliminary Report." *BMC Neurology* 16 (1): 12-016-0536-0.

Sankai, Y. 2011. "HAL: Hybrid Assistive Limb Based on Cybernics." In *Robotics Research*, edited by M. Kaneko and Y. Nakamura, 25–34. Berlin: Springer.

Sanz-Merodio, D., M. Cestari, J. C. Arevalo, and E. Garcia. 2012. "A Lower-Limb Exoskeleton for Gait Assistance in Quadriplegia." *Conference Proceedings: IEEE International Conference on Robotics and Biomimetics (ROBIO)* December 11–14: 122–127.

Spungen, A. M. 2012. "Walking with an Exoskeleton for Persons with Paraplegia [Abstract]." Interdependence 2012: Global SCI Conference. Vancouver, Canada, May 15, 2012. Abstract 19.

Spungen, A. M., P. K. Asselin, D. B. Fineberg, S. D. Kornfeld, and N. Y. Harel. 2013. "Exoskeletal-Assisted Walking for Persons with Motor-Complete Paraplegia." *STO Human Factors and Medicine Panel Symposium in Milan, Italy* 6: 1–15.

Stein, J. 2009. "e100 NeuroRobotic System." *Expert Review of Medical Devices* 6 (1): 15–19.

Stein, J., K. Narendran, J. McBean, K. Krebs, and R. Hughes. 2007. "Electromyography-Controlled Exoskeletal Upper-Limb-Powered Orthosis for Exercise Training After Stroke." *American Journal of Physical Medicine & Rehabilitation/Association of Academic Physiatrists* 86 (4): 255–261.

Svestkova, O. 2008. "International Classification of Functioning, Disability and Health of World Health Organization (ICF)." *Prague Medical Report* 109 (4): 268–274.

Sylos-Labini, F., V. La Scaleia, A. d'Avella, I. Pisotta, F. Tamburella, G. Scivoletto, M. Molinari et al. 2014. "EMG Patterns during Assisted Walking in the Exoskeleton." *Frontiers in Human Neuroscience* 8: 423.

Tamez-Duque, J., R. Cobian-Ugalde, A. Kilicarslan, A. Venkatakrishnan, R. Soto, and J. L. Contreras-Vidal. 2015. "Real-Time Strap Pressure Sensor System for Powered Exoskeletons." *Sensors (Basel, Switzerland)* 15 (2): 4550–4563.

U.S. Code Chapter 31. 2011. *Assistive Technology for Individuals with Disabilities.* U.S. Constitution and Federal Statutes.

U.S. Food and Drug Administration. 2014. "FDA Allows Marketing of First Wearable, Motorized Device that Helps People with Certain Spinal Cord Injuries to Walk." June 26. http://www.fda.gov/NewsEvents/Newsroom/PressAnnouncements/ucm402970.htm.

U.S. Food and Drug Administration, HHS. 2015. "Medical Devices; Physical Medicine Devices; Classification of the Powered Lower Extremity Exoskeleton; Republication. Final Order; Republication." *Federal Register* 80 (85): 25226–25230.

Van der Loos, H. F. M., D. S. Reinkensmeyer, and E. Guglielmelli. 2015. "Health Care and Rehabilitation Robotics." In *Handbook of Robotics*, edited by B. Siciliano and O. Khatib., 2nd ed., 1624–1665. New York: Springer Business+Media.

Wang, S., L. Wang, C. Meijneke, E. van Asseldonk, T. Hoellinger, G. Cheron, Y. Ivanenko et al. 2015. "Design and Control of the MINDWALKER Exoskeleton." *IEEE Transactions on Neural Systems and Rehabilitation Engineering* 23 (2): 277–286.

West, C. R., K. D. Currie, C. Gee, A. V. Krassioukov, and J. Borisoff. 2015. "Active-Arm Passive-Leg Exercise Improves Cardiovascular Function in Spinal Cord Injury: A Case Report." *American Journal of Physical Medicine & Rehabilitation* 94 (11): e102–e106.

Wolff, J., C. Parker, J. Borisoff, W. B. Mortenson, and J. Mattie. 2014. "A Survey of Stakeholder Perspectives on Exoskeleton Technology." *Journal of Neuroengineering and Rehabilitation* 11: 169.

Yan, T., M. Cempini, C. M. Oddo, and N. Vitiello. 2015. "Review of Assistive Strategies in Powered Lower-Limb Orthoses and Exoskeletons." *Robotics and Autonomous Systems* 64: 120–136.

Yang, A., P. Asselin, S. Knezevic, S. Kornfeld, and A. M. Spungen. 2015. "Assessment of In-Hospital Walking Velocity and Level of Assistance in a Powered Exoskeleton in Persons with Spinal Cord Injury." *Topics in Spinal Cord Injury Rehabilitation* 21 (2): 100–109.

Young, A., and D. Ferris. 2016. "State-of-the-Art and Future Directions for Robotic Lower Limb Exoskeletons." *IEEE Transactions on Neural Systems and Rehabilitation Engineering* January 27. [Epub ahead of print]

Zeilig, G., H. Weingarden, M. Zwecker, I. Dudkiewicz, A. Bloch, and A. Esquenazi. 2012. "Safety and Tolerance of the ReWalk™ Exoskeleton Suit for Ambulation by People with Complete Spinal Cord Injury: A Pilot Study." *The Journal of Spinal Cord Medicine* 35 (2): 96–101.

7

Robotic Systems for Augmentative Manipulation to Promote Cognitive Development, Play, and Education

Kim Adams, Liliana Alvarez, and Adriana Rios*

Contents

* The authors acknowledge Javier Leonardo Castellanos Cruz and Maria Fernanda Gomez for their work on the chapter.

Learning Objectives

After completing this chapter, readers will be able to

1. Discuss the importance of manipulation in child development and the potential of robotic systems to enable augmentative manipulation for children with motor impairments.
2. Apply an assistive technology model for using assistive robotic systems in cognitive assessment, play, or education.
3. List the purposes for which different types of robotic systems are currently used for augmentative manipulation in the literature pertaining to cognitive development, play, and learning for children with motor impairments.
4. Describe evidence that supports the use of robotic systems for augmentative manipulation for the assessment or development of cognitive skills, play, and learning.

Case Studies

Three case studies of children with motor impairments are used to examine these learning objectives.

CASE STUDY 7.1   JOSEPH: COGNITIVE ASSESSMENT NEED

Joseph is a 4-year-old boy with Pelizaeus-Merzbacher disease (PMD). PMD is one of several rare diseases commonly known as leukodystrophies because of the disruption in growth and maintenance of the myelin sheath around the axons of a neuron (Kohlschütter and Florian 2011). Joseph has a special seating system in a manual wheelchair, but he does not propel the wheelchair himself. In addition to having spasticity, Joseph has nystagmus (rapid involuntary movements of the eyes). He is nonverbal, and the extent to which his cognitive skills are compromised remains undetermined. His parents are convinced he understands and knows more than what his pediatrician believes, as they can see him interact with them via nonverbal communication, such as smiling. His occupational therapist (OT) has found it difficult to locate an age-appropriate cognitive test that can provide some insight into Joseph's cognitive skills. For the most part, age-appropriate cognitive tests require the child to respond verbally (e.g., by answering a question) or motorically (e.g., by creating a tower of blocks). Thus, none allows Joseph to demonstrate what he knows. The OT continues to explore ways for Joseph to demonstrate his cognitive skills and work on improving them.

CASE STUDY 7.2   JUAN: PLAY NEED

Juan is a 6-year-old boy with spastic athetoid cerebral palsy (CP) that affects all four limbs, resulting in severe physical limitations in reaching and grasping. He has a pediatric manual wheelchair with a positioning system. He is not able to propel the wheelchair by himself, so his mother usually pushes it. There are no issues with Juan's vision or hearing as reported by his family and therapists. Juan recognizes and can say the words for a few colors and shapes and a few familiar animals and objects. He is not able to read or write. He is able to follow three-step directions. Juan has limited spoken language, so he tries to communicate in other ways using nonverbal communication, such as laughter, head nods and shakes, and words and phrases to express himself; however, sometimes people around him, even his mother, find it difficult to understand what he is saying.

Juan lives in a low-income country, and his family belongs to a low social economic strata. Juan lives with his mother, his aunt, three cousins (an 11-year-old boy, a 9-year-old girl, and an 11-month-old boy), and his grandparents on the second floor of a two-story house. He attends a rehabilitation institution every morning, where he receives physiotherapy, occupational therapy, speech language pathology, and special education services. Juan does not yet attend school, but his mother is looking for one.

Juan's favorite activities are watching movies and listening to music; his favorite place for playing is sitting in his wheelchair. His least-favorite activity is grasping toys, as reported by his mother. When Juan plays with his mother, she reads him storybooks and cuddles him; if the play involves toys, she chooses the toys for play. She tends to decide how to play with those toys and to initiate play themes.

Principles

Independent manipulation is instrumental for children's cognitive development, and it enables participation in play and academic activities. It also provides a way for demonstrating acquired skills, which is important because, typically, new opportunities for cognitive development will be available only if adults acknowledge that previous milestones were reached.

Cognitive Development

Children develop cognitive, perceptual, and social skills through motor experience (Flanagan, Bowman, and Johansson 2006; McCarty, Clifton,

CASE STUDY 7.3   JULIA: EDUCATION NEED

Julia is a 10-year-old girl with spinal muscular atrophy that affects all four limbs, leading to severe physical limitations in reaching and grasping. She has a power wheelchair with a custom seating-and-positioning system. She controls her wheelchair using a joystick located at her right hand. Her school desk is customized with a slot for her joystick, so she can drive up to the desk. There are no issues with Julia's vision and hearing, as reported by her teacher. Julia is verbal. She uses an iPad mini™ attached to her wheelchair and positioned directly in front of her using a Modhose iPad Adjustable Cradle™ mounting system. Julia moves her right finger supported by her left hand to access the iPad. She cannot press hard enough to engage the home button, but she can press the iPad screen if it is positioned within her range of motion.

Julia is in an integrated grade four classroom and studies the same curriculum as her classmates. An educational assistant provides academic and personal assistance to Julia and other students in the classroom. Julia's education assistant or the other students in class perform most manipulation required in the school activities. Julia's teacher would like Julia to have hands-on experience manipulating the objects the other students are using to make arrays in order to practice the concept of multiplication.

and Collard 2001). Object manipulation, a critical aspect of motor experience, enables the child to acquire the skills required for learning, emergence of symbols, referential communication, and the understanding of relations between objects (Affolter 2004; Bates 1979; Greenfield 1991; McCarty, Clifton, and Collard 2001; Piaget 1954).

Emerging before locomotion, object manipulation is the first means through which the human infant acts on the world. For the first 9 months of life, human infants rely solely on manipulation for independent interaction with the world (Vauclair 1984). Object manipulation also serves as indication that early milestones of cognitive and perceptual development have been reached (Lockman 2005; Vauclair 1984). Through object manipulation, a child progressively starts to relate to objects, explore their properties, and discover how objects can be used to achieve a goal (i.e., tool use, a landmark cognitive skill in infancy) (Lockman 2000). For example, 18-month-old children can choose which hand to use and how to change their grasp when self-feeding if the spoon is placed in an awkward orientation inside a bowl (Keen 2011; McCarty, Clifton, and Collard 1999). The use of objects as tools extends the capability of the child and enhances the child's interactions (St. Amant and Horton 2008). Thus, tool use has been studied from several cognitive theory approaches. Among these theories, perhaps one of the most influential in the field of child development research is Piaget's (1950) genetic epistemology.

Piaget's observations of children's behaviors led to the definition of four stages of cognitive development that have been used to further explore and understand cognition in children (Solaz-Portolésa and Sanjoséb 2008). According to Piaget, the relation between motor experience and cognitive development starts with the sensorimotor stage (Piaget and Inhelder 1969). The sensorimotor stage takes place during the first 2 years of life and is critical for the achievement of cognitive milestones, such as object permanence and means-end analysis. During the first 2 years, the child actively manipulates objects, explores them individually and sequentially, and finally realizes that one object can be used as a means to reach the other (Piaget 1954). For example, a child can use a stick (McCarty, Clifton, and Collard 2001) or a string (Chen, Sanchez, and Campbell 1997) to retrieve an object out of reach. Other approaches and contributions to the study of cognitive development differ in how and to what extent they emphasize the influence of cultural and social interactions on development (e.g., Vygotsky [1978], 1997). However, there is widespread agreement regarding the critical role of motor experience on the cognitive development of children.

Because of the strong relationship between motor skills and cognitive development, early studies suggested that a lack of motor experience can result in cognitive and perceptual delays (Bertenthal and Campos 1987). The assessment of cognitive skills throughout childhood relies heavily on the child's motor and verbal skills as avenues for demonstrating or explaining concepts or engaging in problem solving. Thus, children with physical disabilities can lose opportunities to demonstrate their skills or learn and develop new ones.

Much as powered mobility provides children with physical disabilities with opportunities for independent mobility, robots with adapted interfaces can provide children with motor impairments with opportunities for independent manipulation of objects (Alvarez 2014). Children with disabilities can accomplish manipulative tasks through the use of robots because robots compensate for their functional limitations by decreasing the motor demand of the task (Alvarez 2014). Given that the motor requirements to control the robot can be minimal and can be adapted to a wide range of possible anatomical control sites (Poletz et al. 2010), robots can be used as a tool to explore the cognitive skills of children with disabilities. Through robots, children with severe motor impairments can demonstrate what they know and can further benefit from independent interaction with objects (Alvarez 2014).

Play

Play is one of the occupations of human beings (American Occupational Therapy Association 2014). While work and activities of daily living are defined and labeled by external social conventions, play is defined only by the player's perception (Bundy 1993). This means that an activity is play if the individual's feelings are related to pleasure, flexibility, spontaneity, intrinsic motivation, choice, challenge, internal control, and creativity (Blanche 2008; Skard and Bundy 2008). Parham (2008) reviewed the characteristics of play and proposed that plays activities (1) are intrinsically motivated; (2) are process oriented because play emphasizes the process rather than the product; (3) are related to free choice because the player is free to choose to play; (4) provide enjoyment and pleasure; (5) involve active engagement because the player is active; and (6) are noninstrumental, or are not "serious," which is related to the pretend element of play. During play, children learn about the properties of objects and how to interact with objects and people (Reilly 1974). Play where the child interacts with people is called *social play* (Coplan, Rubin, and Findlay 2006), and play where the child interacts with objects is called *object play* (Gowen et al. 1992). Both types of play interactions have important benefits for children's development, which occurs in a natural way.

Play follows three stages of development driven by cognitive development: *functional* play, *pretend* or *symbolic* play, and *games with rules* (Piaget 1951). Functional play is the type of play in which a child uses the objects according to the function designed for them and as they would be used in reality (e.g., a ball is used as a ball) (Barton 2010). Pretend play, or symbolic play, is a cognitive play skill of representing knowledge, experience, and objects symbolically (Stagnitti and Unsworth 2004). In pretend play, the child uses an object as if it were a different object (e.g., using a block as if it were a car) (Barton 2010). Games with rules involve more structured play, play activities having rules that need to be followed by each player. Thus, at this stage, play also takes on a social aspect (Piaget 1951).

Play is an ideal way for children to discover the world through practice with different objects and experiences (Ferland 2005). In fact, innovative problem solving occurs during play (Sutton-Smith 2001). However, children with motor limitations, such as children with CP, have difficulties engaging in play (Blanche 2008; Missiuna and Pollock 1991), especially play with objects. Due to their physical limitations, children with CP have constraints in engaging in pretend play (Pfeifer et al. 2011) and object play (Gowen et al. 1992) and expressing *playfulness* (Chang et al. 2014; Harkness and Bundy 2001). Children with CP and their families spend more time in activities related to self-care (including rehabilitation) than do typically developing children. This reduces time for family play routines (Brodin 2005; Hinojosa and Kramer 2008; Missiuna and Pollock 1991). With few opportunities for practicing and testing their skills, children can develop a learned helplessness; that is, children assume that they are unable to perform a task by themselves even though they have the required physical abilities (Harkness and Bundy 2001). All of these situations delay not only the child's play and development but also future overall functioning (Missiuna and Pollock 1991).

The need for interventions focused on promoting play in children with motor impairments has been widely stated (Blanche 2008; Chang et al. 2014; Ferland 2005; Missiuna and Pollock 1991; Pfeifer et al. 2011; Ríos-Rincón et al. 2016). Scholars agree that intervention should improve the play experience in a child's life and involve the child's family (Blanche 2008; Brodin 2005; Ferland 2005; Hinojosa and Kramer 2008; Ríos-Rincón et al. 2016). Promoting engagement in free play in children with motor impairment may affect children's overall functioning. Playfulness is an indicator of self-determined behaviors for children with CP with limited self-mobility. Children who are self-determined present behaviors oriented toward meeting personal life goals; these behaviors include identifying desires, actively pursuing interests, making decisions, and solving problems (Chang et al. 2014). This suggests that increasing playfulness may improve children's ability to find creative strategies to make choices and to solve problems (Chang et al. 2014), which in turn can improve their future functioning in home, community, school, and work contexts.

Education

Education programs of study, for instance, in mathematics (Van De Walle, Karp, and Bay-Williams 2010) or science (McCarthy 2005), emphasize the integration of hands-on activities while communicating about concepts. Learning and retention can be improved when actively participating in direct purposeful experiences as opposed to watching demonstrations (Petress 2008). Being actively engaged in classroom activities contributes to children's motivation to learn (Schunk, Meece, and Pintrich 2012).

Children who have physical impairments often cannot engage in academic activities due to limitations in pointing, grasping, or holding the manipulative objects used in the lessons (Eriksson, Welander, and Granlund 2007). Unfortunately, children with physical disabilities may miss the hands-on component of learning, or they may observe their classmates or an educational assistant perform the steps involving manipulation of objects. Increasing the active component of the learning experience for children with disabilities by providing access to manipulation and communication should have a large impact on a child's education.

There is some assistive technology for manipulation in the classroom; for example, a child can use a switch connected to a battery interrupter (Mistrett and Goetz n.d.) to activate electric scissors while a nondisabled student cuts out pictures for an art project. However, these simple tools cannot provide help to involve students with disabilities once school activities become more sophisticated. Children can direct others to do parts of the activities, for example, telling a classmate which objects to measure (Schlosser et al. 2000). However, it can take a long time to give instructions. There are specialized computer programs for students with disabilities to practice language arts and mathematics concepts (i.e., Intellitools distributed by Mayer Johnson, http://www.mayer-johnson .com/intellitools-classroom-suite-v-4). These tools, when available in a classroom, can be useful to actively engage in learning concepts. However, because they are screen based, these activities do not give access to the physical world, and many early learning lessons use real-world physical objects in experiments.

Robots as augmentative manipulation tools can be beneficial for children with physical disabilities to interact with the same objects as their peers in the classroom. Children with severe disabilities have used robots as a tool to do various learning activities (described in the material that follows), and robots have been found to be more motivating than single-switch appliances or computer programs (Cook et al. 2005; Howell, Martz, and Stanger 1996; Plaisant et al. 2000). Developing robots that can be used for augmentative manipulation in education activities can contribute to the hands-on learning of children with physical impairments.

Effect of Others on Children's Exploration, Play, and Learning

The lack of meaningful opportunities for exploration and manipulation may be affected by the perceptions of clinicians, parents, and teachers who limit the number and type of opportunities they afford to the child. Parents of children with physical disabilities often perceive their child as seeking more adult approval and help, being less motivated, and preferring easy and familiar tasks (Blanche 2008; Jennings and MacTurk 1995). This can have an effect on exploration experiences of children; for example, mothers may encourage less exploration by their children with disabilities than mothers of typically developing children with the same cognitive capacity (Jennings and MacTurk 1995).

Parents of children with disabilities have no clear role in children's play (Brodin 2005); that is, parents do not know clearly whether they should take play as an opportunity for training their child in specific needed skills or whether play should be an opportunity for enjoyment that they should facilitate (Brodin 2005). Generally, caregivers and playmates dominate the play, so that children with CP, for example, become more spectators of others' play rather than active players (Blanche 2008; Brodin 2005). This was seen in a study in which mothers of children with severe CP generally decided what to play and how to play when playing with their children (Ríos-Rincón et al. 2016).

Low expectations of teachers can prevent children from thriving in the classroom. Adults who had speech and physical impairments were critical of the special education they received, saying the expectations were not high enough (McNaughton, Light, and Arnold 2002). Several studies have shown that teachers' perception of the abilities of children with disabilities has increased after seeing children's skills when they use robots in playful or academic activities (Cook et al. 2000).

Requirements for Robotic Systems as Augmentative Manipulation Assistive Technologies for Cognitive Development, Play, and Education

Robots can be used as augmentative manipulation systems due to their capability for picking, placing, and exploring objects (Tejima 2000). Among the assistive technologies available for manipulation for cognitive assessment, play, and academic activities, robots are flexible in interactions with the environment; they can do more than one repetitive action, and they can manipulate three-dimensional objects in the real world (Cook et al. 2000, 2002).

However, using the robot as a tool is not the same as manipulating objects with one's hand. Action mediated by a tool can add additional cognitive demands to the task (Keen 2011), which, in the case of augmentative manipulation, can result in poor robot operational competence, which can be confused with poor performance on the task. For example, to perform the robot-mediated tasks discussed in the work of Poletz et al. (2010), children need to understand that pressing the switch causes the robot to move in a certain way or that when using two or more switches the robot can move in sequences that give the child more control over the step-by-step movement of the robot (Cook et al. 2005; Poletz et al. 2010). Thus, robots may decrease the motor demand while increasing the task's cognitive complexity. It is critical to understand the additional cognitive and perceptual demands that the use of the robot imposes on the child. On one hand, this can guide the selection and adaptation of the human–robot interface. On the other hand, robot characteristics and programming can be adapted to match the needs and skills of the child as well as the task and goals.

A theoretical approach to the assessment and quantification of the complexity of children using the robot as a tool, rather than directly manipulating an object with their arm and hand, has been explored (Alvarez, Adams, and Cook 2016). The complexity number hypothesis, first proposed by Van Leeuwen, Smitsman, and Van Leeuwen (1994) for common tools, was used to assess the complexity of a robot-mediated task performed by an infant with a disability; this was compared with the demands encountered by a typically developing infant when using a common tool. Through this approach, the authors established that, from a cognitive and perceptual perspective, there is an increase in complexity of robot-mediated activities over that of simple tools. Far from discouraging the use of robots by young children with disabilities, the complexity of robotic augmentative manipulation systems further supports the fact that by the very interaction with robots, children with physical disabilities can display and develop cognitive skills.

A survey of commercially available robots costing from $250 to $500 was compiled and compared to desirable characteristics of robots for cognitive development, play, and education of children with disabilities (Cook, Encarnação, and Adams 2010). Characteristics included being flexible, robust, safe, easy to use and learn, portable, aesthetically pleasing, and reasonably priced; having an appropriate human–robot interface; and providing various levels of control. Their cost, bulkiness, and nonplayful appearance eliminate assistive robotic manipulators like the ones described in Chapter 3 as candidates for the applications considered here. A review by Cook, Encarnação, and Adams (2010) revealed no commercially available robots that were entirely suitable for use by children with disabilities, but the Lego Mindstorms or the Fischertechnik Robot Explorer™ were found to be appropriate as long as the needed adaptations for an interface to accept children's alternate physical abilities were made.

Critical factors involved in the use of the robots by children to support play have been identified (Besio, Caprino, and Laudanna 2008): factors related to play (functions of play, types of play); factors related to the individual according to the International Classification of Functioning—Children and Youth Version (ICF-CY); factors related to the context according to the ICF-CY; factors related to technology and robotics (approach to technology development, usability, quality of life, and characteristics for autonomous and safe play); and factors related to methodology. Usability considerations (accessibility, universal design, and innovation) and functional aspects of the technology (communication and social interaction, manipulation and mobility) are discussed (Besio, Caprino, and Laudanna 2008). Usability of assistive robots is a major concern (Tsun et al. 2015), especially when considering their use by children who have physical impairments and perhaps concomitant cognitive impairments or delays. Children's success in understanding the use of a robot depends on the flexibility of the robotic system, not only in terms of the degrees of freedom but also related to the capacity of the robotic system to be adjusted to different levels of cognitive demands and motor impairments for the child.

The human–robot interface (cf. Chapter 2) should accommodate the abilities of the child with disabilities. A complete review of the many different ways to access assistive technology, along with a framework for control interface decision making, has been presented (Cook and Polgar 2015). Many of the typical interfaces to assistive technology (e.g., keyboards, joysticks, head gimbals, eye gaze, voice control, or switches) can also be used to control robots. For children with severe disabilities, finding as many avenues of input as possible may be beneficial. However, these additional input channels need to be balanced with keeping the methods of control intuitive. Another issue is that the interfaces can be cognitively demanding. For instance, using *scanning* with switches requires monitoring the options being presented to the user, correctly selecting the desired option, as well as monitoring the robot. Eye tracking requires children to divert attention from the robot to make selections on a computer screen. Another factor to consider is how multiple activities might need to be controlled from the same interface. Controlling the robot from an *augmentative communication device* is one example of using the same interface for multiple purposes (Adams and Cook 2016b). There are other combinations that may be needed (e.g., electronic aids to daily living, wheelchair, mobile robot, or robot arm).

Similar to any other assistive technology, the considerations mentioned should be framed in a model that encompasses the user, the activity to be performed, the technology, the context of use, and the dynamic interactions between these (cf. the Human Activity Assistive Technology [HAAT] model described in Chapter 1). Depending on the complexity of the situation, a team of individuals may be involved in designing, developing, and implementing a robotic intervention. The knowledge and skills of different professionals may be beneficial in assessing the needs and abilities of the children; demands in the environments; cognitive, play, or educational goals; and related activities. Occupational therapists, physical therapists, speech language pathologists, rehabilitation engineers, psychologists, and teachers are potential team members. At the center of the team should be the child and his or her parents, as they are the experts in the personal factors that will influence functioning of the system, for instance, what motivates the child, preferences, and what is feasible in their environment.

Critical Review of the Technology Available

Stationary and mobile robots have been used in play and education by children with disabilities. For instance, the CRS A465™ (Figure 7.1) is a stationary industrial robotic arm approximately the same size as an adult human arm. It is able to (1) rotate about its base; (2) flex and extend at the elbow and shoulder; (3) extend, flex, supinate, and pronate at the wrist; and (4) open and close a gripper. Children operated a CRS robot through three switches to perform play activities (Cook et al. 2000). A Minimover 5 robotic arm (Microbot, Inc.), about half adult human scale, was used to bring a cookie closer, and was controlled by a switch (Cook, Liu, and Hoseit 1990) (that system is now available as the educational robot, Microbot TeachMover [Questech, Inc], Figure 7.2). Lego Mindstorms™ robots can be configured into "robotic arms," made of Lego pieces with a base, an upper arm, a forearm, and a gripper (Figure 7.3). This type of robot was used by a participant to drop, lift, and release a variety of small toys (Schulmeister et al. 2006). A robot arm was assembled from basic components and controlled by voice to pick up blocks and put them into shapes of letters (Lee 2013). Another type of robot, assembled from basic components, is a 3-DOF (degrees of freedom) Cartesian configuration robot with a special gripper for grasping and inserting Lego bricks on a play area, also made of Lego bricks (Kronreif et al. 2007). The first version of this PlayROB system was called the 3DOF Robot system (Prazak et al. 2004). The PlayROB was controlled through a joystick, keyboard, pointing, and sip-puff input devices.

The most common mobile robots that have been used in play and education are Lego Mindstorms robots, which are made of Lego pieces that can be configured like a car with wheels, sometimes with a gripper (Figure 7.4). These robots have been used in studies for the manipulation of small

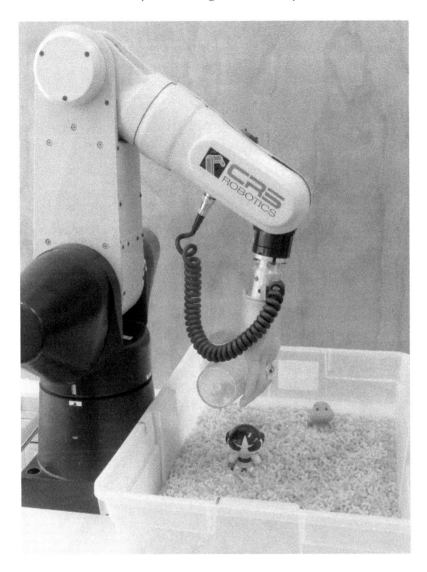

Figure 7.1   A CRS A465, a stationary industrial robotic arm. In the figure, a prosthetic hand is used as a gripper to hold a cup. The robot can be made to dig the cup in the macaroni and collect toys that are buried in the macaroni.

toys, such as dolls, balls, toy cars, and wood blocks, using a gripper or a scoop during semistructured and free-play activities (Encarnação et al. 2014; Poletz et al. 2010; Ríos-Rincón et al. 2016; Schulmeister et al. 2006). Adaptations were necessary for children to operate the robots, such as the design of an infrared remote control adapted for single-switch control of

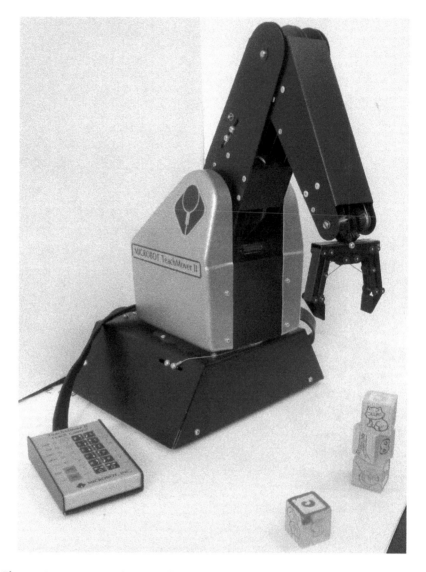

Figure 7.2 A Microbot TeachMover, a half-human size robotic arm with 6 DOF. The robot is poised to move to its right to pick up a block and place it on top of the pile of blocks.

the Lego Mindstorms RCX robots (Poletz et al. 2010; Ríos-Rincón et al. 2016) or the use of a Don Johnston Switch Interface® connected to a computer with a program for controlling Lego Mindstorms NXT robots by BlueTooth (Adams et al. 2015; Ríos-Rincón et al. 2016). Computer-based augmentative communication software has been used to send commands

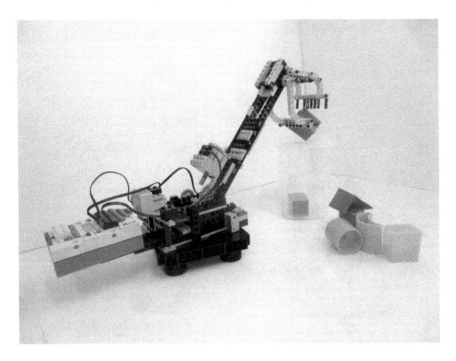

Figure 7.3 A Lego Mindstorms RCX robot configured into a robotic arm. In the figure, the robot is being used to pick up differently shaped objects to put into a bin.

to a program to control Lego NXT robots via trackball and eye gaze (Encarnação et al. 2016). Another method to control the robots, which did not need customized hardware or software, was to train infrared commands for the RCX robot into a communication device (Adams and Cook 2014, 2016b). With this method, children used two switches in scan mode to select robot commands from their device display.

A benefit of using communication devices and computers to control robots is that the same access method that children are used to for accessing the communication device or computer can be used to control the robot. Also, when children are severely impaired, they do not have many anatomical sites with which to control technology. Controlling a robot through a communication device or computer gives children access to robot movements and the other functions of the device or computer. A motivation for using commercial Lego robots is that teachers, therapists, and parents can easily acquire, build, and program them, thus potentially leading to increased opportunities for play and academic activities.

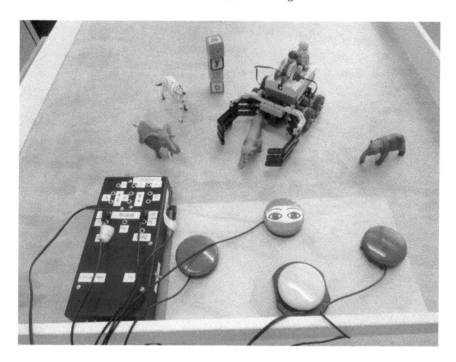

Figure 7.4 A Lego Mindstorms RCX robot configured into a mobile car-like robot. A scoop in front of the robot is being used to move play objects around the play area. A helper can place objects on top of the robot. An adapted remote controller (on the left of the picture) has the same functionality as the original Lego remote control but allows switches to be plugged into it. The push-button switches (on the right of the picture) perform forward (with the symbol of the eyes), left and right, and backward robot movements.

Two low-cost robots are being developed in Brazil for grasping objects or drawing (Ferasoli-Filho et al. 2012). Directional control of the mobile robots is done by tilting the head, read by an accelerometer, and the gripper (or pen) is activated by muscle, read by an electromyography sensor. Robots like this are still in the development stage but would be an important contribution for use in underresourced areas.

Programming the robots requires varying levels of technical expertise. The Lego Mindstorms software is easy to use but can only be used to download programs to the robot to run autonomously. To control the robot in teleoperation mode, some technical programming is needed, and some researchers have made their software available (e.g., http://uarpie.anditec.pt/images/docs/user_manual_iamcat.zip and http://www.rehabresearch.ualberta.ca/assistivetechnology/resources/tools/).

The programming community sometimes makes available useful programs for common platforms, such as the Lego robot, but they are not consistently available (for a list, see the work of Adams and David 2013b). Some robot projects have been designed with the long-term goal of having an easy-to-use programming interface for parents and teachers (Ferasoli-Filho et al. 2012). Most robots used in studies with children with physical impairments have required programming skills to translate input from the user to movements of the robot (e.g., Microsoft® Robotics Developer Studio [Encarnação et al. 2016], LabVIEW in [Adams et al. 2015], or microprocessor programming in [Lee 2013]).

None of the mentioned robots is commercially available as a package ready to be used by children with motor impairments. All of the robotic systems used to promote play and education in children with motor impairments are level 7 or lower according to the technology readiness scale (U.S. Department of Energy 2009). Some of them are prototypes that were completely developed by researchers and used in laboratory settings or real contexts, such as schools or rehabilitation centers. This is the case of the robot arm (Lee 2013) and PlayROB robotic systems (Klein et al. 2011; Kronreif et al. 2007; Marti and Iacono 2011; Prazak et al. 2004). These robotic systems demand the presence of a person with special training to deal with technical issues, which constrains their use in family play routines or in educational settings. Other researchers have used and adapted some commercially available robotic systems, such as the CRS A465 robotic arm (Cook et al. 2000) and the Lego Mindstorms robots (Adams and Cook 2014; Ríos-Rincón et al. 2016; Schulmeister et al. 2006), to be used by children with motor impairments. The adaptations have been focused on the control interfaces. Most robotic systems have been used in laboratory environments or real contexts, such as school or home, and the whole systems are not yet available to be used in the real context by the end users or there is only one prototype that needs to be adjusted for its use by the research team. The Lego Mindstorms robots are the only ones tested in children's homes and operated by children's families (Ríos-Rincón et al. 2016).

Critical Review of Available Utilization Protocols

Utilization Protocols to Assess Cognitive Skills

The performance of children with disabilities when executing robot-mediated play activities designed to elicit particular cognitive skills can be compared to the performance of typically developing children executing the same activities to provide a proxy measure for cognitive development. Typically developing children and children with neuromotor disabilities at the ages of 3, 4, and 5 years old were exposed to four tasks designed to challenge cause and effect, inhibition, laterality, and sequencing skills (Encarnação et al. 2014; Poletz et al. 2010). For each task, children were presented with a specific goal:

1. *Cause and effect*: Children were asked to use the robot to knock over a tower of blocks. To successfully complete the task, children needed to understand that pressing the switch caused the robot to move forward toward the blocks.
2. *Inhibition*: Children were asked to move the robot forward (as in the previous task) and stop at a specific point in the path to pick up a block. To successfully complete the task, children needed to understand that releasing, and thus inhibiting, the pressing action that was previously successful was required.
3. *Laterality*: In this task, children were presented with the robot facing forward, but located midway between two towers of blocks placed at the right and left sides. In addition, children now had three switches instead of one as in the previous tasks. Children were asked to select a tower to knock over; thus, they needed to select the correct switch to make the robot turn and face the chosen tower.
4. *Sequencing*: Complementary to task 3, children needed to press the forward (middle) switch to complete the sequence by which they could knock over the selected tower.

Other robot-mediated activities may be designed to elicit different cognitive skills. Piagetian tasks are often used to gain insight into children's cognitive skills through the child's verbal or motor responses. One example is a conservation task in which children are shown two identical containers filled with the same amount of liquid. After agreeing that they have the same amount, children are shown how the contents of one container are poured into a taller one. Children are then asked whether the containers have the same amount of liquid. Children who cannot yet conserve (typically under the age of 5) will answer no and will identify the taller container as having more liquid. Piaget's conservation task is considered an important cognitive milestone by which children demonstrate that they have reached the cognitive skills that allow them to discern amount from height and focus on the content rather than the shape of the container. A child with physical and speech impairments may have difficulties in expressing his or her answer. A switch-controlled robot can be used by the child to choose between the different answers by driving the robot toward the location at which the child's choice is positioned.

When designing activities to challenge different cognitive skills, it is important to keep in mind that they should be perceived by children as playful activities. In fact, if the activities are meaningless and unappealing to children, the children may underperform and fail to reveal their true cognitive development. Often, the same activity is not engaging for all children, and different activities requiring the same cognitive skills should be prepared to meet each child's preferences. For example, holding down a switch to drive a robot forward to knock over a stack of blocks, to take a flower to a princess, or to feed an animal all require an understanding of cause and effect, and a particular child might prefer one play activity over the others.

Robot Training Protocol

As mentioned, indirect manipulation of objects by controlling a robot is not the same as direct manipulation using one's own hands. In studies where the task was too rigid or too challenging or the interface was too complicated, children had problems understanding how to operate the robot and became passive, frustrated, and uninterested (Besio, Carnesecchi, and Converti 2013; Kronreif et al. 2007; Marti and Iacono 2011; Prazak et al. 2004). Researchers have found that a training-and-practice period is necessary for children to understand how to operate the robot (Adams and Cook 2014; Cook et al. 2000; Ríos-Rincón et al. 2016). This helps to ensure that children will have the operational skills to control the robot to do the activities. This way, the teacher knows if the child is having trouble doing a play or academic task, it is likely due to not understanding the concept, not from lack of knowledge concerning how to control the robot. A protocol for training is available (Adams and Encarnação 2011). The protocol is based on the basic cognitive robot skills mentioned previously (Encarnação et al. 2014; Poletz et al. 2010) and adds tasks with more complexity, such as navigating a slalom course. It includes tests to track the child's progress at using the robot, including the speed and accuracy of using the access method alone and the speed and accuracy of using the access method to control the robot. For a discussion on the use of this protocol with nine children with neuromotor disabilities, please refer to the work of Encarnação et al. (2016).

A framework to describe the competency skills needed to use communication devices to control robots has been proposed (Adams and Cook

2016b). It is based on the competency domains proposed by Light (1989) for using augmentative communication devices: linguistic, operational, social, and strategic competence. In the communication device–robot framework, linguistic competence is knowing what the robot commands will do (e.g., the difference between direct motor control and running a program from a button); operational competence is knowing how to activate the robot commands; social competence is using the robot to interact with others; and strategic competence is knowing when to switch between robot control and communication mode. This framework may also be useful for controlling robots from other types of devices that do not have communication output.

Utilization Protocols to Promote Access to Play

Researchers have designed structured and semistructured play activities to be performed by children using robots. Structured activities have included exploration and cooperative play with an adult. For instance, children were encouraged to hit three switches (using their heads, hands, or legs) in a specific order to perform three sequential tasks: pouring out dry macaroni from a glass, digging up objects, and dumping the objects into a tub with dry macaroni. The design of the activity promoted interaction and turn taking between the child and the researcher (Cook et al. 2000, 2002). Other researchers designed tasks to be performed by a child using a Lego Mindstorms mobile robot and robotic arm through switches. Tasks included activating a song-and-dance program, making the mobile robot move forward to knock over a tower of blocks, dropping a variety of toys, lifting a toy into sight, and rotating the arm closer to the child followed by opening a gripper to release a toy. A prompt hierarchy was developed in case the child did not actively engage in the play activity; the hierarchy progressed from visual prompting (gesture) to full physical and verbal prompting (i.e., researcher hand over child's hand) (Schulmeister et al. 2006).

Other researchers have had a different approach in which the robotic play activities are free-play oriented instead of structured play activities. Children who used the PlayROB were encouraged to freely explore the robot using it to build any structure they wanted with Lego bricks (Kronreif et al. 2007). However, in a second phase of the study, researchers oriented the activity toward a structured play activity. That could be because some participants did not understand the relationship between using the input device and the robot's actions during the free-play phase;

thus, researchers felt they needed to train those children through structured activities (Kronreif et al. 2007; Prazak et al. 2004). Ríos-Rincón et al.
(2016) designed a study in which mother-child dyads were encouraged to
engage in free play with a Lego robot and the child's own toys. A resource
manual was developed to support parents to use robots to promote learning in their children with disabilities through play activities at home. The
robot activities are based on the cognitive skills required for operating a
robot mentioned previously and also encourage free play. The booklet is
available online (http://www.rehabresearch.ualberta.ca/assistivetechnology
/resources/tools/).

Utilization Protocols to Promote Access to Education

The most recent review of educational robots we located was performed
over 10 years ago (Howell 2005). The review presented a historical perspective covering early work from the 1980s that led to present-day robots
for activities of daily living. There were only two robots for augmentative
manipulation in education activities mentioned in the review, and none
of those systems is presently available (Harwin, Ginige, and Jackson 1986;
Howell and Hay 1989; Howell, Martz, and Stanger 1996). From 1986 to
2000, some good progress was made in the area of robots in education
(Eberhart, Osborne, and Rahman 2000; Harwin, Ginige, and Jackson
1988; Howell and Hay 1989; Howell, Martz, and Stanger 1996; Kwee
and Quaedackers 1999; Smith and Topping 1996). The body of work was
impressive in many ways. First, robot use moved out of the laboratory
into classrooms and was tested with actual students, although primarily
case studies with one to seven participants. Children with various physical impairments, including arthrogryposis, muscular dystrophy, and CP
(the most common), tried the systems. Second, some of the stationary
robot arms used had sophisticated vision systems and built-in intelligence
(Harwin, Ginige, and Jackson 1988). Third, the researchers had accommodated severe physical abilities with a wide array of access methods, including switches (Howell and Hay 1989; Kwee and Quaedackers 1999; Smith
and Topping 1996), and some systems were flexible enough to accommodate multiple methods because they were computer based (Harwin,
Ginige, and Jackson 1988; Howell 2005). Trouble using the access methods
was a common concern (Howell and Hay 1989). Finally, the researchers
undertook a number of varied academic tasks, most commonly science lab
activities (Eberhart, Osborne, and Rahman 2000; Howell and Hay 1989),
including sensory inspection (Howell, Martz, and Stanger 1996) and

extinguishing a candle (Kwee and Quaedackers 1999). Other activities included drawing on worksheets to match questions and answers (Smith and Topping 1996) and sorting objects, picking and placing objects, and manipulating the disks for the Tower of Hanoi puzzle (Harwin, Ginige, and Jackson 1988). Unfortunately, the development of robots for manipulation of educational objects lost its momentum, and there has been little research and development in the area lately.

The literature regarding the use of robots for augmentative manipulation by children with physical impairments in academic activities since 2005 is scarce, with only seven studies located. In these recent studies, several robot-mediated educational activities have been performed, showing the flexibility of robots as tools for augmentative manipulation in the classroom. For example, to learn the English letters, children said a letter out loud, and if pronounced correctly, a robot would build the letter in a typesetting plate and the letter would also be displayed on a computer screen (Lee 2013). The authors found that the ideal ages at which children were old enough to understand the system, but not too old to be bored, were 3 and 4 years old.

Being able to control a robot from a communication device to act out a story was motivating for a participant to increase the participant's length of utterance (Adams and Cook 2016b). Often, children who use augmentative communication systems make short utterances, sometimes one word long. A car-like robot and a robot arm were "dressed up" like characters in the story, and the participant moved the robots and spoke their lines.

To write a simple robot program, a participant moved the computer cursor and selected commands in the ROBOLAB program via the participant's communication device (Adams and Cook 2013). The communication device was connected to the computer via a USB cable and operated in mouse emulation mode.

Various mathematics activities have been accomplished using a robot (Adams and Cook 2016b). Building simple puzzles was done by having a puzzle piece placed on top of a mobile robot. The participant then drove the robot to the location where the piece should go and spun the robot into the correct orientation (a helper was needed to insert the piece into the puzzle). A mobile robot was moved along a "board game" while counting spaces. Another numeracy activity was drawing lines between ascending numbers on an enlarged numbered connect-the-dots picture using a marking pen attached to the back of a mobile robot.

A series of studies was performed in which students did mathematics measurement activities: comparing and sorting objects by length (Adams and Cook 2014); measuring the length of objects using nonstandard units, such as paperclips, and then comparing lengths based on the numerical measurement (Adams and Cook 2016b); and measuring using standard centimeter units (Adams and David 2013b). Information about programs to control the robots and instructions for doing the mathematics measurement activities and building NXT and EV3 robots and attachments are available from Adams and David (2013a) and online (http://www.rehab research.ualberta.ca/assistivetechnology/resources/tools/). Simple adaptations were made to the mobile robot to enable the activities (i.e., attaching a ruler to the side of the robot). A method to do a task analysis of the activity and assign parts of the task to the robot, an environmental adaptation, or a helper is available (Adams 2011).

Several robot-mediated language, mathematics, and science and social studies activities have been proposed (Encarnação et al. 2016). In this study, children with neuromotor disabilities used an integrated augmentative manipulation and communication assistive technologies (IAMCAT) system in which a Lego Mindstorms NXT robot was controlled through the computer-based GRID 2 communication software. Many activities were performed, including drawing lines to connect answers; putting story illustrations, letters, or sequences in order; carrying labels for matching words and letters, illustrations, or numbers; or labeling parts of pictures, following pathways on a map, measuring width with non-standard units, or carrying a certain number of items for working with numbers. Instructions, GRID samples, and activities can be found online (http://uarpie.anditec.pt/images/docs/user_manual_iamcat.zip).

Review of User Studies, Outcomes, and Clinical Evidence

Cognitive Assessment

Outcomes of Cognitive Assessment Studies

Several studies have shown that children with disabilities are able to use a robotic system as a tool for augmentative manipulation. Children as young as 7 to 9 months old were able to use an industrial robotic manipulator to bring a cookie closer (Cook, Liu, and Hoseit 1990). Such a finding is consistent with the typical development literature, in which at approximately 9 months children can use objects as tools to retrieve other objects (Claxton, McCarty, and Keen 2009). Cook et al. (2000) reported that children who were unable to directly manipulate objects in their environment were able to use a robotic arm to handle and manipulate objects in a playful scenario. Besides tool use, robot-mediated activities have proven to be a means to demonstrate other cognitive skills, such as cause and effect, inhibition, laterality, and sequencing (Encarnação et al. 2014; Poletz et al. 2010); problem solving and spatial reasoning (Cook et al. 2007, 2011); or conservation (Mainela-Arnold, Evans, and Alibali 2006). These studies showed that cognitive skills revealed by robot use were correlated with the

---

CASE STUDY 7.1 (CONTINUED)   JOSEPH'S COGNITIVE ASSESSMENT NEED

Joseph's OT considers using a robot-adapted version of the conservation task mentioned previously to gain insight into Joseph's current cognitive skills. His OT first considers the human component, as per the HAAT model (cf. Chapter 1). Due to his physical disability, Joseph cannot talk or manipulate objects independently, which limits his ability to make a selection. His nystagmus prevents him from using visual fixation as a reliable response. The OT carefully analyzes the activity and its demands. To participate in the conservation task, Joseph requires a means through which he can reliably and independently express his choice. In addition, his OT wonders whether the limited opportunities afforded to Joseph to independently interact with objects would have limited his ability to develop the cognitive skills required to succeed in the task in the first place. Thus, a gap exists between Joseph's current skills and the demands of the activity, which restricts his participation in the conservation task. The OT concludes that a robotic system for augmentative manipulation could bridge that gap. The OT set up the Microbot TeachMover (as in Figure 7.2), adapted for switch control. The OT placed two switches, one to each side of Joseph's headrest, as she has identified this to be the best site of motor control for Joseph. One switch causes the robot to reach for the container on the left and the other to the container on the right. The OT set up the conservation task and programmed the robot to reach toward the container after a switch selection is made. First, Joseph demonstrated that he understood the concept of laterality by performing the cognitive utilization protocol that required him to knock over stacks of blocks (described previously). After he demonstrated that he could use the appropriate switch to make choices on his left or right side, Joseph was presented with the conservation task. When asked to make a selection, he was able to press the left or right switch to turn the robot toward the response he believed to be the correct one. This provided the OT and parents with unprecedented insight into Joseph's specific cognitive skills and unveiled further potential. Further, after the assessment, the robot could be used as an intervention strategy to help Joseph engage in activities that would increase his understanding of volume, such as pouring water into different size containers. Experiences like these could ultimately improve the mental representations that lead to fully developed conservation skills.

children's developmental age, in line with cognitive development literature. This validates the use of robot-mediated activities as a proxy measure of cognitive development through the comparison of the performance of children with disabilities executing the tasks with that of typically developing children. These studies have also provided the first set of normative data in this regard.

Play

Outcomes of Play Studies

The literature regarding the use of robots to promote play in children with disabilities is scarce. In many studies, play is approached as an activity that promotes or assists the assessment of other skills in the child, such as cognitive development, or play is approached as a motivator during research or therapeutic sessions. This is the case of the robotic applications to assess cognitive skills described in the previous section. Under these two approaches, the play activities were structured and goal oriented; the research team specified the target that the child had to accomplish. Besides the small number of studies that have used robots to promote semistructured activities or free play, the number of participants in each study was also small (between 1 and 10 participants, in the last case all typically developing children). Participants' age ranged from 3 to 11 years. The fact that children younger than 3 years of age were not participants in the studies may be due to the skills required to operate a robot, at least using two switches or more. This can be cognitively demanding for children younger than 4 years of age (Poletz et al. 2010). From a theoretical point of view, an individual experiences pleasure and enjoyment while doing an activity only when there is a balance or a good match between the individual's skills and the challenges of a task (Csikszentmihalyi 2008). Thus, children younger than 4 years of age may not express play behaviors when operating a robot because their cognitive skills may be too low to understand the relationship between the control interface and the robot's movements.

Using robots to promote play in children with motor impairment has been focused mainly on children with a diagnosis of CP, including children with quadriplegia and hemiplegia. This may be due to CP being the most common childhood neurodisability (Eliasson et al. 2006). Other childhood diagnoses related to motor impairments were general developmental delay and transverse spinal cord syndrome (Klein et al. 2011; Prazak et al. 2004). Some studies included children with diagnoses related to cognitive functions, such as global cognitive disability (Kronreif et al. 2007), tuberous sclerosis, and attention deficit/hyperactive disorder, along with children with motor impairments (Marti and Iacono 2011).

Outcomes reported in these studies have consistently been the observation of behaviors such as enjoyment, pleasure, curiosity, active engagement, spontaneity, teasing, and sense of control, all related to play, which occur when children interact with the robot that they are able to operate (Besio, Carnesecchi, and Converti 2013; Cook et al. 2000; Kronreif et al. 2007; Marti and Iacono 2011). Children improve their performance in operating the robot as they practice during play, needing fewer prompts, making fewer errors, and performing the task faster, but they need practice to carry out the most complex tasks (Besio, Carnesecchi, and Converti 2013; Cook et al. 2000; Kronreif et al. 2007; Schulmeister et al. 2006). Other outcomes have been an increase in the child's attention span and frequency of smiles and vocalizations and an improvement in the participant's memory (Schulmeister et al. 2006). Ríos-Rincón and colleagues explored the effects of a robot on mother-child interaction, finding that when children used the robot to access play, mothers tended to decrease their directiveness, allowing the children to be more independent and active during the play interaction (Ríos-Rincón 2014).

Robots have the potential to improve not only children's playfulness and play performance, but also the quality of support of the able-bodied playmates who became more enabling during play. Ríos-Rincón and colleagues explored the use of robots at children's homes in family play routines involving their mothers (Ríos-Rincón et al. 2016). The Lego Mindstorms RCX with an adapted remote control was used by children. The results revealed that the levels of playfulness of all the children, measured using the Test of Playfulness (Bundy 2010), showed a statistically significant increase, and the play performance, measured through the Canadian Occupational Therapy Measure (COPM) (Law et al. 1998), showed a clinically significant improvement according to the COPM manual criteria when the children played with the robot (Ríos-Rincón et al. 2016). The mothers' tendency to direct the play of the child was reduced when the children had access to the robot to play (Ríos-Rincón 2014).

Adams and colleagues investigated the type of play (no play, functional, and pretend) expressed by typically developing children while playing in two conditions: with and without a robot (Adams et al. 2016). A coding system according to Barton's taxonomy of pretend play (Barton 2010)

CASE STUDY 7.2 (CONTINUED)   JUAN'S PLAY NEED SOLUTION

Juan had the physical ability to activate four Jelly Bean switches, so these were utilized to operate a Lego Mindstorms RCX car-like vehicle. The switches were plugged into an adapted remote control, based on the original commercial Lego remote control with switch jacks wired to the remote control circuit board (as in Figure 7.4). The forward switch was located close to Juan's forearm. A right turn switch was attached to the wheelchair's right-hand side using a mounted arm and a left turn switch was attached to the wheelchair's left-hand side, both of them to be hit using Juan's head movements. A backward switch was located on an adapted footrest attached to the wheelchair to be activated by Juan's left foot. Juan had four training sessions in the use of the switches to make the robot move and carry objects. Once he was able to operate the robot, Juan and his mother were encouraged to play together. During the robotic sessions, he made many vocalizations, trying to tell his mom about what he was doing and what he required from her to do what he wanted with the robot and the toys. He explored what to do with the robots and his toys and showed great creativity; for example, he asked his mother to put a toy car, which was about five times bigger than the robot, on top of the robot; initially, his mother refused to do it, but he insisted. When Juan's mother placed the toy on the robot, the robot was able to carry it for a short distance. Thus, the child showed that he was able to explore an object's physical property (weight) while playing with the robot. He also asked his mother to build a pile of plastic donuts so he could hit the pile with the robot to make them fall down. Then, he modified the activity and asked his mother to put the pile of donuts on top of the robot. He designed different strategies to make the donuts fall down, for example, making the robot hit the board edge and making the robot oscillate (forward and backward) to destabilize the pile of toy donuts. During the robotic sessions, Juan used the robot as a tool that supported his independence and participation during free play. Compared to sessions without the robot, he was more responsive, more active, and less compliant in following his mother's lead; he provided ideas for the play activity and was able to lead the play.

was developed and implemented to code the different levels of play (no play, functional play, and pretend play). The results revealed that the scenarios elicited play at the expected developmental levels for the no-robot condition but not for the robot condition. It was also found that children presented a higher percentage of pretend play without the robot than with the robot for both conventional toys and unstructured materials. Researchers hope to use these results to use the robotic scenarios as a proxy of play development in children with motor impairment (Adams et al. 2016).

Education

Outcomes of Education Studies

As mentioned, a literature search revealed only seven recent user studies reporting the use for academic activities of robots for augmentative manipulation by children with physical impairments. The sample sizes in these studies with children with disabilities were very small, with two studies being case studies (Adams and Cook 2013, 2016a), two being a series of case studies (Adams and Cook 2014, 2016b; Adams, David, and Helmbold 2016, in review), and one study having nine participants (Encarnação et al. 2016, in press). The age of the case study participants was between 10 and 14 years, and the study with nine participants worked with young children, 3 to 6 years old. The studies have included children with CP (Adams and Cook 2013; Encarnação et al. 2016), traumatic brain injury, and global development delay (Encarnação et al. 2016). In addition, 20 participants 2 to 5 years old without disabilities used an augmentative manipulation robot to test the system before planned trials with children with disabilities (Lee 2013).

Determining the outcomes to track in order to evaluate the benefits of robot intervention is in the exploratory stages, and studies have included many varied outcomes. One outcome is children's engagement in the robotic system (Lee 2013), or satisfaction with the robot compared to other ways of doing activities, for example, measuring with the robot compared to watching a teacher do the measuring (Adams and Cook 2014, 2016b; Adams and David 2013a). In general, children have preferred to do the manipulation themselves with the robot, except when measuring long objects, which took a long time.

Another outcome studied was children's skill of using the robot or access method to perform activities. The robot competency skills framework described previously (Adams and Cook 2016b) can be used to frame these outcomes. For instance, robot operational skill was tracked as the amount of distance a robot "game piece" traveled outside the board game pathway compared to the distance within the board game pathway (Adams and Cook 2016b). In another study, the operational skill of using the scanning access method to control the cursor to do robot programming was tracked. In this case, poor operational control resulted in a number of unwanted cursor movements and long task times (Adams and Cook 2013). Linguistic competency using the communication device voice output was tracked in a study in which the participant used her communication device to move the robot and say the lines for the characters in the story; the participant generated utterances two and three words long, which were longer than her usual one-word utterances in normal conversation (Adams and Cook 2016b).

Participation in the curriculum is another outcome. For example, the "run" command from the Lego robot remote control was trained into a participant's communication device, allowing her to run the robot programs of the other students in a science class where students were learning to program Lego robots (Adams and Cook 2013). In this way, the participant had a central role in the classroom as she tested her classmates' robot programs. In work by Encarnação et al. (2016), all the children in the class did the same activity, but the children with disabilities did the activity with the integrated augmentative manipulation and communication robotic system. Participation in these studies was alongside other students in the classroom. Participation in the curriculum can also be done in one-on-one sessions. For example, in the study reported by Adams and Cook (2013), programming of the participant's own car-like mobile robot was performed in pull-out sessions due to the level of support needed by the student to do the required tasks. Likewise, gaining experience performing hands-on mathematics activities, including puzzles, number games, or connect-the-numbered dots pictures, was done in one-on-one sessions (Adams and Cook 2016b).

Robot use has enabled teachers to evaluate children's understanding against the standard curriculum rubrics. Success or failure of saying an English letter appropriately was observed when children used a robot (Lee 2013). In addition, teachers have assessed student's mathematical procedures and concepts (Adams and Cook 2014, 2016a) and discovered gaps in students' knowledge, which the students' teaching team attributed to the students not previously having "hands-on" experience in the activities.

Teacher opinion of robot system use was another outcome studied. Stakeholders have indicated that robots in the classroom have a role, with obvious benefits to the children with disabilities and the class, but they are leery of required technical support, even with the simple Lego robot (Adams and Cook 2014; Encarnação et al. 2016). In one study, teachers thought that using the robot was the most effective way for the students to show what they know compared to other methods of manipulating objects in class, i.e., observing a teacher doing manipulation and responding to her questions, or telling the teacher using their communication devices how to manipulate the objects (Adams and David 2013a). The teachers in the classrooms in the work of Encarnação et al. (2016) thought that a robot

CASE STUDY 7.3 (CONTINUED)   JULIA'S EDUCATION NEED

The intended mathematics activity for Julia was to practice with multiplication by making arrays representing statements. For instance, there are four ducks on the pond, each with two feet; how many feet in total are there? Other students in the class placed 1-in. (2.54-cm) square blocks into tightly packed arrays with the required rows and columns and then counted them. Julia has the physical ability to point to and lightly press items on a touch screen, as long as it is positioned within her reach. Because she already had the iPad mini mounted on her wheelchair, options to control a robot through the iPad mini were explored. Lego provides a free download Robot Commander app to control the Lego NXT and EV3 robots. Only the Lego EV3 is controllable from the iPad products. Julia performed a trial of one of the built-in Robot Commander interfaces to control the EV3 and gripper. Several adaptations to the robot, environment, and the app were needed. For instance, rather than using a gripper, which made the blocks shift at an angle when it closed, a scoop built to the size of the blocks was used (Figure 7.5). Grid paper was placed in a box so that Julia could push the

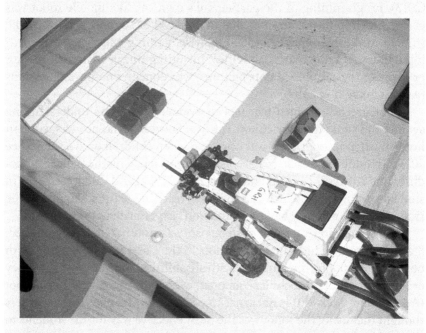

Figure 7.5 A Lego Mindstorms EV3 robot used by Julia to put blocks into arrays to study multiplication. The scoop in the front of the robot was designed so the blocks would fit without spinning. The array of two rows with three objects in each row represents the multiplication equation $3 \times 2 = 6$.

blocks up to the edge of the box to line them up. Julia had trouble using the joystick in the Robot Commander interface to control the robot. When she tried to move the joystick forward she moved it a little to the side as well, which caused the robot to make a large turn. The app allows one to make their own interfaces, so another interface was made with a slider that controlled a motor. The left and right motors for the robot wheels were given the same signal (by making a wire that split one signal to two); thus, only straight forward and backward were possible. The activity was accomplished by Julia with a little assistance from a helper. After placing a block, Julia would request another and ask for the robot to be repositioned one column over, so she could proceed to place the next block. Julia reported that she preferred using the robot over using a screen-based app on her iPad to do the arrays. The teacher expressed that she was confident in assessing Julia's understanding of the multiplication concept when Julia used the robot to manipulate the blocks into arrays.

system was useful and had a positive impact on children with disabilities and the classmates and other teachers. However, they found it difficult to manage the extra time required by children with disabilities to complete the activities. According to Adams and Cook (2016a), teachers felt that some measuring activities were too complex for the children to perform (e.g., measuring a curved surface).

Future Directions

Available research has shown that robot use by children with physical impairments has the potential for many positive outcomes, but further studies are needed to examine the benefits and challenges of using robots for cognitive development, play, and educational activities. Current evidence is mostly based on case studies in which children used the robotic systems for a short period of time in relatively artificial conditions (in a lab or at school but with a research team present). Thus, the level of clinical evidence about the effects of robotics interventions on developmental outcomes in cognitive development, play, and education is low. In the area of assistive technology, single-case research designs (which when carefully designed provide higher evidence than case studies) are recommended and appropriate due to the heterogeneity of the population and the individualized interventions required (Ottenbacher and Hinderer 2001). There is the need to conduct single-case research design studies for longer periods of time in a natural setting (home, classroom, and community) to raise the levels of evidence about the effects of the robotic systems.

Other areas of play and education should be examined. For instance, the use of augmentative manipulation robotic systems has been shown to have positive effects on mother-child interaction during free play (Ríos-Rincón et al. 2016). Further research should focus on the effects of robotic interventions on other interactions, such as those of a child with motor impairments with other family members (e.g., fathers, siblings, and cousins) and peers with and without disabilities during free-play activities. In the area of education, experimental results relating to the expected outcomes in the programs of study that are taught in the schools will truly align with what is actually happening in the classroom. Assessment instruments that evaluate outcomes of the interventions should be created.

Studies should be widely disseminated and translated into easily accessible resources to increase awareness of potential benefits among stakeholders such as parents, therapists, educators, researchers, and funding agencies (Cooper et al. 1999; Tejada et al. 2007). Resources and databases for parents and therapists that integrate robotic play should be created and evaluated. More resources for teachers who integrate the robotic tools directly with curriculum materials are needed (Cooper et al. 1999; Tejada et al. 2007).

Technical development is needed to develop appropriate, robust, easy-to-use assistive robots for children with physical impairments. The only robots used in studies with children that are presently commercially available are the Lego robots, and although they are inexpensive, safe, and flexible, they have limitations. They are fragile and require frequent minor adjustments; they have limited payloads; and limited environmental sensing and navigation capabilities may limit the degree of autonomy that can be achieved (Cook, Encarnação, and Adams 2010).

Standard robot control software is needed to enable the use of the same program across robotic systems (Howell, Martz, and Stanger 1996). The open source Robotics Operating System (ROS) has gained some ground in the last few years and could be a useful tool for programmers. However, if robots are to be useful at home and in hospitals and the classroom, the user interface must be simple. Another approach is to have a wide range of applications for a common robotic platform (Cooper et al. 1999). When an appropriate robot is commercially available, it enables researchers to build technology and strategies with it; this is the situation with the MANUS robotic arm, which evolved over decades to become the iArm (Brose et al. 2010) (cf. Chapter 3).

Guidelines for reproducing or emulating previously utilized prototypes could increase effort into researching and developing assistive robotics for children. A template has been proposed for facilitating the understanding of the various interdependent hardware and software components of a typical assistive robot for children with cognitive disabilities (Tsun et al. 2015). The authors gave a concrete example of how it was used in development of a robotic system for children, but no evidence of other researchers using it was found. Although not specifically proposed for development of augmentative manipulation systems, the basic concepts could be applied.

There are various interfaces that can be used to interact with assistive technologies, but the control interfaces most commonly used in the robot studies discussed were switches, followed by touch screens, motion detection, and joysticks. The lower cost and availability of innovative controls should be pursued, such as eye tracking or brain-computer interfaces. Recent innovations in intelligent techniques to switch between items to be controlled with few input signals could be beneficial, for instance, to switch between robot controls and augmentative communication software or between forward movement of a robot and turns (Pilarski et al. 2012).

Many recent technological developments can potentially facilitate children's functioning in tasks. For example, now that vision systems have decreased in cost, they could be beneficial tools for detecting objects of interest in the environment so the robot can autonomously interact with them. In addition, the human technology interface can be made to better reflect the environmental situation (e.g., detecting if objects are hard or soft). With the robotic systems available today, the user is able to experience picking and placing objects. But, the interfaces do not provide the sensation of feeling different textures or allow children to move an object in order to be able to see it from different perspectives and explore all its features; children do not feel the different weights of different objects or freely explore the object. The activities performed have been structured, mainly because of the technical limitations of the robotic systems. Independent exploration is important for cognitive and perceptual development. There are tactile sensors available that require some sort of additional device to relay the information to the body (i.e., a pad attached to the upper arm). Kinesthetic touch information can be fed back to the user through the robotic interface, providing a richer manipulative experience, and could require less time to set up the system (Atashzar et al. 2016; Jafari, Adams, and Tavakoli 2015).

In addition, as children become more proficient using the robots with experience, it is important that they continue to be challenged to take on as much of the task as appropriate. The level of autonomy of the robotics system could adapt automatically to the user's capabilities by using machine learning capabilities.

More than 10 years ago, Howell (2005) predicted that it will take years to develop an easy-to-use, cost-effective, and reliable assistive robot for home and classroom use, and once developed, it will take more time to develop appropriate activities. The need is still present, as there have been recent calls to develop appropriate robots for children with disabilities (Cook, Encarnação, and Adams 2010). Significant advances have been made in robotics for activities of daily living (Brose et al. 2010) and robots for seniors (Broadbent, Stafford, and MacDonald 2009; further described in Chapter 9 of this book) as far as commercializing systems and addressing safety and usability concerns. It is hoped this momentum will carry into the development of robotics for children with physical disabilities to manipulate play and learning objects because the benefits to children could be significant.

STUDY QUESTIONS

1. List the HAAT components for each case study.
2. Discuss the impact of motor skills on the cognitive development of young children.
3. Based on Joseph's case, design an activity in which Joseph could use a robot to demonstrate his cognitive skills (assessment).
4. Based on your response to question 3, adapt the activity demands so that Joseph can use the robot to further develop that skill (intervention).
5. What are the most common features of play as an occupation?
6. Define these types of play: functional play, pretend play, and object play.
7. How does physical impairment affect children's engagement in play alone and with others?
8. Explain why promoting play in children with motor impairment is important for their functioning.
9. Based on Juan's case, design an activity in which Juan could use a robot to engage in play with family members.
10. How does physical impairment affect children's engagement in education?
11. Based on Julia's case, design an activity in which Julia could use a robot to do an addition problem or a division problem.
12. What are some features that have made Lego Mindstorms robotic systems feasible to use in children's real educational contexts?
13. Name some factors that should be addressed to facilitate the adoption of robots in homes and schools.
14. What are some new technologies that may be beneficial for children using robots for cognitive assessment, play, or education?

References

Adams, K. "Access to math activities for children with disabilities by controlling Lego robots via augmentative and alternative communication devices." Doctoral dissertation, Faculty of Rehabilitation Medicine, University of Alberta, 2011.

Adams, K., and A. Cook. "Programming and controlling robots using scanning on a speech generating communication device: A case study." *Technology and Disability* 25 (2013): 275–286.

Adams, K., and A. Cook. "Access to hands-on mathematics measurement activities using robots controlled via speech generating devices: Three case studies." *Disability and Rehabilitation: Assistive Technology* 9, no. 4 (2014): 286–298.

Adams, K., and A. Cook. "Performing mathematics activities with non-standard units of measurement using robots controlled via speech generating devices: Three case studies." *Disability and Rehabilitation: Assistive Technology* March 15 (2016a): 1–13. [Epub ahead of print]

Adams, K., and A. Cook. "Using robots in 'hands-on' academic activities: A case study examining speech-generating device use and required skills." *Disability and Rehabilitation: Assistive Technology* no. 11 (2016b): 433–443.

Adams, K., and B.-L. David. *Making Hands-on Activities for Everyone: Math and the Lego Mindstorms Robot*. Edmonton, Alberta: Alberta Teacher's Association Library, 2013a.

Adams, K., and B.-L. David. "Methods of manipulation for children with severe disabilities to do hands-on math activities: Robot, directing, guiding." Presentation at the RESNA conference, Bellevue, WA, June, 2013b.

Adams, K., and P. Encarnação. "A training protocol for controlling lego robots via speech generating devices." In: *Everyday Technology for Independence and Care—AAATE 2011*, G.J. Gelderblom, M. Soede, L. Adriaens, and K. Miesenberger (eds.). Assistive Technology Research Series, vol. 29. Amsterdam: IOS Press, 2011: 517–525.

Adams, K., A. Ríos, L. Becerra, and P. Esquivel. "Using robots to access play at different developmental levels for children with severe disabilities: A pilot study." Presentation at the RESNA Conference, Denver, CO, June, 2015.

Adams, K., A. Rios Rincon, L. Becerra, J. Castanellos, M. Gomez, A.M. Cook, and P. Encarnação. "An exploratory study of children's pretend play when using a switch-controlled assistive robot to manipulate toys." Manuscript submitted for review, 2016.

Affolter, F. "From action to interaction as primary root for development." In: *Movement and Action in Learning and Development: Clinical Implications for Pervasive Developmental Disorders*, I. Stockman (ed.). San Diego, CA: Elsevier, 2004: 169–199.

Alvarez, L. "A robot journey into developmental pathways: Exploring cognitive skills of young children with motor impairments." Doctoral dissertation, Faculty of Rehabilitation Medicine, University of Alberta, 2014.

Alvarez, L., K. Adams, and A. Cook. "Quantifying the complexity of using robots as augmentative manipulation tools: An affordances perspective." Manuscript submitted for review, 2016.

American Occupational Therapy Association. "Occupational therapy practice framework: Domain and process (3rd ed.)." *The American Journal of Occupational Therapy* 68, Supplement 1 (2014): s1–s48.

Atashzar, F., N. Jafari, M. Shahbazi, H. Janz, M. Tavakoli, Rajni Patel, and K. Adams. "Telerobotics-assisted platform for enhancing interaction with physical environments designed for people living with cerebral palsy." *Journal of Medical and Rehabilitation Robotics, Special Issue on Rehabilitation Robotics* (2016).

Barton, E. "Development of a taxonomy of pretend play for children with disabilities." *Infants and Young* 23, no. 4 (2010): 247–261.

Bates, E. "The biology of symbols: Some concluding thoughts." In: *The Emergence of Symbols: Cognition and Communication in Infancy*, by E. Bates, L. Benigni, I. Bretherton, L. Camaioni, and V. Volterra. New York: Academic Press, 1979: 315–370.

Bertenthal, B.I., and J.J. Campos. "New directions in the study of early experience." *Child Development* 58, no. 3 (1987): 560–567.

Besio, S., F. Caprino, and E. Laudanna. "Profiling robot-mediated play for children with disabilities through ICF-CY: The example of the European Project IROMEC." Paper presented at the 11th International Conference on Computers Helping People with Special Needs—ICCHP'0, Linz, Austria, July 9–11, 2008.

Besio, S., M. Carnesecchi, and R.M. Converti. "Prompt-fading strategies in robot mediated play sessions." In: *Assistive Technology: From Research to Practice*, P. Encarnação, L. Azevedo, G. J. Gelderblom, A. Newell, and N.-E. Mathiassen (eds.). Vilamoura, Algarve, Portugal: IOS Press, 2013: 143–149.

Blanche, E.I. "Play in children with cerebral palsy: Doing with-not doing to." In: *Play in Occupational Therapy for Children*, D. Parham and L. Fazio (eds.). St. Louis, MO: Mosby Elsevier, 2008: 375–393.

Broadbent, E., R. Stafford, and B. MacDonald. "Acceptance of healthcare robots for the older population: Review and future directions." *International Journal of Social Robotics* 1, no. 4 (2009): 319–330.

Brodin, J. "Diversity of aspects on play in children with profound multiple disabilities." *Early Child Development and Care* 175, no. 7 and 8 (2005): 635–646.

Brose, S.W., D.J. Weber, B.A. Salatin, G.G. Grindle, H. Wang, J.J. Vazquez, and R.A. Cooper. "The role of assistive robotics in the lives of persons with disability." *American Journal of Physical Medicine & Rehabilitation* 89, no. 6 (2010): 509–521.

Bundy, A. "Assessment of play and leisure: Delineation of the problem." *American Journal of Occupational Therapy* 47, no. 3 (1993): 217–222.

Bundy, A. "Test of playfulness (ToP)." Version 4.2. Manual revised 11/10. Lidcombe: Unpublished document, 2010.

Chang, H.-J., L.A. Chiarello, R.J. Palisano, M.N. Orlin, A. Bundy, and E.J. Gracely. "The determinants of self-determined behaviors of young children with cerebral palsy." *Research in Developmental Disabilities* 35 (2014): 99–109.

Chen, Z., R.P. Sanchez, and T. Campbell. "From beyond to within their grasp: The rudiments of analogical problem solving." *Developmental Psychology* 33, no. 5 (1997): 790–801.

Claxton, L.J., M.E. McCarty, and R. Keen. "Self-directed action affects planning in tool-use tasks with toddlers." *Infant Behavior and Development* 32, no. 2 (2009): 230–233.

Cook, A., K. Adams, N. Harbottle, and C. Harbottle. "Using Lego robots to estimate cognitive ability in children who have severe disabilities." Presented at the RERC State of the Science Conference and Coleman Institute Annual Conference, Broomfield, CO, October, 2007.

Cook, A. M., K. Adams, J. Volden, N. Harbottle, and C. Harbottle. "Using Lego robots to estimate cognitive ability in children who have severe physical disabilities." *Disability and Rehabilitation. Assistive Technology* 6, no. 4 (2011): 338–346.

Cook, A. M., B. Bentz, N. Harbottle, C. Lynch, and B. Miller. "School-based use of a robotic arm system by children with disabilities." *IEEE Transactions on Neural Systems and Rehabilitation Engineering* 13, no. 4 (2005): 452–460.

Cook, A., P. Encarnação, and K. Adams. "Robots: Assistive technologies for play, learning and cognitive development." *Technology and Disability* 22, no. 3 (2010): 127–145.

Cook, A., K. Howery, J. Gu, and M. Meng. "Robot enhanced interaction and learning for children with profound physical disabilities." *Technology and Disability* 13, no. 1 (2000): 1–8.

Cook, A.M., K.M. Liu, and P. Hoseit. "Robotic arm use by very young children." *Assistive Technology: The Official Journal of RESNA* 2, no. 2 (1990): 51–57.

Cook, A., M.Q.-H. Meng, J.J. Gu, and K. Howery. "Development of a robotic device for facilitating learning by children who have severe disabilities." *IEEE Transactions on Neural Systems and Rehabilitation Engineering* 10, no. 3 (2002): 178–187.

Cook, A., and J.M. Polgar. *Assistive Technologies: Principles and Practices.* 4th ed. Philadelphia: Elsevier, 2015.

Cooper, M., D. Keating, W. Harwin, and K. Dautenhahn. "Robots in the classroom— Tools for accessible education." Presented at the AAATE Conference, the 5th European Conference for the Advancement of Assistive Technology, Dusseldorf, Germany, September, 1999.

Coplan, R., K. Rubin,., and L. Findlay. Social and nonsocial play. In: *Play from Birth to Twelve: Contexts, Perspectives, and Meaning,* D. Fromberg and D. Bergen (eds.). New York: Garland, 2006: 75–86.

Csikszentmihalyi, M. *Flow the Psychology of Optimal Experience.* New York: Harper Perennial, 2008.

Eberhart, S.P., J. Osborne, and T. Rahman. "Classroom evaluation of the Arlyn Arm Robotic Workstation." *Assistive Technology* 12 (2000): 132–143.

Eliasson, A.C., S.L. Krumlinde, B. Rösblad, E. Beckung, M. Arner, A.M. Öhrvall, and P. Rosenbaum. "The Manual Ability Classification System (MACS) for children with cerebral palsy: Scale development and evidence of validity and reliability." *Developmental Medicine and Child Neurology* 48 (2006): 549–554.

Encarnação, P., L. Alvarez, A. Rios, C. Maya, K. Adams, and A. Cook. "Using virtual robot mediated play activities to assess cognitive skills." *Disability and Rehabilitation: Assistive Technology* 9, no. 3 (2014): 231–241.

Encarnação, P., T. Leite, C. Nunes, M. Nunes da Ponte, K. Adams, A. Cook, A. Caiado et al. "Using assistive robots to promote inclusive education." *Disability and Rehabilitation: Assistive Technology* April 26 (2016): 1–21. [Epub ahead of print]

Eriksson, L., J. Welander, and M. Granlund. "Participation in everyday school activities for children with and without disabilities." *Journal of Developmental and Physical Disabilities* 19 (2007): 485–502.

Ferasoli-Filho, H., M.A. Corbucci Caldeira, R. Pegoraro, S.F. dos Reis Alves, C. Valadão, and T. Freire Bastos-Filho. "Use of myoelectric signals to command mobile entertainment robot by disabled children: Design and control architecture." Paper presented at the Biosignals and Biorobotics Conference (BRC), January, 2012.

Ferland, F. *The Ludic Model:Play, Children with Physical Disabilities and Occupational Therapy.* 2nd ed. Translated by P. Aronoff and H. Scott. Ottawa: CAOT Publications ACE, 2005.

Flanagan, J.R., M.C. Bowman, and R.S. Johansson. "Control strategies in object manipulation tasks." *Current Opinion in Neurobiology* 16, no. 6 (2006): 650–659.

Gowen, J.W., N. Jonhson-Martin, B. Davis Goldman, and B. Hussey. "Object play and exploration in children with and without disabilities: A longitudinal study." *American Journal of Mental Retardation* 97 (1992): 21–38.

Greenfield, P. "Language, tools and brain: The ontogeny and phylogeny of hierarchically organized sequential behavior." *Behavioral and Brain Sciences* 14, no. 4 (1991): 531–551.

Harkness, L., and A. Bundy. "The test of playfulness and children with physical disabilities." *The Occupational Therapy Journal of Research* 21, no. 2 (2001): 73–89.

Harwin, W., A. Ginige, and R. Jackson. "A potential application in early education and a possible role for a vision system in a workstation based robotic aid for physically disabled." *Interactive Robotic Aids—One Option for Independent Living: An International Perspective* 37 (1986): 18–23.

Harwin, W., A. Ginige, and R. Jackson. "A robot workstation for use in education of the physically handicapped." *IEEE Transactions on Biomedical Engineering* 35, no. 2 (1988): 127–131.

Hinojosa, J., and P. Kramer. "Integrating children with disabilities into family play." In: *Play in Occupational Therapy for Children*, D. Parham and L. Fazio (eds.). St. Louis, MO: Mosby Elsevier, 2008: 321–334.

Howell, R. "Robotic devices as assistive and educational tools for persons with disabilities." In: *Handbook of Special Education Technology Research and Practice*, D. Edyburn, K. Higgins, and R. Boone (eds.). Whitefish Bay, WI: Knowledge by Design, 2005: 849–862.

Howell, R., and K. Hay. "Software-based access and control of robotic manipulators for severely physically disabled students." *Journal of Artificial Intelligence in Education* 1, no. 1 (1989): 53–72.

Howell, R., S. Martz, and C. A. Stanger. "Classroom applications of educational robots for inclusive teams of students with and without disabilities." *Technology and Disability* 5 (1996): 139–150.

Jafari, N., K. Adams, and M. Tavakoli. "Haptic telerobotics: Application to assistive technology for children with disabilities." Paper presented at the Rehabilitation Engineering and Assistive Technology Society of North America (RESNA) Annual Conference, Denver, CO, June, 2015.

Jennings, K., and R. MacTurk. "The motivational characteristics of infants and children physical and sensory impairments." In: *Mastery Motivation: Origins, Conceptualization and Applications*, R. Macturk and G. Morgan (eds.). Norwood, NJ: Ablex, 1995: 201–220.

Keen, K. "The development of problem solving in young children: A critical cognitive skill." *Annual Review of Psychology* 62 (2011): 1–21.

Klein, T., G.J. Gelderblom, L. de Witte, and S. Vanstipelen. "Evaluation of short term effects of the IROMEC robotic toy for children with developmental disabilities." Presented at IEEE International Conference on Rehabilitation Robotics. ETH Zurich Science City, Switzerland, June–July, 2011.

Kohlschütter, A., and F. Eichler. "Childhood leukodystrophies: A clinical perspective." *Expert Review of Neurotherapeutics* 11, no. 10 (2011): 1485–1496.

Kronreif, G., M. Kornfeld, B. Prazac, S. Mina, and M. Fürst. "Robot assistance in playful environment—User trials and results." *IEEE International Conference on Robotics and Automation* September (2007): 2898–2903.

Kwee, H., and J. Quaedackers. "Pocus Project: Adapting the control of the Manus manipulator for persons with cerebral palsy." Paper presented at the ICORR '99: International Conference on Rehabilitation Robotics, Stanford, CA, July 1999.

Law, M., S. Baptiste, A. Carswell, M.A. McColl, H. Polatajko, and N. Pollock. *The Canadian Occupational Performance Measure*. 3rd ed. Ottawa: CAOT Publications ACE, July, 1998.

Lee, Hou Tsan. "Voice controlled typesetting robot of alphabets for children learning." *Journal of Information Technology and Application in Education* 2, no. 1 (2013): 47–54.

Light, J. "Toward a definition of communicative competence for individuals using augmentative and alternative communication systems." *AAC Augmentative and Alternative Communication* 5, no. 2 (1989): 137–144.

Lockman, J.J. "A perception-action perspective on tool use development." *Child Development* 71, no. 1 (2000): 137–144.

Lockman, J.J. "Tool use from a perception–action perspective: Developmental and evolutionary considerations." In: *Stone Knapping: The Necessary Conditions for a Uniquely Hominid Behaviour*, V. Roux and B. Bril (eds.). Cambridge, UK: McDonald Institute for Archaeological Research, (2005): 319–330.

Mainela-Arnold, E., J.L. Evans, and M.W. Alibali. "Understanding conservation delays in children with specific language impairment: Task representations revealed in speech and gesture." *Journal of Speech, Language, and Hearing Research: JSLHR* 49, no. 6 (2006): 1267–1279.

Marti, P., and I. Iacono. "Learning through play with a robot companion." In: *Everyay Technology for Independence and Care*, G.J. Gelderblom, M. Soede, L. Adriaens, and K. Miesenberger (eds.). Assistive Technology Research Series, vol. 29. Amsterdam: IOS Press, 2011: 526–533.

McCarthy, C. B. "Effects of thematic-based, hands-on science teaching versus a textbook approach for students with disabilities." *Journal of Research in Science Teaching* 42, no. 3 (2005): 245–263.

McCarty, M.E., R.K. Clifton, and R.R. Collard. "Problem solving in infancy: The emergence of an action plan." *Developmental Psychology* 35, no. 4 (1999): 1091–1101.

McCarty, M.E., R.K. Clifton, and R. Collard. "The beginnings of tool use by infants and toddlers." *Infancy* 2, no. 2 (2001): 233–256.

McNaughton, D., J. Light, and K.B. Arnold. "'Getting your wheel in the door': Successful full-time employment experiences of individuals with cerebral palsy who use augmentative and alternative communication." *AAC Augmentative and Alternative Communication* 18 (2002): 59–76.

Missiuna, C., and N. Pollock. "Play deprivation in children with physical disabilities: The role of the occupational therapist in preventing secondary disability." *American Journal of Occupational Therapy* 45, no. 10 (1991): 882–888.

Mistrett, S., and A. Goetz. "Playing with switches." Center for Assistive Technology, University at Buffalo. n.d. http://letsplay.buffalo.edu/products/switches.doc.

Ottenbacher, K.J., and S.R. Hinderer. "Evidence-based practice: Methods to evaluate individual patient improvement." *American Journal of Physical Medicine and Rehabilitation* 80, no. 10 (2001): 786–796.

Parham, L. "Play in occupational therapy." In: *Play in Occupational Therapy for Children*, L. Parham and L. Fazio (eds.). St. Louis, MO: Mosby Elsevier, 2008: 3–39.

Petress, Ken. "What is meant by 'active learning'?" *Education* 128, no. 4 (2008): 566.

Pfeifer, L.I., A.M. Pacciulio, C.A. Dos Santos, J.L. Stagnitti, and K.E. Dos Santos. "Pretend play of children with cerebral palsy." *Physical and Occupational Therapy in Pediatrics* 31, no. 4 (2011): 390–402.

Piaget, J. *The Psychology of Intelligence*. London: Taylor & Francis, 1950.

Piaget, J. *Play, Dreams and Imitation*. New York: Norton, 1951.

Piaget, J. *The Construction of Reality in the Child*. London: Routledge, 1954.

Piaget, J., and B. Inhelder. *The Psychology of the Child*. New York: Basic Books, 1969.

Pilarski, P. M., M. R. Dawson, T. Degris, J. P. Carey, and R. S. Sutton. "Dynamic switching and real-time machine learning for improved human control of assistive biomedical robots." Paper presented at 2012 4th IEEE RAS and EMBS International Conference on the Biomedical Robotics and Biomechatronics (BioRob), Rome, June, 2012.

Plaisant, C., A. Druin, C. Lathan, K. Dakhane, K. Edwards, J. M. Vice, and J. Montemayor. "A storytelling robot for pediatric rehabilitation." Paper presented at the ASSETS'00, Arlington, VA, November, 2000.

Poletz, L., P. Encarnação, K. Adams, and A. Cook. "Robot skills and cognitive performance of preschool children." *Technology and Disability* 22 (2010): 117–126.

Prazak, B., G. Kronreif, A. Hochgatterer, and M. Fürts. "A toy robot for physically disabled children." *Technology and Disability* 16 (2004): 131–136.

Reilly, M. *Play as Exploratory Learning: Studies of Curiosity Behavior*. Beverly Hills, CA: Sage, 1974.

Ríos-Rincón, A.M. "Playfulness in children with severe cerebral palsy when using a robot." PhD dissertation, University of Alberta, Edmonton, 2014.

Ríos-Rincón, A.M., K. Adams, J. Magill-Evans, and A. Cook. "Playfulness in children with severe cerebral palsy when using a robot." *Physical and Occupational Therapy in Pediatrics* 36, no. 3 (2016). http://www.tandfonline .com/doi/abs/10.3109/01942638.2015.1076559.

Schlosser, R., D. McGhie-Richmond, S. Blackstien-Adler, P. Mirenda, K. Antonius, and P. Janzen. "Training a school team to integrate technology meaningfully into the curriculum: Effects on student participation." *Journal of Special Education Technology* 15, no. 1 (2000): 31–44.

Schulmeister, J., C. Wiberg, K. Adams, N. Harbottle, and A. Cook. "Robot assisted play for children with disabilities." Paper presented at RESNA Conference, Atlanta, May, 2006.

Schunk, D.H., J.R. Meece, and P.R. Pintrich. *Motivation in Education: Theory, Research, and Applications*. Toronto: Pearson Higher Education, 2012.

Skard, G., and A. Bundy. "Test of playfulness." In: *Play in Occupational Therapy for Children*, L.D. Parham and L.S. Fazio. St, Louis, MO: Mosby Elsevier, 2008: 71–93.

Smith, J., and M. Topping. "The introduction of a robotic aid to drawing into a school for physically handicapped children: A case study." *British Journal of Occupational Therapy* 59, no. 12 (1996): 565–569.

Solaz-Portolésa, J.J., and V. Sanjoséb. "Piagetian and neo-Piagetian variables in science problem solving: Directions for practice." *Ciências & Cognição* 13 (2008): 192–200.

St. Amant, R., and T.E. Horton. "Revisiting the definition of animal tool use." *Animal Behavior* 75 (2008): 1199–1208.

Stagnitti, K., and C. Unsworth. "The test–retest reliability of the Child-Initiated Pretend Play Assessment." *American Journal of Occupational Therapy* 58 (2004): 93–99.

Sutton-Smith, B. *The Ambiguity of Play*. London: Harvard University Press, 2001.

Tejada, S., N. Traft, M. Hutson, H. Bufford, M. Dooner, J. Hanson, G. Mauer et al. "Educational robots: Three models for the research of learning theories and human–robot interaction." Presented at the AAAI Workshop WS, Boston, July, 2007.

Tejima, N. "Rehabilitation robotics: A review." *Advanced Robotics* 14, no. 7 (2000): 551–564.

Tsun, M.T.K., L.B. Theng, H.S. Jo, and P.T. Hang Hui. "Robotics for assisting children with physical and cognitive disabilities." In: *Assistive Technologies for Physical and Cognitive Disabilities*, L.B. Theng (ed.). Hershey, PA: Medical Information Science Reference/IGI Global, 2015: 78–120.

U.S. Department of Energy. *Technology Readiness Assessment Guide*. Washington, DC: Office of Management, 2009.

Van De Walle, J.A., K.S. Karp, and J.M. Bay-Williams. *Elementary and Middle School Mathematics: Teaching Developmentally*. 7th ed. Boston: Allyn and Bacon, 2010.

Van Leeuwen, L., A. Smitsman, and C. Van Leeuwen. "Affordances, perceptual complexity, and the development of tool use." *Journal of Experimental Psychology* 20, no. 1 (1994): 174–191.

Vauclair, J. "Phylogenetic approach to object manipulation in human and ape infants." *Human Development* 27 (1984): 321–328.

Vygotsky, L. "Interaction between learning and development." In: *Readings on the Development of Children*. New York: Freeman, 29–36. Original work published in Vygotsky, L.S. *Mind and Society*. Cambridge, MA: Harvard University Press, 1978 (1997): 79–91.

8

Social Assistive Robots for Children with Complex Disabilities

Cathy Bodine, Levin Sliker, Michael Marquez, Cecilia Clark, Brian Burne, and Jim Sandstrum

Contents

Learning Objectives

After completing this chapter, readers will be able to

1. Describe socially assistive robots (SARs) and their clinical use with children who have disabilities.
2. Characterize pioneering SARs and current state of the science.

3. Explain applications and limitations of machine-based learning and how it applies to SAR design and development.
4. Describe the methodology used to define clinical intervention objectives and how to incorporate those assessment components in SAR applications.

Principles

Play Is Fundamental

Play has been described as the most important "work" of being a child (Glenn et al. 2013). Children learn cognitive, social, motor, and linguistic skills by manipulating objects in the context of play (Cardon 2011; Lee, Song, and Shin 2001; Roussou 2004). Play offers young children the opportunity to create, imitate, imagine, and practice while interacting with their environment. Participating in play for all children is extremely important, but children with physical, sensory, or intellectual and developmental disabilities (IDD) cannot always access the same opportunities as typically developing (TD) children. They may not have the physical ability to reach for or manipulate a toy or may have diminished awareness of a toy to begin with due to visual or hearing deficits. Because of cognitive or other limitations, the quality of play and learning of skills may be compromised for children with disabilities (Hamm, Mistret, and Goetz-Ruffino 2006; Musselwhite 1986; Porter, Hernandez-Reif, and Jessee 2007; Robins, Ferrari, and Dautenhahn 2008). Children with cognitive or other severe disabilities, such as **autism spectrum disorder (ASD)**, cannot experience or explore the world like other children, and these limitations can lead to further developmental delays during formative learning years. The lack of independent discovery and exploration of the environment can negatively affect learning and social interaction outcomes for children with cognitive disabilities (Brodin 1999).

Toys have an essential role in enhancing play skills because children are naturally attracted to them. Toys may have greater impact for children with severe disabilities when they have educational value or when a child can use them for learning purposes (Brodin 1999; Hamm, Mistret, and Goetz-Ruffino 2006; Lathan et al. 2001). Brodin stated that children with disabilities, particularly when they are young, have to be "lured into, tempted, persuaded and sometimes nagged at in order to actively engage themselves in objects or people. They need exciting opportunities, not only as much, but much more than ordinary children" (Brodin 1999, 31).

Toys that are adapted to provide multisensory input and allow for repetitive interaction can provide an exciting opportunity for a child with a disability (Hamm, Mistret, and Goetz-Ruffino 2006; Porter, Hernandez-Reif, and Jessee 2007).

Socially Assistive Robots

Socially assistive robots (SARs) are at the forefront of new technologies designed to generate therapeutic benefit for children with complex disabilities because, like toys, they can be designed to be socially engaging and fun for children. SARs assist the child through social interaction while creating measurable growth in learning and rehabilitation (Chang et al. 2007; Feil-Seifer, Skinner, and Matarić 2007; Lindblom and Ziemke 2006; Šabanović, Michalowski, and Caporael 2007; Tanaka, Cicourel, and Movellan 2007).

A robotic system has the ability to sense the environment, process that information, and perform actions based on the input received. Robots may facilitate discovery and enhance opportunities for play, learning, and cognitive development in children with a wide range of impairments. The use of robots in play situations can also help track changes in cognitive development and may contribute to improved cognitive comprehension (Encarnação et al. 2014; Lee, Song, and Shin 2001). Within this context, robots are generally characterized as either assistive or interactive. An assistive robot (AR) gives aid or support to a human user. Interactive robots are typically designed to entertain or to form a social bond with an individual. When this interaction is mainly social, they are termed socially interactive robots (SIR). Feil-Seifer and Matarić explained the importance of this distinction by defining what features characterize "socially assistive" and how these features affect the human participant. Specifically, they suggested that SARs represent "robotic systems whose primary purpose is to provide assistance and measureable progress in rehabilitation, learning or convalescence through the establishment of close and effective interaction" (Feil-Seifer and Matarić 2005, 466). This description differs from that for SIRs in that the goal is to provide assistance to the user and not simply establish a social connection as for the SIR. A SAR represents the intersection of assistive and interactive robotics. The SAR's goal of providing assistance to human users is similar to ARs, but the assistance is through *social interaction* (Besio 2002). Put simply, SARs seek to replicate or modify, but not replace, the benefits (therapeutic/educational) that stem from the relationship between a caregiver, peer, or the individual(s) with a disability. An effective SAR must interact with its environment, exhibit social behavior, and focus its attention and communication on the user to help him or her achieve desired goals (Matarić et al. 2009; Tapus, Tapus, and Matarić 2009).

The SARs have been primarily used to mediate social interactions for children with ASD (Costa et al. 2013; Dickerson, Robins, and Dautenhahn 2013; Feil-Seifer and Matarić 2008a,b, 2009b; Ferrari, Robins, and Dautenhahn 2009; Robins et al. 2005, 2012). They have also been used therapeutically for adults with dementia (Felzmann et al. 2015; Marti et al. 2006; Šabanović et al. 2013; Tapus, Tapus, and Matarić 2009; Wada et al. 2008) and individuals undergoing poststroke rehabilitation (Matarić et al. 2007, 2009; Swift-Spong et al. 2015; Tapus, Tapus, and Matarić 2007). Rabbitt, Kazdin, and Scassellati (2015) provided a review of SAR use in mental health interventions, including ASD, and gave recommendations for clinical interventions employing SARs. They emphasized the importance of thinking about SARs as supplements to, not replacement of, human care providers.

Using SARs that interact with children with a complex disability presents a unique set of challenges (Dautenhahn 2007). Children with complex disabilities are often nonverbal, with a range of sensory or cognitive impairments, or can have a variety of neuromuscular conditions that affect fine and gross motor patterns, movement, and posture (Collins 2007; Cook et al. 2002; Hartshorne et al. 2013). In addition, studies that analyzed neuroplasticity have found that the ideal age for therapeutic intervention is before 7 years, so the target demographic can be very young (Lane and Schaaf 2010).

For many children, especially those with ASD, emotion detection or affect recognition can be extremely challenging. The American Psychiatric Association identified ASD as a range of "neurodevelopmental conditions characterized by persistent significant impairment in the social-communication domain along with restricted, repetitive patterns of behavior, interests and activities" (2013, 50). ASD is generally recognized during early development and may coexist with other conditions, such as genetic syndromes, IDD, and seizure disorders (American Psychiatric Association 2013). Constraints may include limited/nonverbal communication, difficulty with visual tracking, and fine motor impairment (Centers for Disease Control and Prevention 2013; Lindblom and Ziemke 2006; Marti 2012; Risley, Ramey, and Washington 2012; Seelye et al. 2012; Stansfield, Dennis, and Larin 2012; Zhang 2012).

Use of SARs as a therapeutic tool for children with ASD is one of the most widely recognized applications for SARs. This is due in large part because SARs are at the nexus between inanimate objects or toys and humans whose attempts at social engagement are often stressful for a child with ASD (Scassellati, Admoni, and Matarić 2012). However, developing a SAR that is appropriately initiatory and responsive to a child with ASD is challenging because these children do not present a homogeneous group. To create an effective SAR requires the work of many disciplines. This means that engineers designing a SAR must work with children with ASD, their clinicians, and caregivers and vice versa. Research on the effectiveness of available SARs, while expanding rapidly, is still of inconsistent quality and somewhat limited (Pennisi et al. 2016; Scassellati, Admoni, and Matarić 2012).

Cabibihan et al. (2013) reviewed the design features of available SARs and how these robots were used during therapeutic sessions with children with ASD. From the design perspective, they categorized requirements based on appearance, functionality, safety requirements, autonomy, modularity, and adaptability (Cabibihan et al. 2013, 618). They also looked at the types of behaviors targeted in therapy by various clinicians. These behaviors included imitation, eye contact, joint attention, turn-taking, emotion recognition and expression, self-initiated interactions, and triadic interactions. They concluded that SARs were used to achieve a variety of therapeutic intentions. Among them are assisting in the diagnosis of ASD; as a friendly playmate; as a behavior-eliciting agent; as a social mediator; as a social actor; and as a personal therapist (Cabibihan et al. 2013). Table 8.1 provides a summary overview of SARs and their components used for investigational research as well as those that are commercially available today. Each of these devices has been used to address therapeutic intervention goals for children with complex disabilities.

Socially assistive robots are intended to be an extension of the therapist across the ASD spectrum. Therefore, the SAR must utilize affective feedback to initiate and encourage interaction while responding to affective cues from the child to maintain an interaction. The SAR must be capable of detecting and expressing a variety of affective states. SARs such as Kismet rely on a combination of speech and facial expression to determine affect (Lin and Schmidt 2015). The haptic sensors of Pleo provide a sense of touch and human warmth (Park and Lee 2014). Humanoid SARs used in ASD therapy, including Zeno (Salvador, Silver, and Mahoor 2015), KASPAR (Wainer et al. 2014), and NAO (Tapus et al. 2012), utilize a variety of facial or postural expressions to provide affective feedback.

While a variety of cameras, microphones, and sensors are used to detect emotion in these robots, all were designed to mimic human-human interaction. Kismet's eye gaze effectively relays the focus of the SAR's attention.

TABLE 8.1 Summary Table for Investigational and Commercial SARs for ASD

Robot		Vision System	Auditory System	Mobility System	Technology Readiness Level (TRL)	Development Status
1	Bobus	Infrared	None	Wheeled base	7	Investigational (University of Sherbrooke)
2	Child-centered Adaptive Robot for Learning in an Interactive Environment (CHARLIE)	Mono	1 speaker	2-DOF head and arms	7	Investigational (University of South Carolina)
3	C-Pac	Infrared	Speaker	Wheeled base	7	Investigational (University of Sherbrooke)
4	Diskcat	None	Speaker	Wheeled base	7	Investigational (University of Sherbrooke)
5	Facial Automation for Conveying Emotions (FACE)	Mono	None	32-DOF facial movement	7	Investigational (University of Pisa)
6	Humanoid for Open Architecture Platform (HOAP)-2	Stereo	None	25-DOF with humanoid legs	9	Commercial (Fujitsu Laboratories)
7	Infanoid	Foveated stereo	None	24-DOF torso	7	Investigational (Japan)
8	Interactive Robotic Social Mediators as Companions (IROMEC)	RGB-D	Microphones and speaker	Wheeled base	7	Investigational (European Union)

(Continued)

TABLE 8.1 (CONTINUED) Summary Table for Investigational and Commercial SARs for ASD

Robot		Vision System	Auditory System	Mobility System	Technology Readiness Level (TRL)	Development Status
9	Jumbo	Infrared	Speaker	Wheeled base with moving trunk	7	Investigational (University of Sherbrooke)
10	KASPAR	None	Speaker	8-DOF head, 3-DOF arms (2)	7	Investigational (University of Hertfordshire)
11	Keepon	Stereo	Microphone	4-DOF (turn, nod, rock, bob)	7	Investigational (Carnegie Mellon University)
12	Kismet	Foveated stereo	Microphone and speaker	15-DOF expressive face	7	Investigational (Massachusetts Institute of Technology)
13	Labo-1	Infrared	Speaker	4-wheel base	7	Investigational (University of Hertfordshire)
14	Lego Mindstorms® NTX	None	Microphone	Wheeled base	6	Investigational
15	Maestro	Infrared	Speaker	Wheeled base	7	Investigational (University of Sherbrooke)
16	Milo	RGB-D	8 microphones and speaker	18-DOF with legs	9	Commercial (Robokind)
17	NAO	Stereo	4 directional microphones and loudspeakers	25-DOF with humanoid legs	9	Commercial (Aldebaran Robotics)
18	Pekee	Infrared	None	3-wheel base	9	Commercial (Wany Robotics)

(Continued)

TABLE 8.1 (CONTINUED)   **Summary Table for Investigational and Commercial SARs for ASD**

Robot	Vision System	Auditory System	Mobility System	Technology Readiness Level (TRL)	Development Status
19	QueBall (formerly Roball) (Figure 8.1)	None	Speaker	2-DOF sphere	9	Commercial (Que Innovations)
20	Leka	None	Speaker	2-DOF sphere	9	Commercial preordering now available (Leka)
21	Robota	Infrared	2 speakers	5-DOF (2 legs, 2 arms, 1 head)	9	Investigational (Federal Polytechnic School in Lausanne)
22	Tito	Mono	Microphone and speaker	Wheeled base	7	Investigational (University of Sherbrooke)
23	Triadic Relationship EVOking Robot (TREVOR)	None	None	3-DOF arms	7	Investigational (Brigham Young University)
24	Troy	None	Speaker	4-DOF arms, 2-DOF head	7	Investigational (Brigham Young University)
25	Buddy	Mono	Microphone and speaker	Wheeled base	8	Presale

Note: TRLs in this table refer to the robotic platform itself and not to its application in therapy of children with ASD. ASD, degrees of freedom.

KASPAR and Zeno utilize several motors to change between three facial expressions. The Huggable uses speech and tone to express a variety of affective states, including curiosity, happiness, and sadness (Santos 2012). The underlying principles of affective interaction of these SARs are rooted in developmental psychology and are designed to promote an intuitive experience (Scassellati, Admoni, and Matarić 2012). The following sections provide background on available technologies that may be incorporated into SARs for children with complex disabilities.

Critical Review of the Technology Available

"SARs are used to communicate, express and perceive emotions, maintain social relationships, interpret natural cues and develop social competencies" (Cabibihan et al. 2013, 595). To adhere to these principles (a SAR that is socially engaging, interactive, and attractive to the child with ASD or other neurodevelopmental impairments), developers must consider a wide range of robotic capabilities and the integration of these features. They must also consider the intent of the therapeutic intervention (Dautenhahn 2007). The following sections describe the technologies that enable these principles to be met.

As is evident from Table 8.1, most SARs applied in ASD are investigational. Some of these have been specifically developed for use with children on the ASD spectrum. Others are off the shelf robots developed for entertainment, hobbyists, or developers that have been applied in ASD research. There appear to be five commercially available robots developed specifically for clinical or educational use in ASD: Milo (http://www.robokindro bots.com/), QueBall (http://www.queinnovations.com/) (Figure 8.1), Leka (http://leka.io/), Ask NAO (https://asknao.aldebaran.com/) (Figure 8.2), and Buddy (http://www.bluefrogrobotics.com/en/buddy-your-companion -robot/). The last, Buddy, is being applied in ASD but was not specifically designed for that population. These robots differ dramatically in structure, aim, and overall design. Milo and NAO are human-like robots capable of changing facial features, speaking, and reacting to a child's movements through tactile, voice, and visual sensors. QueBall and Leka are in the shape of a ball that includes colored lights, touch sensors, and sound generation. Children play with QueBall or Leka on the floor, chasing it and touching it for different effects. A suite of games is available. Buddy is designed as a companion robot that is mobile, has sensors similar to home security systems, and provides some typical home computer applications, such as calendar and alarm clock.

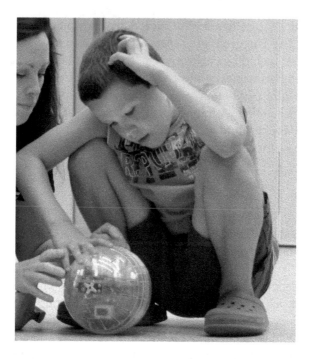

Figure 8.1   QueBall (formerly Roball).

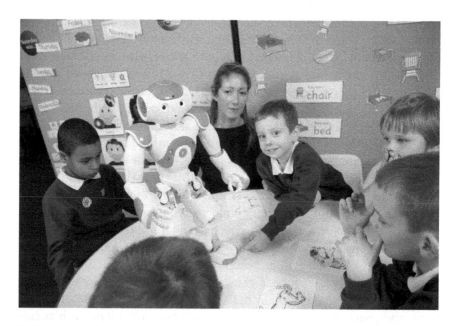

Figure 8.2   The NAO robot.

Because the commercially available sector of robots for ASD is so small, we describe characteristics that SARS should exhibit based on a relatively large body of developmental research. Most of the research has been based on the investigational robots listed in Table 8.1.

Power Systems

All SARs need power, and careful consideration is needed to ensure the SAR is fully powered, safe, and efficient. There are several options when considering power for robotic systems. The most common power systems include shore power (both alternating current and direct current), and energy storage devices (e.g., batteries). Some of the most important considerations for ensuring adoptability include safety, convenience, time, monetary cost, and energy capacity (i.e., energy density). Table 8.2 summarizes the most common battery types used in robotics. Battery types are grouped into one of two categories, disposable or rechargeable, and given a description or rating for safety, convenience, operating time (ranked), monetary cost, and energy density. The ranked operating time is directly correlated to the energy density. The description for monetary cost takes into consideration the cost of a single battery and whether there is a recurring cost (e.g., disposable batteries). The safety descriptions are derived from the Material Safety Data Sheet (MSDS) for each battery type. The convenience rating is defined as Bad, OK, Good, and Excellent (from least to most convenient). Convenience is an overall score that takes into account the benefits and drawbacks of safety, monetary cost, and operating time. In general, the more convenient a battery is, the less likely the technology that utilizes it would be abandoned. For example, cobalt lithium ion batteries receive an Excellent convenience score because there is only an up-front cost, and the batteries have the longest operating time (i.e., largest energy density). On the other hand, silver oxide batteries receive a Bad convenience rating because a single unit has a very high cost, and the disposable nature of these batteries results in a high recurring cost. In this case, the high cost outweighs the relatively high operating time and safety ratings.

A critical issue with all battery-powered technology is the relatively short life span available when compared to shore power. When battery life is not long enough for a therapy session, the typical solution is to utilize multiple batteries. When using rechargeable batteries, this involves charging batteries during the use of others. When using disposable batteries, this involves replacing (potentially frequently) batteries. While this can be sustainable, it incurs a higher cost due to the need for multiple batteries

TABLE 8.2 Adoptability Considerations for Different Battery Types

	Battery Type	Safety	Convenience	Operating Time (Ranked)	Monetary Cost	Energy Density (Wh/kg)
Rechargeable	Lead acid	Flammable gas during charging	OK	1	Up front	40
	NiCd	No hazard during normal use	OK	2	Up front	62
	NiMH	No hazard during normal use	OK	3	Up front	89
	Manganese Li-ion	Potential fire hazard	Good	5 (tie)	Up front	107
	Phosphate Li-ion	Potential fire hazard	Good	5 (tie)	Up front	107
	Cobalt Li-ion	Potential fire hazard	Excellent	8	Up front	162
Disposable	Silver oxide	No hazard during normal use	Bad	7	Continuous and high	130
	Alkaline	No hazard during normal use	OK	6	Continuous	110
	Zinc-carbon	No hazard during normal use	Bad	4	Continuous	92

(especially when using disposable ones) and chargers. Furthermore, if a patient or caregiver continually forgets to recharge (or purchase more disposable) batteries in between sessions, then SAR abandonment rates can increase (O'Rourke et al. 2014). Because rechargeable batteries are the most convenient power source for SARs, there is a need to automate the recharging process to maximize adoptability. Hasan et al. (2015) developed a wireless power transfer (WPT) system that can recharge SARs without human intervention. With the integration of WPT systems that eliminate the need to remember to recharge a battery, ease of use could increase and perhaps adoptability of SARs would increase as well.

SAR Mobility Systems

Mobility can be an integral or peripheral aspect of a SAR. Two investigational SARs used in the treatment of ASD are KASPAR and Zeno (eventually commercialized as Milo) (Pennisi et al. 2016). Interventions are focused on human-like interaction, so both SARs are excellent with conversation and expression but, beyond arm gestures, do not move about the room. On the other end of the spectrum, NAO has 25 degrees of freedom and can mimic human gestures, including walking, sitting, and dancing (Shamsuddin et al. 2012). SAR mobility, like all other components, is yet another tool that must be effectively tailored to the appropriate demography. Early results from pilot testing completed in the fall of 2015 at the University of Colorado by a team led by the first author of this chapter (Figure 8.3) suggested that

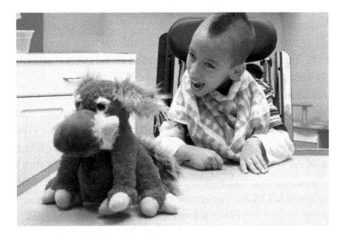

Figure 8.3 Jayden and Glus, University of Colorado Denver (2015).

toddlers with severe cerebral palsy (CP) do not require the complexity of a 25-degree-of-freedom system for engagement.

In a comparative study of 22 children between the ages of 7 and 13, 11 with high-functioning ASD and 11 neurotypical children, researchers compared the influence of incorporating robotic gestures along with facial expressions of happiness, sadness, anger, disgust, fear, surprise, and neutrality to determine recognition predictions. The Zeno robot (a previous version of Milo) was used in this study. Although there were no differences between the two groups for recognizing basic emotions, the children with ASD were significantly impaired when recognizing fear when the robotic gestures were added. Both groups showed variability, both positively and negatively, when asked to predict emotions when gestures were included with the basic emotional facial states. The authors pointed out that it would be important to further "investigate whether the children can truly identify the emotional meaning connected to the label and visual cue" (Salvador, Silver, and Mahoor 2015, 6132).

SAR Vision Systems

We use vision to interact with the world around us. Our eyes allow us to detect objects, plan routes, gauge communication, and generally provide the capability to assess our environment. Similarly, SARs equipped with an effective sense of perception can enhance therapeutic applications for children with complex disabilities (Tapus et al. 2012). At a minimum, the vision systems enable the SAR to engage with the child in an interactive manner (Vázquez et al. 2014).

The SAR vision systems have specific and various levels of capability requirements. For example, a robot designed to follow a line only requires reflective sensors to visualize its task. A SAR that relies on facial cues for affect recognition requires an advanced camera vision system (Zeng et al. 2009). This utilization of cameras to acquire images and perform analysis to determine an outcome is termed *machine vision*. Traditionally, SAR machine vision supplements affect recognition (e.g., Kismet robot) (Breazeal and Aryananda 2002) and navigation (e.g., NAO robot) (Gillesen et al. 2011) and enhance the interactivity of play by tracking objects and positioning the SAR in an engaged orientation.

The systems listed in Table 8.1 provide a wide range of utility for SAR machine vision. Table 8.3 provides an overview of machine vision subsystems and a list of SARs that use them.

TABLE 8.3   SAR Machine Vision Subsystems

Camera System	Description	Characteristics, Applications	SARs
Mono	Single camera	Limited spatial recognition, 2-D landmark detection/tracking	CHARLIE, FACE, Tito
Stereo	Dual-camera system with a shared field of view	Enhanced depth perception, 3-D landmark detection/tracking	HOAP-2, Keepon, NAO
Foveated stereo	4-camera systems common, 2 fields of view with different focal points	Stereo vision in multiple fields of view	Infanoid, Kismet
Infrared	Infrared transmitter and receiver used together	Ideal field-of-view depth tracker, commonly used for indoor mapping	Bobus, C-Pac, Jumbo, Labo-1, Maestro, Pekee, Robota
Red Green Blue-Depth (RGB-D)	Infrared with optical camera system	Facial and skeletal tracking	IROMEC, Milo
Laser	Range detection from a spinning laser source	Outdoor mapping, automated vehicles	None
Motion capture	Optical cameras and reflective sensors	Skeletal tracking	None
Ultrasound	Ultrasonic transmission/reception	Proximity detection	IROMEC
Radar	Radio frequency	Dynamic computations, range finding	None

Note: 2-D, two dimensional; 3-D, three dimensional.

SAR Auditory Systems

The SARs focus on interaction between an individual and the robot. For auditory interaction, two-way speech communication is the medium of choice. Speech is the predominant mode of communication among humans. Using speech, we can effectively convey thoughts and emotions. Robots can use speech synthesis as an output mode to communicate with a child and speech recognition as a means of capturing the utterances of the child. Even as infants, babies are quickly able to recognize and interpret tonal cues from their parents (Snow 1972). These verbal cues can be critical for SAR-child interaction as they can be used to engage the child as a social mediator or as a facilitator in social exchanges (Diehl 2003; Diehl et al. 2012).

Other Sensor Capabilities

A wide variety of remaining tools and sensors are available to integrate within a SAR. It is only necessary to determine the most effective modes of engagement. For example, if a certain child is relatively mobile and affectionate, that child may be more engaged with a SAR that has the ability to sense touch with tactile sensors, such as Roboskin (Billard et al. 2013). Perhaps another child who is nonverbal with limited mobility and cognitive impairments might benefit from a myoelectric sensor to connect muscle activity directly to the SAR. Other sensors include electronic noses (Loutfi and Coradeschi 2006), force plates to determine the direction of lean (Kudoh, Komura, and Ikeuchi 2006), reflective sensors for refined skeletal tracking (Mbouzao 2013), and heart rate monitors to track mood (Appelhans and Luecken 2006). The key is to capitalize on the modes of communication best represented by the SARs' demographic.

Affect Recognition

Interaction between individuals involves more than speaking and hearing; a key component of human communication is emotional intelligence, the ability to recognize someone's emotional state and respond. This involves not only listening, but also recognizing the social cues of facial expression, voice intonation, body positioning, and physiological reactions. To enhance human-computer interaction through use of SARs, all of these elements must come together to enable the robot to accurately recognize the user's affective state. For these interactions, affect should be considered as an innate sensation that may not consciously register, while an individual's feelings and emotions are based on this sensation, which is then made conscious (feeling) and dramatized (emotion) (Gunes and Piccardi 2009). This definitive connection between affect and emotion is why multiple modalities are important in human-SAR interaction to ensure that each individual's affective state is accurately recognized and used as an input for future robot behavior.

Recognizing affective state involves multiple capabilities, such as visual recognition, voice recognition, and posture recognition. Incorporating these modalities and using them concurrently greatly benefits a robot's ability to determine a child's affective state and to respond appropriately. For example, if a robot behavior elicits a frustrated or angry response from the child, the robot should recognize the child's reaction and then alter its behavior to keep the child engaged and willing to learn. Affect recognition is crucial for SARs because a child who becomes upset when using the robot is much less likely to continue interacting, making the SAR an inadequate therapeutic tool (Dautenhahn 2007).

In one of the earliest reported studies on affect recognition, Liu et al. (2007) compared the results of computer-based psychophysiological analysis (anxiety, engagement, and liking) with therapists and parent reports of the affect of three "high-functioning" teenagers diagnosed with ASD. An 83% agreement between the machine classifications and the therapists' reports was obtained (Liu et al. 2007).

Multimodal Systems

Using robots to accurately determine human affect is an area of extensive research. Giving a robot the task of identifying a child's affective state is no small feat. There may always be some form of error, but this error can be minimized through a common technique that utilizes multimodal systems (Jiang and Zhang 2015; Leo et al. 2015; Liu et al. 2007; Liu, Zhang, and Yadegar 2011; Ranatunga et al. 2011; Salvador, Silver, and Mahoor 2015).

A multimodal system (Figure 8.4) is a program or algorithm that takes into account several different aspects (modalities) of an individual and combines them to make a sound inference. The most common modalities used include facial features, gesture and body movement, and audio or vocal expression. Each of these modalities can include a significant number of factors themselves. For example, facial feature modalities may include eye movement, mouth deformations, and eyebrow movement. Body movement modalities might focus on self-touch, reaching toward

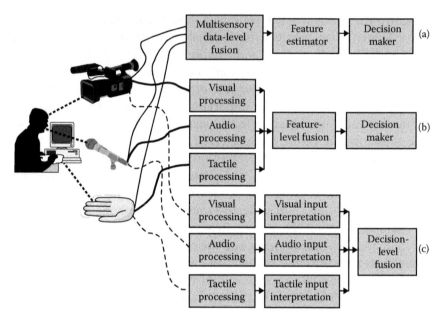

Figure 8.4 Fusion of multiple sensing modalities. (a) Data-level fusion integrates raw sensory data. (b) Feature-level fusion combines features from individual modalities. (c) Decision-level fusion combines data from different modalities at the end of the analysis. (Pantic, M, and LJM Rothkrantz. 2003. "Toward an affect-sensitive multimodal human-computer interaction." *Proceedings of the IEEE* 91 (9):1370–1390.)

or pulling away from the robot, and general body movement or posture (Panning et al. 2012).

In addition, focusing on vocal expression for a young child with ASD would include volume, frequency of noises, and presence of noises such as laughing, crying, and babbling. All of these modalities, when used in conjunction, aid a robot in determining an individual's affective state by comparing their responses and actions to either an internal database or previously established emotional responses (Chan, Nejat, and Chen 2011; Dautenhahn 2007; Feil-Seifer and Matarić 2009b).

Recognizing the presence of any of these factors is the first step in creating a multimodal system. After recognition, the robot needs to account for the frequency at which these behaviors appear. Rapid signals would be more commonly used for recognizing affective state, as they include facial muscle movement and eye movement. Furthermore, the robot will need to consider the context of the child's movements and vocalizations. Because children with ASD do not always present social behaviors like their TD peers, the robot will need to establish a new baseline norm for each child. This can be demonstrated by using a SAR as a therapeutic tool for a child diagnosed with ASD. The child may not look directly at the robot when the child is happy or angry because the child may not be socially comfortable. Thus, to accurately account for affective state, the robot should have a normalized baseline for any possible conditions the child may have and account for a lack of potential eye contact (Dautenhahn 2007; Scassellati, Admoni, and Matarić 2012).

After determining an individual's actions and comparing any differences from their specific baseline, the modality information needs to be fused to infer the corresponding affective state. Modality fusion can have as great an influence on the system as the modalities used. The level at which information is fused can be the deciding factor on whether the robot can accurately predict affective state, and this fusion can occur at the data level, feature level, or decision level, as shown in the studies discussed next (Bekele et al. 2013; Castellano et al. 2013; Panning et al. 2012; Scassellati, Admoni, and Matarić 2012).

By 2015, affect recognition tools were being used by researchers to better understand how affect recognition could improve or facilitate therapeutic interventions with children with ASD. One of the first of these studies involved the use of machine learning strategies to detect and recognize emotions exhibited by three children with high-functioning ASD. The implemented system used the Milo robot from Robokind™. This pilot study was designed to enable the researchers to test the components of the system in a real-world environment and to verify if the system enabled the children to participate freely in interactions with the SAR. Three children formally diagnosed with high-functioning ASD (ages not provided) were situated in front of the robot and presented with four different robot-produced facial expressions (happiness, sadness, anger, and fear). They were asked to reproduce or imitate the expressions provided by the robot. Of the 60 interactions, in only three cases the system failed to identify the child's expression (in one case, the child's face was not detected due to a wide rotation while imitating the fear expression; in the other two, anger expressions were taken as fear expressions) (Leo et al. 2015).

All of the system attributes mentioned should be considered when developing a SAR for children with neurodevelopmental impairments. The robot should be able to act as a companion for the child while using individualized learning techniques to help them reach a specified developmental goal.

Machine Learning

New models of SARs are becoming increasingly dynamic to continually improve clinical outcomes. To keep up with this demand, SARs need to be able to adapt to their environments and use previous knowledge—from clinician input and prior experience—and dynamic interactions to respond appropriately. To develop such an intelligent system, one of the more powerful aspects is machine learning, which involves the development and improvement of computer models to simulate human learning activities (Wang, Ma, and Zhou 2009).

Learning from both new and old experiences is crucial and has multiple facets that need to be considered and analyzed, something that goes well beyond simple memorization. It may be possible to utilize machine learning to incorporate user input, prior knowledge, and experience to respond to an individual child's behavior and encourage certain responses. Machine learning involves collection and analysis of data or observations, identification of relevant information, and use of this information to predict future behaviors in similar scenarios. In the case of a SAR, an ideal machine learning system would recognize certain behaviors or actions made by the child, determine if this behavior is relevant to the specified goal, and then modify its own behavior to either elicit the same response or obtain a new reaction. Creating more adaptable SARs will ensure that they are both clinician and user friendly (Mead and Matarić 2015). This section expands on this idea to include a background of traditional learning methods and newer methods that have shown promise in SAR development.

Traditional Methods

Machine learning has been a collaborative effort between computer programmers and psychologists since it was first introduced over 60 years ago. Understanding and mimicking the ways humans learn started with basic memorization and presentation of a memorized response. Since then, machine learning has focused on multiple techniques based on three fundamental learning mechanisms:

1. Perceptual Learning: Learning of new objects, categories, and relations, comparable to seeking to improve and grow.
2. Episodic Learning: Learning based on events and information about the event, focusing on change in behavior due to an event.
3. Procedural Learning: Learning based on actions and action sequences to accomplish a task, which is how most machine learning is approached. (Kulkarni 2012, 5)

These learning mechanisms are the approaches by which humans learn, and they have been the basis of machine learning. However, humans are able to adapt to new learning experiences much more deftly than their machine counterparts, which do not come to the same conclusions as quickly or easily.

Machine learning methods include supervised, unsupervised, and semisupervised learning. Supervised learning is the simplest of the three and relies on labeled data. A system makes predictions about the labeled data and is corrected if it predicts incorrectly; the predictions continue until the system has become sufficiently accurate. This learning style is commonly used to create a classifier given certain classified training examples in the form of labeled data sets or for problems regarding regression. Unsupervised learning does not have labeled data and a specific end result. Instead, this learning style is based on visible similarities and differences between data, which are then represented mathematically to either organize the data or reduce redundancy. The third learning style is semisupervised learning, which combines the two previous methods. Here, data are both labeled and unlabeled, and the system is able to combine both to achieve better performance. This learning style is the most flexible method for modeling unlabeled data (Chang 2011; Kulkarni 2012).

Deciding which learning style to use when developing a SAR depends primarily on the functional goals of the SAR. In some cases, the robot will require human assistance and input, but the knowledge and understanding of information is programmed into the robot, as shown in SARs with speech recognition capabilities. The input is directly mapped to a designated output. Another instance may include a dynamic situation with frequent changes in environment or parameters. Instead of writing extensive algorithms to account for every possible scenario, a more robust learning program can be used to predict changes and respond accordingly. Last, and most applicable to SARs for children with developmental disabilities, are situations that cater to the individual. To accomplish this, the robot would be equipped with specific information about each child and how this information influences child-robot interaction.

Emerging Methods
One of the most common and effective learning methods for SARs is reinforcement learning, which relies on a balance between exploitation and exploration. With this learning method, the robot relies on exploiting known information and exploring the environment and individual behaviors to make appropriate decisions. Reinforcement learning strongly

mimics the way children learn by combining dynamic learning methods with supervised learning. For example, Mead and Matarić (2015) are working to develop a unified framework of multimodal communication and proxemics (human–robot location/orientation to each other). In their work, they are combining machine-based models of social signals and how these might be perceived or interpreted by both the human and the SAR. This helps the robot to know where to locate itself in proximity to the child and how to modulate its speech and gestures to accommodate the social signals and communication provided by the child. Although the work is in the early stages, it is an exciting and interesting approach to facilitating social engagement, particularly for children with ASD.

Reinforcement learning systems are able to interact with the environment in discrete time steps when the robot is able to make an observation and relate it to a corresponding action. Unlike supervised learning, however, there is no specific predetermined input/output relation that the robot needs to recognize. Rather, reinforcement learning relates the observation to a reward and set of possible actions. After an action is chosen, the system moves on to the next time step with a new reward based on the change in state and a new set of actions. The goal of the system is to collect as much reward as possible by selecting the most efficient actions. Because of the way the method is designed, it considers the complete goal-oriented problem when making decisions and can be easily modified (Sutton and Barto 1998).

In 2005, Mitsunaga et al. aspired to develop a robot with the capability to adapt to individual communication preferences. In this study, the reinforcement algorithm was equipped with parameters of normal discomfort signals. In testing, the robot communicated with 15 human subjects (typically developed adults) for up to 30 minutes and mostly adapted its communication preferences by noting behaviors that resulted in discomfort signals from the human and then implemented new behaviors to minimize these signals. Using the given parameters caused the robot to reach the comfort levels of most participants within 15–20 minutes or about 10 iterations. It was concluded that changing the parameters within a reinforcement learning algorithm caused a variation in success rates, as parameters were labeled with unequal importance for successful interaction, causing the "important" parameters to converge more quickly than their "less-important" counterparts (Mitsunaga et al. 2005).

Machine Learning and Early Intervention
Learning from clinician and parental input (which specific goals need to be met) and incorporating these data into decision making is crucial

for the success of a SAR. Using this knowledge in real-world environments to elicit a desired response from the child can significantly improve clinical outcomes. For example, a clinician working to elicit vocal engagement behaviors from a child can incorporate information about how the child responds to physical closeness to the SAR, and the parents' knowledge of the types of output a child responds to can be used to initiate SAR-child engagement (Robins, Dautenhahn, and Dickerson 2009).

Adaptability through machine learning makes the SAR more capable of working one on one with the child, so it may be used in home therapy. Clinical intervention techniques can be used as input for the robot to make decisions. Using reinforcement learning allows the robot to focus on the overall goal for the child, no matter what it may be, and interact with the child in a way to help them reach that goal. Using machine learning, the robot can emulate clinician behaviors following objectives set by the clinician until they reach the desired goal. Because the clinician sets the pattern with the robot, these play activities can be used to reinforce clinical intervention sessions (Allievi et al. 2014; Basu and Clowry 2015).

The SARs that are able to sustain engagement can be a valuable therapeutic tool for children with complex disabilities. The clinical target determines which characteristics would be most beneficial for the SAR, as each child is different. For example, one should keep in mind any auditory, visual, spatial perception, or language impairments, as each of these has an effect on their interaction (Michaud, Duquette, and Nadeau 2003). Each child has his or her own individual needs, so the SAR should either be relatively customizable or cover as large a range of impairments as possible. The remainder of this section provides a comparative example by describing design considerations for children with ASD and children with CP. Children with ASD are considered because studies have shown that SARs can be effective therapeutic tools for these children. This is then compared to CP to show that SARs can have both major similarities and differences between various developmental disorders (Robins et al. 2012; Syrdal et al. 2014).

Using SARs to bridge the gap between no communication and normal communication has been a frequently explored therapy tool (Bosseler and Massaro 2003; Boucher 2003; Feil-Seifer and Matarić 2009a; Ferrari, Robins, and Dautenhahn 2009; Light et al. 1998; Robins, Dautenhahn, and Dickerson 2009; Tapus et al. 2012). For these children, maintaining their attention and prompting them to interact a certain way has been accomplished through significant design considerations, including the following:

1. Attraction: Children with ASD often respond better if they can see electrical or mechanical components, so creating a robot that exposes some of the inner mechanisms can be beneficial (Salter, Davey, and Michaud 2014). Conversely, designing a robot with human features can also attract the child's attention and help the child adjust to interacting with people while interacting with a robot (Robins, Dautenhahn, and Dickerson 2009).
2. Adaptability: Each child will respond differently, so having a robot that can adapt to personality types would be the most beneficial method for interaction (Salter, Davey, and Michaud 2014).
3. Maintaining Interaction: Keeping the child engaged for an extended period of time allows the robot to have greater therapeutic benefit. If the child engages the toy but quickly leaves it or becomes disinterested, the child will be less likely to benefit from the SAR (Robins et al. 2012; Salter, Davey, and Michaud 2014).
4. Routine Movements: Children with ASD can sometimes become locked in to a particular repetitive movement. A SAR can counter this by mimicking this routine movement and slowly prompting them into more typical behaviors (Salter, Davey, and Michaud 2014).
5. Simplistic Design: Robots are much more simplistic than humans when it comes to communication, which may be a contributing factor regarding successful robot interaction for children with ASD. Keeping the design relatively simple may help the child focus on communication or performing a given task to reach a specified goal (Salter, Davey, and Michaud 2014).

Like ASD, CP encompasses a wide range of developmental delays. However, in addition to focusing on mediating social and communication interactions, children with CP can use SARs to reach physical, sensory, and cognitive developmental milestones and receive therapeutic interaction that they may not be regularly able to access. For this reason, the design considerations for this type of SAR may include the following:

1. *Attraction*: SAR therapy for children with CP can occur at a very early age, so the robot needs to reflect the cute, endearing models that attract young children. This may include bright colors, soft fur, large eyes, or blinking lights (Howard 2013).
2. *Adaptability*: Like with ASD, a SAR for children with CP will need to be able to adapt to a child's individual needs. This adaptability can help maintain interaction while providing the best therapeutic experience for the child (Calderita et al. 2013).

3. *Repetitive Movement*: To reach a developmental milestone, the child will most likely need to have consistent practice making a designated movement. This can be accomplished by designing a SAR to encourage a child, through play, to repeat this movement until the child reaches a specified therapeutic goal, such as reaching across midline (Howard 2013; Robins et al. 2012).

4. *Simplistic Design*: Making the robot endearing to children will be important, but the robot should not become overwhelming. The design should be simple for the child as well as for the parents so they may use the SAR as a therapeutic tool at home. Making a complicated device could end up frustrating the child and parents, preventing them from accessing the benefits of the robot (Ljunglöf et al. 2011).

Comparing just a few of the many available design considerations for the two populations shows that, in both cases, SARs need to be individually customizable, even while targeting a specific audience. Not only do specifics of developmental disorders have a significant range, but also the differences between individual children of any disorder are just as vast.

Robotics Safety Standards

In addition to the design considerations mentioned, SARs must be safe to use. Current guidelines for robot safety include the International Organization for Standardization standard, *ISO 13482 International Standard: Robots and Robotic Devices—Safety Requirements for Personal Care Robots* (please refer to Chapter 1). The proper selection of an effective robotics safety system is based on hazard analysis of the operation involving a particular SAR. Among the factors for consideration in such an analysis are tasks a robot is programmed to perform, the startup and the programming procedures, environmental conditions and location of the robot, requirements for corrective tasks to sustain normal operations, human errors, and possible SAR malfunctions.

Critical Review of the Available Utilization Protocols

Pennisi et al. (2016) addressed the question, "Can social robots be a useful tool in autism therapy?" (p. 165). Following an extensive review of the literature that resulted in the identification of 998 studies focused on SARs and ASD, 179 articles fit their criteria for inclusion in the final analysis. For each of the included studies, they posed 10 specific questions. These questions centered on the use of a SAR for eliciting social behaviors, joint attention, imitation, task performance, language use, and reduction of repetitive and stereotypical movements during SAR interactions as compared to human interactions. The authors concluded that, in general, the results are promising. SARs were used as attractors and mediators or as measurement tools. They reported the greatest clinical success occurred when the robots were used in free or semistructured interactions. They also noted the need to improve study designs. Questions remained regarding whether gender, IQ, or age of the participants affected outcomes and whether generalization to other settings occurred (Pennisi et al. 2016).

The Adaptive Systems Research Group at the University of Hertfordshire has developed a humanoid robot named KASPAR. The SAR was developed using an open source platform to enable engineers to continuously create new controllers and algorithms. However, there was recognition of the need to create a system that could be easily used by nontechnical personnel. To test this concept, they developed a pilot project using KASPAR in an early childhood center specializing in children between the ages of 2 and 6 with complex social and communication disorders. KASPAR has been used at the center with children in groups as large as eight. Although the study is ongoing, researchers have learned a great deal about important features of the SAR as well as motivating factors for the adults to implement the SAR in their day-to-day routines. In particular, ease of use (usability) is a key component for professionals. Suggestions, such as creating a troubleshooting manual for nontechnical users, were quickly adopted by the research team. Motivation to use the SAR transitioned from a theoretical perspective to recognition of enhanced child-robot and child-adult interactions that occurred in situ (Syrdal et al. 2014).

Team members from the Autism Treatment Center of Dallas and the Callier Center for Communication Disorders at University of Texas–Dallas have implemented a research-based curriculum designed for children in elementary and middle school who have been diagnosed with ASD. Titled Robots4Autism, the curriculum is structured around common social interactions and situations that occur in the everyday world. The modules make use of the SAR Milo (Figure 8.5) and a tablet, creating a safe space to educate the children and provide practice. Evidence to date suggests children with higher-functioning autism are engaging more with the SAR than children with lower-functioning autism (specifics not available). In all cases, the children were more engaged with Milo and their teachers than when the SAR was not present (Rollins 2016).

Golliot et al. (2015) designed an experimental protocol to evaluate the use of QueBall in diagnosing ASD for children from 2 to 5 years of age.

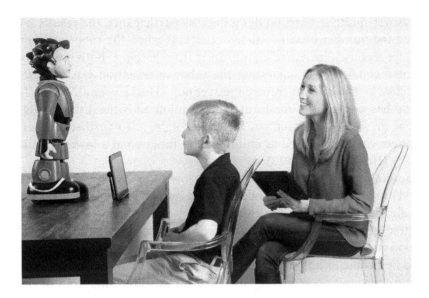

Figure 8.5   The Milo robot.

They began by observing children reacting to and playing with QueBall. They added a touch game in which each time the child touched one of the sensors, the robot changed or played a different sound or both. Sounds of interest to the child such as nursery rhymes were used to calm the children. An iPad interface was developed for programming and data collection. Thirty-one trials with 16 children were done over a period of 12 weeks. Using this process, six tests were developed to facilitate executing the games and collecting data: interaction with different colors and sounds, turn-taking, verbal imitation, motion imitation, ability to ask for help, and presence of stereotyped behaviors. Trials were conducted in a Snoezelen room with QueBall, the child, and a clinician. The lighting was minimal, and there were no other stimulating objects. The clinician used the iPad to enter the child's response to the programmed interactions in the six games.

A research group in the Netherlands implemented a question-asking protocol for school-aged children with ASD. In this study, they used an applied behavior analysis (ABA) intervention conducted by a robot and compared it to the same intervention conducted by a human trainer. The goal was to determine if the children would be more responsive to the SAR or to the human in promoting self-initiated questions. Six male children with a diagnosis of ASD, between the ages of 8 and 14 years with a full-scale IQ above 80, participated in the study. Using a combined crossover multiple-baseline design across participants, the results indicated the number of self-initiated questions when the robot or human trainer was used increased significantly from baseline. Both groups performed equally well, suggesting the robot intervention was at least as effective as the human trainer intervention (Huskens et al. 2013). This study has possibilities for future intervention activities using SARs as social mediators. The authors highly recommended further studies of younger children as well as children who function at a lower cognitive ability (Huskens et al. 2013).

Several investigators have developed closed-loop systems in which the child's interaction with a robot and with a human is monitored and stimuli are altered based on the child's response. Bekele et al. (2014) used a custom head-tracking system mounted in a baseball cap to monitor the child's gaze direction to evaluate the use of joint attention prompts delivered by a robot or human. Zheng et al. (2014) used a Microsoft Kinect for gesture recognition in a study of imitation skill learning. Both of these studies used the NAO robot.

The joint attention study involved a total of 12 children (six with ASD, six TD) with an age range for the ASD group of 2.78–4.9 years and 2.18–4.96 years for the TD group (Bekele et al. 2014). Four quasi-randomized total blocks of joint attention tasks were presented by the human administrator (two blocks) and NAO robot (two blocks). The total time that children's gaze was directed toward the region of interest was computed. All participants spent a higher percentage of time looking toward the robot compared to the human administrator, but all groups required higher levels of prompting to successfully orient within robot-administered trials. Children with ASD also spent significantly more time looking at the humanoid robot than the human administrator.

The gesture imitation task involved gestures taught by human or robot (NAO). Five children with ASD (age in years $m = 3.93$, $SD = 0.68$) and five TD children (age $m = 3.88$, $SD = 0.39$) participated in the study. The ASD group spent 18% more time attending to the robot as compared to attending to the human therapist. The TD group spent equal attention to the robot and therapist and was more successful in imitating the gestures than the ASD group. The ASD group was far more successful imitating the target gestures during the robot session than in the human session.

One of the key components of any implementation protocol is the ability to measure progress of participants and the specific impact of a SAR feature. Investigators from around the world are eagerly exploring how SARs might be used to facilitate acquisition of sensory, communication, physical, and cognitive skill sets for children with complex disabilities, particularly children with ASD. However, as Scassellati, Admoni, and Matarić (2012) described, the field is rapidly growing, and multiple disciplines are involved, each focusing on their particular area of strength (computational science, mechanical and electrical engineering, robot control, human–robot interaction, social psychology, and clinical research). Developing a common language to facilitate understanding among groups has the potential to be helpful and to ensure the needs of children are met.

The International Classification of Functioning, Disability, and Health (ICF) and its children and youth version (ICF-CY) (World Health Organization 2001) is a conceptual framework offering a paradigm and taxonomy of human functioning that can be used to guide holistic and interdisciplinary approaches to assessment and intervention. In settings serving children and youth with disabilities, the ICF-CY can provide comprehensive documentation.

Implementation of the ICF-CY in early intervention, special education, and habilitation settings builds on the adoption of a dimensional framework for practice and corresponding applications in assessment and intervention practices. An important priority in such applications is the identification and development of instruments and assessment tools that can provide evidence for assigning severity levels to ICF-CY codes (Simeonsson 2009).

Besio, Caprino, and Laudanna (2008) implemented the ICF-CY protocol as a resource in the European project Interactive Robotic Social Mediators as Companions (IROMEC). The SAR team, covering six countries in Europe, used the ICF-CY during the early concept generation phase, development of play scenarios and environmental components. From this, they set up a methodological framework that could be used as a validation guide for future studies. The key ingredient is the placement of the child as the center of the proposed intervention. Use of the ICF-CY assisted the development team to determine which tasks and items should be included in the development of the SAR (Besio, Caprino, and Laudanna 2008).

McDougall and Wright (2009) described how the ICF-CY could be used in combination with Goal Attainment Scaling (GAS), an individualized measure of change determined by a family-centered team, to connect the various phases of the therapeutic process for consistent, collaborative, well-directed, and accountable clinical care. The article discusses how the use of GAS facilitated translation of clients' identified needs into distinct, measurable goals set collaboratively by clients, their families, and service providers. Examples of integrated GAS goals set for the various components of the ICF-CY were provided. The utility of GAS as a measure of clinical outcomes for individual clients was also discussed. Used in combination, the ICF-CY and GAS can serve to coordinate, simplify, and standardize assessment and outcome evaluation practices for individual clients receiving pediatric rehabilitation services (McDougall and Wright 2009). Although this model has yet to be applied to SAR research, it presents a potentially useful construct.

A study by Adolfsson et al. (2011) was part of a larger work to develop an authentic measure consisting of code sets for self- or proxy report of child participation. The aim was to identify common everyday life situations of children and youth based on measures of participation. The study was descriptive in nature and involved several stages: first, a systematic search of the literature to find articles presenting measures for children and youth with disabilities, identifying measures in selected articles, linking items in included measures to the ICF-CY, analyzing content in measures presented as performance and participation, and identifying aggregations of ICF-CY codes across these measures. A large number of measures for children and youth with disabilities was identified, but only 12 fulfilled the inclusion criteria. Measures presented as performance covered all the ICF-CY Activities and Participation chapters, whereas measures presented as participation covered five of nine chapters. Three common everyday life situations emerged from the measures: moving around, engagement in play, and recreation and leisure (Adolfsson et al. 2011). Again, this model for determining level of child participation holds promise for future SAR research.

Another protocol, Every Move Counts (http://www.everymovecounts.net /index.html), represents the completion of a 33-month Innovative Research Grant awarded by the National Institutes of Health and funded through the National Institutes for the Neurologically and Communicatively Disordered. Ninety-one children and 41 speech/language pathologists, teachers, and occupational therapists from seven different sites participated in the implementation and validation of the Every Move Counts approach (Korsten, Foss, and Berry 2007). At the University of Colorado, use of the Every Move Counts methodology has been incorporated into SAR research and development. Working with clinicians with extensive experience with children who have complex disabilities, this methodology enables our SAR to closely model the incremental physical and cognitive changes our clinicians are working to elicit. Early pilot results suggest this model is proving useful, and efforts are under way to expand this model (Bodine 2016).

Each child's developmental needs are broad, deep, and complex, radiating into all aspects of physical, sensory, and cognitive performance. One proposition implicit in the occupational performance model (Chapparo and Ranka 1996) is that the role of player, with its associated play behaviors and component elements, is a primary occupational role of children. Of the broad categories of occupational performance, play is particularly limited in most children with IDDs (Bourke-Taylor and Pallant 2013). Children with multiple sensory, motor, and intellectual disabilities have difficulty developing and engaging in play behaviors. Whereas school and self-maintenance tasks can be taught in a systematic fashion, play does not appear to change in response to similar instructional strategies. Various researchers have found that cognitive, sensorimotor, and perceptual component deficits are not able to account for deficient play performance in populations of children with multiple developmental disabilities. Moreover, current assessment tools available to therapists are unable to describe play patterns and play deficits in children with developmental disorders (Bundy 1997; Seligman and Darling 2009). Behaviors that appear to interfere most often with their ability to perform play and school tasks include diminished attention to the environment, high levels of stereotyped or self-absorbed behavior, passivity, lack of initiative, and poor self-expression (Nelson 2003).

Therapists who work with children who have disabilities adopt different approaches to direct intervention to improve play responses. These include the following three approaches: First, the most traditional form of therapy advocates the development of adaptive play skills through the use of play tasks that are directed by the therapist (Rubin et al. 2014). Second, therapists who work specifically with children who have visual and hearing impairments apply additional visual and auditory stimulation during play occupations to assist the child to be more aware of and responsive to the environment (Barton et al. 2015). Third, therapists employ added touch and movement stimulation that is embedded in play occupations through the use of sensory integrative procedures (Jenvey 2013; Smith, Mruzek, and Mozingo 2015; Zimmer et al. 2012). In addition, children seek play during solitary times, and it is during this type of play that environmental properties are learned and mastery of the environment during play is reinforced (Jenvey 2013; Logan et al. 2015). Aspects of frameworks such as these have the potential to improve the development of effective SAR therapeutic intervention models. Also key is the full inclusion of experienced clinicians and families to ensure adoption of a SAR as a viable clinical support (Scassellati, Admoni, and Matarić 2012).

Review of User Studies, Outcomes, and Clinical Evidence

Interest in clinical outcomes research following implementation of SARs with children who have complex disabilities such as ASD is growing.

However, the research to date has focused more on the development of various robotic capabilities designed to elicit behaviors such as body awareness (Costa et al. 2013); communication (Robins, Dautenhahn, and Dickerson 2009); cognition (Chan, Nejat, and Chen 2011; Feil-Seifer and Matarić 2009b); social interaction (Breazeal and Scassellati 2000; Robins 2005; Robins et al. 2012); and play facilitation (Robins, Ferrari, and Dautenhahn 2008). To date, minimal research has been published that has been designed to measure the effectiveness of these interventions (Pennisi et al. 2016). There is, however, a growing body of work that suggests SARs have the potential to generate desired clinical outcomes, particularly for children with ASD.

A case in point is the Aurora project. In a single-subject case study evaluation of three children aged 6 to 16, diagnosed as having "low-functioning autism," the robot KASPAR was used to investigate the effect of the SAR on the children and a co-present adult. The investigators were also interested in evaluating the robot's ability to mediate interactions between children with ASD who did not typically interact and others. Interestingly, the children were able to generalize their behaviors with KASPAR (touching, visual regard) to co-present others. The authors concluded that children who were low functioning could benefit from the SAR and were able to demonstrate important interactional competencies (Robins, Dautenhahn, and Dickerson 2009).

Kim et al. (2013) examined the social behaviors of twenty-four 4- to 12-year-old children with ASDs during interactions with three different "partners": (1) another adult human, (2) a touch screen computer game, and (3) a social dinosaur robot. They found "that children with ASD spoke more, in general, while interacting with a social robot than with another adult or a novel, touch screen computer game" (p. 1046). These results indicate that robots can potentially affect social and communication skills for children with ASD, ultimately affecting their ability to interact socially. The major increase in speech by the children with ASD was directed at the "confederate" adult who was helping the child, not toward the robot itself. Thus, the robot enhanced the useful social behavior of interaction with another person rather than just social interaction with objects.

Returning to the Pennisi et al. (2016) meta-analysis of available research related to ASD and SARs mentioned previously in this chapter, the authors approached their analysis from a clinical perspective. They looked at study design, participant characteristics, ASD symptom severity, and any neuropsychological measures tested and the experimental results. They concluded that, of 28 studies that met their criterion for inclusion, there were some generalizations that could be made regarding ASD and the use of

SARs as an intervention method. "1. Participants with ASD often had better performances in *robot conditions* (RC) rather than in *human condition* (HC); 2. In some cases, ASD patients had, toward robots, behaviors that *typically developing* (TD) patients normally had toward human agents; and 3. To benefit the positive effects of the use of robot in therapy, higher levels of stimulation were better than lower levels of stimulation" (Pennisi et al. 2016, 173).

The authors also reported that, when it came to SARs, the NAO robot was the most widely used to date. NAO is classified as a humanoid robot able to move around, dance, talk, and engage interactively with humans. Based on the overarching conclusions drawn by Pennisi et al. (2016), the NAO also embodies those characteristics described by the authors as generalizable. Over 7,000 units have been sold worldwide since it became available (Tomizawa 2016).

One interesting study using NAO focused on the proprioceptive, visual, and kinematic profiles of 13 participants (ages not well defined), including both children and adults attending two care centers in France (Chevalier et al. 2016). The investigators hypothesized that mitigated behavioral response (hyporeactivity) to visual motion and overreliance on proprioceptive information are linked in individuals with ASD to integrating social cues and engaging in successful interactions. They recognized that individuals diagnosed with ASD also have motor, sensory, and visual impairments often overlooked in the diagnosis of ASD. Profiles of each participant were first developed using a virtual motion setup with a stable and unstable platform. With these data, the authors were able to observe a close relationship between postural behaviors/movement sensitivity and visual sensation seeking. During the second part of the study, the participants were greeted by NAO, who asked their names and then asked them if he should dance for them and continued the engagement as long as possible. Participants' gaze direction and gestures were then analyzed, which confirmed their hypothesis. Social engagement was decreased for subjects with increased visual motion and overreliance on proprioceptive information (Chevalier et al. 2016). While this study could benefit from a clearer description of the subjects and the methodology, it suggests a link that should be further explored as we investigate clinical outcomes with the use of SARs.

A study in the United Kingdom explored tactile interactions of children with ASD with the humanoid robot KASPAR (Robins, Amirabdollahian, and Dautenhahn 2013). The authors hypothesized that a tactile robot could serve as a mediator between a child with ASD and another person. They suggested that "a robot with tactile applications could allow a child with ASD to feel safe and build confidence in tactile interaction where they can explore touch in a playful way that could be completely under their control" (p. 89). Fourteen children were recruited to participate in this study (ages and other demographics not provided). They were invited to engage with KASPAR, and all sessions were video recorded. Touch events were recorded as grasp, touch, stroke, poke, and pinch, and touch pressure was recorded by the robot as light, medium, or tight. The results, as predicted by the authors, were extremely varied, and each child was highly individualistic. The authors concluded the need for and potential benefit of creating play scenarios and robots that were flexible and responsive to the many individualized responses of children with ASD (Robins, Amirabdollahian, and Dautenhahn 2013).

Hanson et al. (2012) investigated the use of realistic human-like robots with adults and children with ASD. Two robots were used. One was a realistic, human-size, female robot with an expressive face, and the other was a predecessor of Milo called Zeno. The participants interacted with both robots and found them engaging and not frightening. They also responded with interest to the robot, answering the robot's questions and verbalizing in response to the robot's actions. Participants with ASD also displayed increased social engagement with people. Their behaviors included increased affect, eye contact, verbalization, and several instances of theory of mind by showing concern for the feeling of others.

In a pilot study centered on reducing social anxiety and improving social/vocational skills in adolescents with ASD, Kaboski et al. (2015) conducted a summer robotics camp. In this pilot study, the authors recruited eight adolescents (12–17 years old) with ASD and eight TD matched pairs to attend one of two consecutive week-long camps (3 hours/day for 5 consecutive days). Because all of the participants had a distinct interest in learning to program a robot, the authors focused on social skills performance rather than acquisition of social skills. Camp facilitators were not informed that any of the children were diagnosed with ASD. All participants received the same social/vocational training. Participant pairs worked together to learn to program the NAO robot and then signed up to test out their programming with a camp facilitator. Results at the end of the week were compared to pretest scores of self-reported social anxiety, social skills, and knowledge of robots and robotics. The ASD group demonstrated a significant reduction in self-reported anxiety. In fact, the ASD group came very close to reaching the "non–socially anxious" score on the Social Anxiety Scale Adolescent. Social skills did not increase significantly for those with ASD. All of the participants (16) demonstrated a significant improvement on their knowledge of robots and robotics. Although this was an unusual implementation of a SAR for ASD research, the investigators correctly pointed out that it was indeed possible to conduct an ASD study without disclosing the diagnosis to TD peers. They also pointed out the intervention itself resulted in a reduction in social anxiety of the adolescents with ASD and interventions such as this should receive a great deal of further study (Kaboski et al. 2015).

Future Directions

Today's SARs represent a fusion of the best of engineering, clinical, and caregiver support addressing the educational, social-emotional, cognitive, sensory, and motor interventional needs of children with complex disabilities (Shic and Goodwin 2015). However, there is much yet to learn. A key issue lies in working to improve the quality of the research itself.

While there is a goodly amount of rich description in available studies, limited quantitative data are available. To date, the vast majority of the studies involved a small number of subjects, and demographic information is not always available. Inclusion/exclusion criteria are also lacking in many of the studies, as are careful descriptions of the methods used to conduct the study. Study replication would be extremely difficult in all but a handful of the available publications. The external validity, or how well we can apply the research to other settings, is also limited. Most of the reported findings are exploratory, making it even more difficult to extrapolate findings (Diehl et al. 2012; Pennisi et al. 2016; Scassellati, Admoni, and Matarić 2012).

How can we improve the research? Scassellati, Admoni, and Matarić (2012) discussed the need for research groups to collaborate more effectively with "respect to participant pools and experimental methods, largely owing to geographical distance between research groups and the lack of affordable commercial autism-relevant robot platforms" (p. 286). In many studies, the investigators conducted a one-time experiment. Children with ASD vary from hour to hour and day to day. For example, changes in routine are often upsetting and response to stimuli can fluctuate based on the individual child and their environment. Repeated exposure to a robot can and often does elicit differing responses. Engineers with limited human subject experience would benefit from working with seasoned applied clinical researchers. Likewise, clinicians unfamiliar with technology should seek to collaborate with roboticists who can facilitate proper use of the SAR. It is important to consider these and many other factors when designing a study. If we are to improve the research and move to a solid base with which we can deploy SARs in a meaningful intervention, we must work together to improve the available data (Diehl et al. 2012; Pennisi et al. 2016; Scassellati, Admoni, and Matarić 2012).

Key features of SARs are their physical appearance and actions. When it comes to ASD therapy, currently available robots are very different. Some are humanoid (Milo), while others are animal-like (Keepon), or machine-like (Leka). Because there are few robots commercially available (and affordable), many research groups create their own version of a SAR. This influences available features and behaviors of the robots (Scassellati, Admoni, and Matarić 2012).

Because the field of robotics employs a diverse group of investigators, findings are often published in engineering journals, where most clinicians do not think to look (Diehl et al. 2012). In addition, many clinicians and certainly most families do not recognize the important role they serve in providing feedback to engineers laboring to create a clinically relevant ASD.

What is exciting about the use of SARs for children with ASD and other complex disabilities is their immediate potential. Sensors, actuators, and processing capabilities are improving rapidly. Combined with today's hardware, SARs are quickly expanding in their ability to interact effectively with humans. Two promising developments are under way. The first involves the use of high-level commands from the interventionist. This enables the clinician to incorporate his or her therapeutic objectives within the robot's behavioral sequences and eliminates the need for the therapist to physically direct the robot's actions. Also, robot controllers are now able to recognize human behavior and respond to that behavior, creating a truly interactive companion/therapist (Bekele et al. 2013; Ranatunga et al. 2011; Scassellati, Admoni, and Matarić 2012; Warren et al. 2015).

Today's scientists and engineers are learning a great deal about using technology to mediate social interactions, support educational goals, and improve cognitive and sensory abilities, thus leading to improved clinical outcomes (Chan, Nejat, and Chen 2011; Feil-Seifer and Matarić 2009b; Ranatunga et al. 2011). However, there is a great deal of research that is needed to truly understand the clinical relevance and promise of SARs for children with ASD and other complex disabilities.

"What is crucial for the successful integration of robots in clinical therapy, as well as subsequent acceptance of the approach by the greater ASD community, will be thoughtful collaboration between the clinical and technological fields" (Diehl et al. 2014, 415). Diehl et al. concluded that it will be important to determine the following (p. 416):

1. If the presence of a co-robot therapist enhances outcomes over and above existing empirically supported diagnostic and therapeutic approaches (incremental validity)
2. How individual characteristics of the robot and the child affect therapeutic outcomes (predictive validity)
3. The most effective roles of the robot in a session, such as whether a robot is effective as a co-therapist working alongside a human therapist and whether the use of a robot as the lone therapist is possible (or even desirable)
4. The importance of the autonomy of the robot, for example, how much does it benefit therapeutic outcomes and broad application of the robot if the robot can respond on its own, rather than responding based on the input of a human
5. The most effective ways to implement this approach in real clinical settings, such as schools, hospitals, and nonprofit centers that provide services to individuals with ASD (ecological validity)

STUDY QUESTIONS

1. How are SARs being used clinically for children with disabilities?
2. What features of SARs make them appropriate for use with children with ASD?
3. What is the current state of the science of SARs?
4. What are the applications and limitations of machine-based learning, and how do these apply to SARs?
5. How could SARs be used to supplement clinical interventions for children with complex disabilities?
6. How would you design clinical intervention objectives using NAO?
7. What clinical information is necessary to complement the engineering design of a SAR?
8. How important is the role of family in the adoption and integration of a SAR at home?

References

Adolfsson, Margareta, Johan Malmqvist, Mia Pless, and Mats Granuld. 2011. "Identifying child functioning from an ICF-CY perspective: Everyday life situations explored in measures of participation." *Disability and Rehabilitation* 33 (13–14):1230–1244.

Allievi, Alessandro G, Tomoki Arichi, Anne L Gordon, and Etienne Burdet. 2014. "Technology-aided assessment of sensorimotor function in early infancy." *Frontiers in Neurology* 5:197.

American Psychiatric Association. 2013. *Diagnostic and Statistical Manual of Mental Disorders (DSM-5®)*. Washington, DC: American Psychiatric Association.

Appelhans, Bradley M, and Linda J Luecken. 2006. "Heart rate variability as an index of regulated emotional responding." *Review of General Psychology* 10 (3):229.

Barton, Erin E, Brian Reichow, Alana Schnitz, Isaac C Smith, and Daniel Sherlock. 2015. "A systematic review of sensory-based treatments for children with disabilities." *Research in Developmental Disabilities* 37:64–80.

Basu, Anna P, and Gavin Clowry. 2015. "Improving outcomes in cerebral palsy with early intervention: New translational approaches." *Frontiers in Neurology* 6: 24.

Bekele, Esubalew, Julie A Crittendon, Amy Swanson, Nilanjan Sarkar, and Zachary E Warren. 2014. "Pilot clinical application of an adaptive robotic system for young children with autism." *Autism* 18 (5):598–608.

Bekele, Esubalew T, Uttama Lahiri, Amy R Swanson, Julie A Crittendon, Zachary E Warren, and Niladri Sarkar. 2013. "A step towards developing adaptive robot-mediated intervention architecture (ARIA) for children with autism." *IEEE Transactions on Neural Systems and Rehabilitation Engineering* 21 (2):289–299.

Besio, Serenella. 2002. "An Italian research project to study the play of children with motor disabilities: The first year of activity." *Disability and Rehabilitation* 24 (1–3):72–79.

Besio, Serenella, Francesca Caprino, and Elena Laudanna. 2008. "Profiling robot-mediated play for children with disabilities through ICF-CY: The example of the European project IROMEC." In Klaus Miesenberger, Joachim Klaus, Wolfgang Zagler, and Arthur Karshmer (eds.), *Computers Helping People with Special Needs: 11th International Conference, ICCHP 2008, Linz, Austria, July 9–11, 2008. Proceedings.* Berlin: Springer, pp. 545–552.

Billard, Aude, Annalisa Bonfiglio, Giorgio Cannata, Piero Cosseddu, Torbjorn Dahl, Kerstin Dautenhahn, Fulvio Mastrogiovanni et al. 2013. "The ROBOSKIN Project: Challenges and results." In Vincent Padois, Philippe Bidaud, and Oussama Khatib (eds.), *Romansy 19—Robot Design, Dynamics and Control: Proceedings of the 19th CISM-Iftomm Symposium.* Vienna: Springer, pp. 351–358.

Bodine, Cathy. 2016. "Early developmental skills acquisition and socially assistive robotics (SARS): A pilot investigation of effectiveness." To be submitted.

Bosseler, Alexis, and Dominic W Massaro. 2003. "Development and evaluation of a computer-animated tutor for vocabulary and language learning in children with autism." *Journal of Autism and Developmental Disorders* 33 (6):653–672.

Boucher, Jill. 2003. "Language development in autism." *International Journal of Pediatric Otorhinolaryngology* 67 (Suppl 1):s159–163.

Bourke-Taylor, Helen, and Julie F Pallant. 2013. "The assistance to participate scale to measure play and leisure support for children with developmental disability: Update following Rasch analysis." *Child: Care, Health and Development* 39 (4):544–551.

Breazeal, Cynthia, and Lijin Aryananda. 2002. "Recognition of affective communicative intent in robot-directed speech." *Autonomous Robots* 12 (1):83–104.

Breazeal, Cynthia, and Brian Scassellati. 2000. "Infant-like social interactions between a robot and a human caregiver." *Adaptive Behavior* 8 (1):47–72.

Brodin, Jane. 1999. "Play in children with severe multiple disabilities: Play with toys—A review." *International Journal of Disability, Development and Education* 46 (1):25–34.

Bundy, Anita C. 1997. "Play and playfulness: What to look for." In LD Parham and LS Fazio (eds.), *Play in Occupational Therapy for Children*. St. Louis, MO: Mosby, pp. 52–66.

Cabibihan, John-John, Hifza Javed, Marcelo Ang Jr., and Sharifah Mariam Aljunied. 2013. "Why robots? A survey on the roles and benefits of social robots in the therapy of children with autism." *International Journal of Social Robotics* 5 (4):593–618.

Calderita, Luis Vicente, Pablo Bustos, Cristina Suárez Mejías, Felipe Fernández, and Antonio Bandera. 2013. "Therapist: Towards an autonomous socially interactive robot for motor and neurorehabilitation therapies for children." Proceedings of the 7th International Conference on Pervasive Computing Technologies for Healthcare, May 5–8, Venice, Italy.

Cardon, Teresa A. 2011. "Caregiver perspectives about assistive technology use with their young children with autism spectrum disorders." *Infants and Young Children* 24 (2):153.

Castellano, Ginevra, Iolanda Leite, André Pereira, Carlos Martinho, Ana Paiva, and Peter W McOwan. 2013. "Multimodal affect modeling and recognition for empathic robot companions." *International Journal of Humanoid Robotics* 10 (1):1350010.

Centers for Disease Control and Prevention. 2013. "Cerebral palsy." http://www.cdc.gov/ncbddd/cp/index.html.

Chan, Jeanie, Goldie Nejat, and Jingcong Chen. 2011. "Designing intelligent socially assistive robots as effective tools in cognitive interventions." *International Journal of Humanoid Robotics* 8 (1):103–126.

Chang, Yi-Fan. 2011. "An overview of machine learning." http://www.slideshare.net/drcfetr/an-overview-of-machine-learning.

Chang, Yao-Jen, Tsen-Yung Wang, Shin-Kai Tsai, and Yen-Yun Chu. 2007. "Social computing on online wayfinding training for individuals with cognitive impairments." Presented at World Conference on E-Learning in Corporate, Government, Healthcare, and Higher Education, October, Quebec City, Canada.

Chapparo, Christine, and Judy Ranka. 1996. "Definition of terms." In Christine Chapparo and Judy Ranka (eds.), *Occupational Performance Model (Australia)*. Monography 1. Sydney: Occupational Performance Network, pp. 58–60.

Chevalier, Pauline, Brice Isableu, Jean-Claude Martin, and Adriana Tapus. 2016. "Individuals with autism: Analysis of the first interaction with NAO robot based on their proprioceptive and kinematic profiles." In T Borangiu (ed.), *Advances in Robot Design and Intelligent Control: Proceedings of the 24th International Conference on Robotics in Alpe-Adria-Danube Region (RAAD)*. Cham, Switzerland: Springer International, pp. 225–233.

Collins, Belva C. 2007. *Moderate and Severe Disabilities: A Foundational Approach.* Upper Saddle River, NJ: Pearson Education.

Cook, Albert M, Max QH Meng, Jason J Gu, and Kathy Howery. 2002. "Development of a robotic device for facilitating learning by children who have severe disabilities." *IEEE Transactions on Neural Systems and Rehabilitation Engineering* 10 (3):178–187.

Costa, Sandra, Hagen Lehmann, Ben Robins, Kerstin Dautenhahn, and Filomena Soares. 2013. "'Where is your nose?': Developing body awareness skills among children with autism using a humanoid robot." Presented at the Sixth International Conference on Advances in Computer-Human Interactions, March, Nice, France.

Dautenhahn, Kerstin. 2007. "Socially intelligent robots: Dimensions of human–robot interaction." *Philosophical Transactions of the Royal Society of London B: Biological Sciences* 362 (1480):679–704.

Dickerson, Paul, Ben Robins, and Kerstin Dautenhahn. 2013. "Where the action is: A conversation analytic perspective on interaction between a humanoid robot, a co-present adult and a child with an ASD." *Interaction Studies* 14 (2):297–316.

Diehl, Joshua J, Charles R Crowell, Michael Villano, Kristin Wier, Karen Tang, and Laurel D Riek. 2014. "Clinical applications of robots in autism spectrum disorder diagnosis and treatment." In B Patel, R Preedy, and R Martin (eds.), *Comprehensive Guide to Autism.* New York: Springer, pp. 411–422.

Diehl, Joshua J, Lauren M Schmitt, Michael Villano, and Charles R Crowell. 2012. "The clinical use of robots for individuals with autism spectrum disorders: A critical review." *Research in Autism Spectrum Disorders* 6 (1):249–262.

Diehl, Sylvia F. 2003. "Autism spectrum disorder: The context of speech-language pathologist intervention." *Language, Speech & Hearing Services in Schools* 34 (3):177–179.

Encarnação, Pedro, Liliana Alvarez, Adriana Rios, Catarina Maya, Kim Adams, and Al Cook. 2014. "Using virtual robot mediated play activities to assess cognitive skills." *Disability and Rehabilitation: Assistive Technology* 9(3): 231–241.

Feil-Seifer, David, and Maja J Matarić. 2005. "Defining socially assistive robotics." Presented at ICORR 2005. 9th International Conference on Rehabilitation Robotics, June 28–July 1, Chicago.

Feil-Seifer, David J, and Maja J Matarić. 2008a. "B3IA: An architecture for autonomous robot-assisted behavior intervention for children with autism spectrum disorders." IEEE Proceedings of the International Workshop on Robot and Human Interactive Communication, August, Munich, Germany.

Feil-Seifer, David J, and Maja J Matarić. 2008b. "Robot-assisted therapy for children with autism spectrum disorders." Presented at Refereed Workshop Conference on Interaction Design for Children: Children with Special Needs, Chicago.

Feil-Seifer, David J, and Maja J Matarić. 2009a. "Toward socially assistive robotics for augmenting interventions for children with autism spectrum disorders." In Oussama Khatib, Vijay Kumar, and George J Pappas (eds.), *Experimental Robotics: The Eleventh International Symposium*. Springer Tracts in Advanced Robotics, 54. Berlin: Springer, pp. 201–210.

Feil-Seifer, David, and Maja J Matarić. 2009b. "Towards the integration of socially assistive robots into the lives of children with ASD." Presented at Human–Robot Interaction '09, March, San Diego, CA.

Feil-Seifer, David, Kristine Skinner, and Maja J Matarić. 2007. "Benchmarks for evaluating socially assistive robotics." *Interaction Studies* 8 (3):423–439.

Felzmann, Heike, Kathy Murphy, Dympna Casey, and Oya Beyan. 2015. "Robot-assisted care for elderly with dementia: Is there a potential for genuine end-user empowerment?" Proceedings of ACM/IEEE International Conference on Human–Robot Interaction Workshops, March, Portland, OR.

Ferrari, Ester, Ben Robins, and Kerstin Dautenhahn. 2009. "Therapeutic and educational objectives in robot assisted play for children with autism." Presented at the 18th IEEE International Symposium on Robot and Human Interactive Communication, September 27–October 2, Toyama, Japan.

Gillesen, Jan CC, EI Barakova, Bibi EBM Huskens, and Loe MG Feijs. 2011. "From training to robot behavior: Towards custom scenarios for robotics in training programs for ASD." IEEE International Conference on Rehabilitation Robotics (ICORR) 2011:5975381.

Glenn, Nicole M, Camilla J Knight, Nicholas L Holt, and John C Spence. 2013. "Meanings of play among children." *Childhood* 20 (2):185–199.

Golliot, Julie, Raby-Nahas Catherine, Mark Vezina, Yves-Marie Merat, Audrée-Jeanne Beaudoin, Mélanie Couture, Tamie Salter et al. 2015. "A tool to diagnose autism in children aged between two to five old: An exploratory study with the robot QueBall". In *Proceedings of the Tenth Annual ACM/IEEE International Conference on Human–Robot Interaction Extended Abstracts (HRI'15 Extended Abstracts)*. New York: ACM, pp. 61–62.

Gunes, Hatice and Massimo Piccardi. 2009. "Automatic temporal segment detection and affect recognition from face and body display." *IEEE Transactions on Systems, Man, and Cybernetics, Part B (Cybernetics)* 39 (1):64–84.

Hamm, Ellen, Susan G Mistret, and Amy Goetz-Ruffino. 2006. "Play outcomes and satisfaction with toys and technology of young children with special needs." *Journal of Special Education Technology* 21 (1):29–35.

Hanson, David, Daniele Mazzei, Carolyn Garver, Arti Ahluwalia, Danilo De Rossi, Matt Stevenson, and Kellie Reynolds. 2012. "Realistic humanlike robots for treatment of ASD, social training, and research; shown to appeal to youths with ASD, cause physiological arousal, and increase human-to-human social engagement." Proceedings of the 5th International Conference on Pervasive Technologies Related to Assistive Environments (PETRA), June, Crete, Greece. http://www.faceteam.it/wp-content/uploads/2012/07/PETRA-2012_Realistic -Humanlike-Robots-for-ASD.pdf.

Hartshorne, Timothy S, Alyson Schafer, Kasee K Stratton, and Tasha M Nacarato. 2013. "Family resilience relative to children with severe disabilities." In Doroth S Becvar (ed.), *Handbook of Family Resilience*. New York: Springer, pp. 361–383.

Hasan, Nazmul, Isaac Cocar, Thomas Amely, Hongjie Wang, Regan Zane, Zeljko Pantic, and Cathy Bodine. 2015. "A practical implementation of wireless power transfer systems for socially interactive robots." 2015 IEEE Energy Conversion Congress and Exposition (ECCE), September 20–24, Montreal.

Howard, Ayanna M. 2013. "Robots learn to play: Robots emerging role in pediatric therapy." Presented at the Twenty-Sixth International FLAIRS Conference, January, St. Pete Beach, FL.

Huskens, Bibi, Rianne Verschuur, Jan Gillesen, Robert Didden, and Emilia Barakova. 2013. "Promoting question-asking in school-aged children with autism spectrum disorders: Effectiveness of a robot intervention compared to a human-trainer intervention." *Developmental Neurorehabilitation* 16 (5):345–356.

International Organization for Standardization (ISO). 2014. *ISO 13482 International Standard: Robots and Robotic Devices—Safety Requirements for Personal Care Robots.* Geneva: ISO.

Jenvey, Vickii B. 2013. "Play and disability." In RE Tremblay, M Boivin, and R DeV Peters (eds.), *Encyclopedia on Early Childhood Development*. Montreal, QC, Canada: CEE CD/SKC-ECD, pp. 1–5.

Jiang, Ming, and Li Zhang. 2015. "Big data analytics as a service for affective humanoid service robots." *Procedia Computer Science* 53:141–148.

Kaboski, Juhi R, Joshua J Diehl, Jane Beriont, Charles R Crowell, Michael Villano, Kristin Wier, and Karen Tang. 2015. "Brief report: A pilot summer robotics camp to reduce social anxiety and improve social/vocational skills in adolescents with ASD." *Journal of Autism and Developmental Disorders* 45 (12):3862–3869.

Kim, Elizabeth S, Lauren D Berkovits, Emily P Bernier, Dan Leyzberg, Frederick Shic, Rhea Paul, and Brian Scassellati. 2013. "Social robots as embedded reinforcers of social behavior in children with autism." *Journal of Autism and Developmental Disorders* 43 (5):1038–1049.

Korsten, Jane Edgar, Teresa Vernon Foss, and Lisa Mayer Berry. 2007. *Every Move Counts Clicks and Chats: Sensory-Based Strategies for Communication and Assistive Technology.* Vol. 1. Kansas City, MO: EMC.

Kudoh, Shunsuke, Taku Komura, and Katsushi Ikeuchi. 2006. "Stepping motion for a human-like character to maintain balance against large perturbations." Proceedings 2006 IEEE International Conference on Robotics and Automation, May, Orlando, FL.

Kulkarni, Parag. 2012. *Reinforcement and Systemic Machine Learning for Decision Making.* New York: Wiley, pp. 1–21.

Lane, Shelly J, and Roseann C Schaaf. 2010. "Examining the neuroscience evidence for sensory-driven neuroplasticity: Implications for sensory-based occupational therapy for children and adolescents." *American Journal of Occupational Therapy* 64 (3):375–390.

Lathan, Corina, Jack Maxwell Vice, Michael Tracey, Catherine Plaisant, and Allison Druin. 2001. "Therapeutic play with a storytelling robot." Presented at CHI '01 Extended Abstracts on Human Factors in Computing Systems, April, Seattle, WA.

Lee, Haejung, Rhayun Song, and Heajong Shin. 2001. "Caregiver burnout." In EA Capetuzi, ML Malone, PR Katz and MD Mezey (eds.), *The Encyclopedia of Elder Care*. New York: Springer, pp. 114–116.

Leo, Marco, Marco Coco, Pierluigi Carcagni, Cosimo Distante, Massimo Bernava, Giovanni Pioggia, and Giuseppe Palestra. 2015. "Automatic emotion recognition in robot-children interaction for ASD treatment." Proceedings of the IEEE International Conference on Computer Vision Workshops, December, Santiago, Chile.

Light, Janice, Barbara Roberts, Rosemarie Dimarco, and Nina Greiner. 1998. "Augmentative and alternative communication to support receptive and expressive communication for people with autism." *Journal of Communication Disorders* 31:153–180.

Lin, Yingzi, and David Schmidt. 2015. "Wearable sensing for bio-feedback in human robot interaction." In Subhas C Mukhopadhyay (ed.), *Wearable Electronics Sensors*. New York: Springer, pp. 321–332.

Lindblom, Jessica, and Tom Ziemke. 2006. "The social body in motion: Cognitive development in infants and androids." *Connnection Science* 18 (4):333–346.

Liu, Changchun, Karla Conn, Nilanjan Sarkar, and Wendy Stone. 2007. "Affect recognition in robot assisted rehabilitation of children with autism spectrum disorder." Proceedings of the 2007 IEEE International Conference on Robotics and Automation, April 10–14, Rome.

Liu, Xiaoqing, Lei Zhang, and Jacob Yadegar. 2011. "An intelligent multi-modal affect recognition system for persistent and non-invasive personal health monitoring." Presented at 2011 IEEE 22nd International Symposium on Personal, Indoor and Mobile Radio Communications, September 11–14, Toronto.

Ljunglöf, Peter, Britt Claesson, Ingrid Mattsson Müller, Stina Ericsson, Cajsa Ottesjö, Alexander Berman, and Fredrik Kronlid. 2011. "Lekbot: A talking and playing robot for children with disabilities." Presented at the 2nd Workshop on Speech and Language Processing for Assistive Technologies, July, Edinburgh.

Logan, Samuel W, Melynda Schreiber, Michele Lobo, Breanna Pritchard, Lisa George, and James Cole Galloway. 2015. "Real-world performance: Physical activity, play, and object-related behaviors of toddlers with and without disabilities." *Pediatric Physical Therapy* 27 (4):433–441.

Loutfi, Amy, and Silvia Coradeschi. 2006. "Smell, think and act: A cognitive robot discriminating odours." *Autonomous Robots* 20 (3):239–249.

Marti, Patricia. 2012. "Materials of embodied interaction." Presented at the 14th ACM International Conference on Multimodal Interaction, October 22–26, Santa Monica, CA.

Marti, Patrizia, Margherita Bacigalupo, Leonardo Giusti, Claudio Mennecozzi, and Takanori Shibata. 2006. "Socially assistive robotics in the treatment of behavioural and psychological symptoms of dementia." Presented at the First IEEE/RAS-EMBS International Conference on Biomedical Robotics and Biomechatronics, February 20–22, Pisa, Italy.

Matarić, Maja J, Jon Eriksson, David J Feil-Seifer, and Carolee J Winstein. 2007. "Socially assistive robotics for post-stroke rehabilitation." *Journal of Neural Engineering and Rehabilitation* 4 (5).

Matarić, Maja, Adriana Tapus, Carolee Winstein, and Jon Eriksson. 2009. "Socially assistive robotics for stroke and mild TBI rehabilitation." *Studies in Health Technology and Informatics* 145:249–262.

Mbouzao, Boniface. 2013. "Quantitative assessment of human motion capabilities with passive vision monitoring." MSc thesis, Ottawa, ON, Canada: University of Ottawa.

McDougall, Janette, and Virginia Wright. 2009. "The ICF-CY and goal attainment scaling: Benefits of their combined use for pediatric practice." *Disability and Rehabilitation* 31 (16):1362–1372.

Mead, Ross, and Maja J Matarić. 2015. "Toward robot adaptation of human speech and gesture parameters in a unified framework of proxemics and multi-modal communication." Presented at the Workshop on Machine Learning for Social Robotics, ICRA, May 26–30, Seattle, WA.

Michaud, François, Audrey Duquette, and Isabelle Nadeau. 2003. "Characteristics of mobile robotic toys for children with pervasive developmental disorders." Presented at the IEEE International Conference on Systems, Man and Cybernetics, October 5–8, Washington, DC.

Mitsunaga, Noriaki, Christian Smith, Takayuki Kanda, Hiroshi Ishiguro, and Norihiro Hagita. 2005. "Robot behavior adaptation for human–robot interaction based on policy gradient reinforcement learning." Presented at the 2005 IEEE/RSJ International Conference on Intelligent Robots and Systems (IROS 2005), August 2–6, Edmonton, AB, Canada.

Musselwhite, Caroline R. 1986. *Adaptive Play for Special Needs Children: Strategies to Enhance Communication and Learning.* Austin, TX: Pro Ed.

Nelson, Charles A. 2003. "Neural development and lifelong plasticity." In RM Lerner, F Jacobs, and D Wertlieb (eds.), *Handbook of Applied Developmental Science.* Thousand Oaks, CA: Sage, 31–60.

O'Rourke, Pearl, Ray Ekins, Bernard Timmins, Fiona Timmins, Siobhan Long, and Eugene Coyle. 2014. "Crucial design issues for special access technology; A Delphi study." *Disability and Rehabilitation: Assistive Technology* 9(1):48–59.

Panning, Axel, Ingo Siegert, Ayoub Al-Hamadi, Andreas Wendemuth, Dietmar Rösner, Jane Frommer, Gerald Krell, and Brend Michaelis. 2012. "Multimodal affect recognition in spontaneous HCI environment." *2012 IEEE International Conference on Signal Processing, Communication and Computing (ICSPCC),* August 12–15, pp. 430–435.

Pantic, Maja, and Leon JM Rothkrantz. 2003. "Toward an affect-sensitive multimodal human-computer interaction." *Proceedings of the IEEE* 91 (9):1370–1390.

Park, Eunil, and Jaeryoung Lee. 2014. "I am a warm robot: The effects of temperature in physical human–robot interaction." *Robotica* 32 (01):133–142.

Pennisi, Paola, Alessandro Tonacci, Gennaro Tartarisco, Lucia Billeci, Liliana Ruta, Sebastiano Gangemi, and Giovanni Pioggia. 2016. "Autism and social robotics: A systematic review." *Autism Research* 9 (2):165–183.

Porter, Maggie L, Maria Hernandez-Reif, and Peggy Jessee. 2007. "Play therapy: A review." *Early Child Development and Care* 179 (8):1025–1040.

Rabbitt, Sarah, Alan Kazdin, and Brian Scassellati. 2015. Integrating socially assistive robotics into mental healthcare interventions: Applications and recommendations for expanded use. *Clinical Psychology Review* 35:35–46.

Ranatunga, Isura, Jartuwat Rajruangrabin, Dan O Popa, and Fillia Makedon. 2011. "Enhanced therapeutic interactivity using social robot Zeno." Proceedings of the 4th International Conference on Pervasive Technologies Related to Assistive Environments, May 25–27, Crete, Greece.

Risley, Todd R, Sharon Landesman Ramey, and Julie Washington. 2012. "Building pre-reading skills: Discussing research-based strategies for developing language and pre-reading skills in young children." http://www.readingrockets .org/webcasts/1002/?trans=yes#transcript.

Robins, Ben. 2005. "A humanoid robot as assistive technology for encouraging social interaction skills in children with autism." PhD thesis, Hatfield, UK: University of Hertfordshire.

Robins, Ben, Kerstin Dautenhahn, and Paul Dickerson. 2009. "From isolation to communication: A case study evaluation of robot assisted play for children with autism with a minimally expressive humanoid robot." Presented at the Second International Conferences on Advances in Computer-Human Interactions, February 1–7, Cancun, Mexico.

Robins, Ben, Kerstin Dautenhahn, Ester Ferrari, Gernot Kronreif, Barbara Prazak-Aram, Patrizia Marti, Iolanda Iacono et al. 2012. "Scenarios of robot-assisted play for children with cognitive and physical disabilities." *Interaction Studies* 13 (2):189–234.

Robins, Ben, Kerstin Dautenhahn, René Te Boekhorst, and Aud Billard. 2005. "Robotic assistants in therapy and education of children with autism: Can a small humanoid robot help encourage social interaction skills?" *Universal Access in the Information Society* 4:105–120.

Robins, Ben, Ferrari, Ester, and Dautenhahn, Kerstin. 2008. "Developing scenarios for robot assisted play." Presented at the 17th IEEE International Symposium on Robot and Human Interactive Communication, August 1–3, Munich, Germany.

Robins, Ben, Farshid Amirabdollahian, and Kerstin Dautenhahn. 2013. "Investigating child-robot tactile interactions: A taxonomical classification of tactile behaviour of children with autism towards a humanoid robot." Presented at the Sixth International Conference on Advances in Computer-Human Interactions (ACHI), February 24–March 1, Nice, France.

Rollins, Pamela. 2016. "Robokind: Advanced social robots." http://www.robokin drobots.com/robots4autism-home/social-skills-curriculum/.

Roussou, Maria. 2004. "Learning by doing and learning through play: An exploration of interactivity in virtual environments for children." *Computers in Entertainment (CIE)* 2 (1):10–10.

Rubin, Daniela A, Kathleen S Wilson, Lenny D Wiersma, Jie W Weiss, and Debra J Rose. 2014. "Rationale and design of active play@ home: A parent-led physical activity program for children with and without disability." *BMC Pediatrics* 14 (1):41.

Šabanović, Selma, Marek P Michalowski, and Linnda R Caporael. 2007. "Making friends: Building social robots through interdisciplinary collaboration." Proceedings of AAAI 2007 Spring Symposium on Multidisciplinary Collaboration for Socially Assistive Robotics, March 26–28, Palo Alto, CA.

Šabanović, Selma, Casey C Bennett, Wan-Ling Chang, and Laszlo Huber. 2013. "PARO robot affects diverse interaction modalities in group sensory therapy for older adults with dementia." Presented at the 2013 IEEE International Conference on Rehabilitation Robotics (ICORR), June 24–26, Seattle, WA.

Salter, Tamie, Neil Davey, and François Michaud. 2014. "Designing and developing QueBall, a robotic device for autism therapy." Presented at 2014 RO-MAN: The 23rd IEEE International Symposium on Robot and Human Interactive Communication, August 25–29, Edinburgh.

Salvador, Michelle J, Sophia Silver, and Mohammad H Mahoor. 2015. "An emotion recognition comparative study of autistic and typically-developing children using the Zeno robot." Presented at the 2015 IEEE International Conference on Robotics and Automation (ICRA) May 26–30, Seattle, WA.

Santos, Kristopher B. 2012. "The Huggable: A socially assistive robot for pediatric care." Master of science thesis, Cambridge, MA: Massachusetts Institute of Technology (830533394).

Scassellati, Brian, Henny Admoni, and Maja Matarić. 2012. "Robots for use in autism research." *Annual Review of Biomedical Engineering* 14 (1):275–294.

Seelye, Adriana M, Maureen Schmitter-Edgecombe, Barnan Das, and Diane J Cook. 2012. "Application of cognitive rehabilitation theory to the development of smart prompting technologies." *IEEE Reviews in Biomedical Engineering* 5:29–44.

Seligman, Milton, and Rosalyn Benjamin Darling. 2009. *Ordinary Families, Special Children: A Systems Approach to Childhood Disability*. New York: Guilford Press.

Shamsuddin, Syamimi, Hanafiah Yussof, Luthffi Idzhar Ismail, Salina Mohamed, Fazah Akhtar Hanapiah, and Nur Ismarrubie Zahari. 2012. "Initial response in HRI—A case study on evaluation of child with autism spectrum disorders interacting with a humanoid robot NAO." *Procedia Engineering* 41:1448–1455.

Shic, Frederick, and Matthew Goodwin. 2015. "Introduction to technologies in the daily lives of individuals with autism." *Journal of Autism and Developmental Disorders* 45 (12):3773–3776.

Simeonsson, Rune J. 2009. "ICF-CY: A universal tool for documentation of disability." *Journal of Policy and Practice in Intellectual Disabilities* 6 (2): 70–72.

Smith, Tristram, Daniel W Mruzek, and Dennis Mozingo. 2015. "Sensory integration therapy." In RM Foxx and JA Mulick (eds.), *Controversial Therapies for Autism and Intellectual Disabilities: Fad, Fashion, and Science in Professional Practice*, 2nd ed. New York: Routledge, p. 247.

Snow, Catherine E. 1972. "Mothers' speech to children learning language." *Child Development* 43 (2):549–565.

Stansfield, Sharon, Carole Dennis, and Hélène Larin. 2012. "WeeBot: A novel method for infant control of a robotic mobility device." Presented at the 2012 IEEE International Conference on Robotics and Automation, May 14–18, St. Paul, MN.

Sutton, Richard S, and Andrew G Barto. 1998. *Reinforcement Learning: An Introduction*. Cambridge, MA: MIT Press.

Swift-Spong, Katelyn, Elaine Short, Eric Wade, and Maja J Matarić. 2015. "Effects of comparative feedback from a Socially Assistive Robot on self-efficacy in post-stroke rehabilitation." Presented at the 2015 IEEE International Conference on Rehabilitation Robotics (ICORR), August 11–14, Singapore.

Syrdal, Dag Sverre, Hagen Lehmann, Ben Robins, and Kerstin Dautenhahn. 2014. "KASPAR in the wild—Initial findings from a pilot study." Presented at AISB 2014–50th Annual Convention of the AISB, April 1–4, London.

Tanaka, Fumihide, Aaron Cicourel, and Javier R Movellan. 2007. "Socialization between toddlers and robots at an early childhood education center." *Proceedings of the National Academy of Sciences* 104 (46):17954–17958.

Tapus, Adriana, Andreea Peca, Amir Aly, Cristina Pop, Lavinia Jisa, Sebastian Pintea, Alina S Rusu et al. 2012. "Children with autism social engagement in interaction with NAO, an imitative robot—A series of single case experiments." *Interaction Studies* 13 (3):315–347.

Tapus, Adriana, Cristian Tapus, and Maja J Matarić. 2007. "Hands-off therapist robot behavior adaptation to user personality for post-stroke rehabilitation therapy." Presented at the IEEE International Conference on Robotics and Automation (ICRA), April 10–14, Rome.

Tapus, Adriana, Cristian Tapus, and Maja J Matarić. 2009. "The use of socially assistive robots in the design of intelligent cognitive therapies for people with dementia." Presented at the IEEE International Conference on Rehabilitation Robotics, June 23–26, Kyoto, Japan.

Tomizawa, Fumihide. 2016. "Cool robots." https://www.aldebaran.com/en/cool-robots/nao.

Vázquez, Marynel, Aaron Steinfeld, Scott E Hudson, and Jodi Forlizzi. 2014. "Spatial and other social engagement cues in a child-robot interaction: Effects of a sidekick." Proceedings of the 2014 ACM/IEEE International Conference on Human–Robot Interaction, March 3–6, Bielefeld, Germany.

Wada, Kazuyoshi, Takanori Shibata, Toshimitsu Musha, and Shin Kimura. 2008. "Robot therapy for elders affected by dementia." *IEEE Engineering in Medicine and Biology* 27 (4):53–60.

Wainer, Jacques, Ben Robins, Farshid Amirabdollahian, and Kerstin Dautenhahn. 2014. "Using the humanoid robot KASPAR to autonomously play triadic games and facilitate collaborative play among children with autism." *IEEE Transactions on Autonomous Mental Development* 6 (3):183–199.

Wang, Hua, Cuiqin Ma, and Lijuan Zhou. 2009. "A brief review of machine learning and its application." ICIECS 2009. International Conference on Information Engineering and Computer Science, December 19-20, Wuhan, China.

Warren, Zachary, Zhi Zheng, Shuvajit Das, Eric M Young, Amy Swanson, Amy Weitlauf, and Nilanjan Sarkar. 2015. "Brief report: Development of a robotic intervention platform for young children with ASD." *Journal of Autism and Developmental Disorders* 45 (12):3870–3876.

World Health Organization. 2001. *International Classification of Functioning, Disability and Health: ICF.* Geneva: WHO.

Zeng, Zhihong, Maja Pantic, Glenn I Roisman, and Thomas S Huang. 2009. "A survey of affect recognition methods: Audio, visual, and spontaneous expressions." *IEEE Transactions on Pattern Analysis and Machine Intelligence* 31 (1):39–58.

Zhang, Zhengyou. 2012. "Microsoft Kinect sensor and its effect." *IEEE Computer Society* April–June:1–10.

Zheng, Zhi, Shuvajit Das, Eric M Young, Amy Swanson, Zachary Warren, and Nilanjan Sarkar. 2014. "Autonomous robot-mediated imitation learning for children with autism." Proceedings of the 2014 IEEE International Conference on Robotics & Automation (ICRA), May 31–June 7, Hong Kong.

Zimmer, Michelle, Larry Desch, Lawrence D Rosen, Michelle L Bailey, David Becker, Timothy P Culbert, Hilary McClafferty et al. 2012. "Sensory integration therapies for children with developmental and behavioral disorders." *Pediatrics* 129 (6):1186–1189.

9

Robots Supporting Care for Elderly People

Sandra Bedaf, Claire Huijnen,
Renée van den Heuvel, and Luc de Witte

Contents

Learning Objectives
After completing this chapter, readers will be able to

1. Describe problematic activities of elderly people that hinder their **independent living**.
2. Describe robotic solutions to assist elderly people in those activities.
3. Explain a robotics framework that is used to classify robots supporting care for elderly people.
4. Describe specific robots, illustrating different areas within the proposed robotics framework.

Principles

Aging-Related Challenges

The Western population is aging. In 2014, the percentage of people aged 65+ in Europe was 18.5% (Eurostat 2016). Per 100 persons of working age (15–64 years old), 28.1 persons were aged 65+. Twenty years ago, this number was lower, with 21.6 persons aged 65+ per 100 persons of working age. The elderly population is expected to continue to grow in the upcoming years not only in Europe, but also in many countries all over the world. Most elderly people are healthy and participate actively in society, but a substantial number have chronic diseases or other conditions that hinder them in daily life. For those, the performance of everyday tasks may become difficult, challenging, or even impossible due to the negative consequences of their decreasing abilities. Different kinds of solutions are being created for people who are (becoming) impaired in their capabilities for independent living in the hope of regaining or sustaining their independence. Examples are informal or formal care. However, social structures are changing, which results in informal caregivers being less inclined or able to provide care. In addition, professional caregivers are unable to answer the growing demand for home care as societies are facing an increasing shortage of care staff (Cameron and Moss 2007). For those who are unable to continue to live at home, institutional arrangements for dependent living are offered. It is known that the causes of institutionalization of an elderly person are complex (Miller and Weissert 2000). However, institutionalized care is often a final recourse due to its high costs and because elderly people usually prefer to stay at home as long as possible. "Aging in place" is also the best solution from the societal point of view.

Assistive technology (AT) can play a major role in supporting elderly people in their daily life. AT, such as (powered) wheelchairs, stair lifts, and in general home accessibility adaptations, have come a long way in supporting individuals in their independence (Vlaskamp, Soede, and Gelderblom 2011) and are increasingly becoming accepted. A new field within AT that emerged from the ongoing development of technology is robotics, which has the potential to support care and independence in many ways (Bekey et al. 2006). The technological developments of robotics are promising; however, only a limited number of care robots designed for elderly people have become commercially available (Bedaf, Gelderblom, and De Witte 2015). It seems that the envisioned role of the robots and the type of tasks they perform are often primarily guided by technical feasibility and to a lesser degree by the target users' needs (Butter et al. 2008).

When developing a robot supporting care for elderly people, it is important to know which activities are most likely to threaten independent living when it becomes difficult. Bedaf et al. (2014) made an inventory of these activities based on a systematic literature search and focus group sessions with older people and formal and informal caregivers. The International Classification of Functioning, Disability, and Health (ICF) (World Health Organization 2001) of the World Health Organization, which provides a structured taxonomy for the description of human functioning, was adopted to group the variety of activities found in this study. The ICF domains mobility, self-care, and social isolation seemed to be the most problematic and threatening for the independence of elderly people (Bedaf et al. 2014). However, no single activity could be selected as the main activity resulting in institutionalization. One needs to take into consideration that this study by Bedaf et al. (2014) focused on elderly people with no cognitive decline even though there is a growing number of elderly people who experience problems in this area. For this group, probably a different set of activities would prove to be a threat to independent living, as they would likely experience more problems related to cognitive decline (e.g., need for reminders to take medication).

In general, a robot is an embodied system that can be programmed to perform different automated tasks involving physical movement or force exertion (see Chapter 1). Looking at the three problematic activity domains mentioned and considering the expected problems with people with cognitive decline, robots can support a number of these tasks, but for other tasks, it is more questionable. For example, several activities within the domains self-care (e.g., washing, toileting, dressing, and eating) and mobility (e.g., climbing stairs, lifting and carrying objects) involve physical movement or force exertion. These activities may therefore be interesting for a robotic system. The third problematic domain, social isolation, or the provision of reminders may be less suitable for solution by a robotic system as there is most likely no need for physical movement or force exertion. There are already several (low-cost) non-robotic Information and Communication Technology (ICT) technologies available to support social interaction (e.g., Skype, tele-home care systems), and it is easier to place a tablet in every room than to create an expensive tablet on wheels that can navigate through the house without problems. Nevertheless, there are exceptions, such as the seal-like social robot PARO (PARO Robots 2014), which also addresses social isolation and has received some attention (Gelderblom et al. 2010).

A Framework for Robotics Supporting Care for Elderly People

The domain of robots for the care of elderly people is broad and includes many different robots with varying goals and intentions, as shown in a number of earlier reviews on socially assistive robots (SARs) for care of elderly people (Bedaf, Gelderblom, and De Witte 2015; Bemelmans et al. 2012; Broekens, Heerink, and Rosendal 2009; Kachouie et al. 2014). To categorize these different efforts, a care robotics framework is suggested in this chapter that can help to distinguish between the different types of robots and their focus. The framework proposes two dimensions: the level of social interaction on the one hand and the targeted end user on the other hand.

With respect to the first dimension, distinction is made between physically assistive robots (PARs) and SARs. Assistive robots (ARs) are robots that provide aid or support to a human user (Feil-Seifer and Matarić 2005). An adequate definition of a PAR is one that gives aid or support to a human user through physical interaction. SARs share with PARs the goal of assisting human users, but the assistance is provided through social interaction rather than physical interaction. SARs can have a role in assisting people similar to the role guide dogs have for visually impaired people. In short, Feil-Seifer and Matarić (2005) defined an SAR as the intersection of AR and socially interactive robotics (SIRs), which was first used by Fong et al. (2003) to describe robots with the goal to develop close and effective interactions with a human for the sake of interaction itself (also see Chapter 1 for definition of SARs). Because of the emphasis on social interaction, SARs have a similar focus to SIRs. With SARs, however, the robot's goal is to create close and effective interaction with a human user for the purpose of giving assistance and achieving measurable progress in convalescence, rehabilitation, learning, and so on (Fong, Nourbakhsh, and Dautenhahn 2003). As such, SARs can also be seen as a subsection of SIRs. A review of SAR systems concluded that different roles could be distinguished, ranging from companionship to therapeutic play partner, coach, or instructor (Rabbitt, Kazdin, and Scassellati 2015).

An example of a PAR is the mealtime assistance robot My Spoon (http://www.secom.co.jp/english/myspoon/). This robot supports the user physically with the activity of eating without any social interaction. A good example of a SAR (or a SIR) is the interactive seal-like robot PARO. PARO is a therapeutic robot for people with dementia. It can perceive people and its environment, and by interaction with people, it responds as if it is alive.

Both the My Spoon and the PARO focus on the user. However, there are also robots that focus more on (providing support for) the caregivers. This

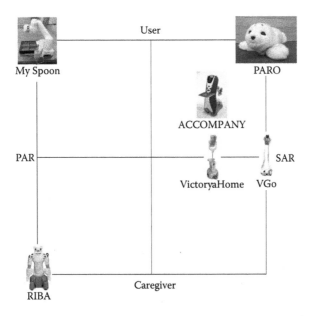

Figure 9.1   Care robotics framework for care of elderly people. (Robot images reproduced with the permission of the ACCOMPANY Project, Focal Meditech BV, the VictoryaHome Consortium, Vecna Technologies, Inc., and RIKEN-TRI.)

is the second dimension in our framework in which a distinction is made between user-oriented robots and caregiver-oriented robots. One example of a caregiver-oriented robot is the RIBA (Robot for Interactive Body Assistance; and its follow-up version, ROBEAR [Robot for Interactive Body Assistance]) (http://rtc.nagoya.riken.jp/RIBA/index-e.html). This robot can crouch down and pick up a patient off the floor, a strenuous action that caregivers must do frequently.

The two dimensions described can be schematically described in a matrix that can function as a framework for positioning different robots for the care of elderly people. In Figure 9.1, some examples of specific robots are positioned in this matrix. These robots are illustrative examples to understand different kinds of support that robots can give. These are discussed in more detail in the remainder of this chapter.

Critical Review of the Technology Available

Even though applications of robotics in health care are not new (Butter et al. 2008), there are not many robotic systems for elderly people that have reached and (successfully) stayed in the market. This section describes available robotic systems with high technology readiness levels (TRLs) that are illustrative of systems in several positions of the care robotics framework in Figure 9.1.

PARO

PARO is an interactive baby seal-like robot developed by Takanori Shibata from the National Institute of Advanced Industrial Science and Technology (AIST; http://www.aist.go.jp/index_en.html) in Japan (Figure 9.2). PARO interacts with people as if it is "alive," moving its head and legs and making sounds (it imitates the voice of a real baby harp seal). PARO is covered with soft natural-feel fur, and the interior contains five types of sensors: tactile, light, audio, temperature, and posture. With these sensors, it can perceive people and its environment. With the light sensor, it can make the distinction between light and dark. By its tactile sensors, PARO feels when it is being stroked or beaten, and posture sensors indicate if it is being held. Finally, it can recognize the direction of voice and words such as its name and greetings with its audio sensor (Bemelmans et al. 2012). In addition to the sensors, PARO has actuators that control the seal's eyelids, back limb, front paw, and neck. PARO is able to learn to behave in the way the user prefers and to respond to its given name. The robot has no

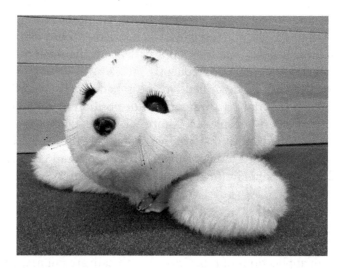

Figure 9.2   PARO seal robot.

mobility capabilities (i.e., it does not move around freely in the environment) and weighs about 2.8 kg (~6.2 lb) (Kachouie et al. 2014).

PARO has been used as a therapeutic robot for people with dementia in Japan and throughout Europe since 2003. According to the manufacturer, "It allows the documented benefits of animal therapy to be administered to patients in environments such as hospitals and extended care facilities where live animals present treatment or logistical difficulties" (PARO Robots 2014).

PARO is one of the few commercially available robots for elderly people that are actually being adopted, used, and implemented in care processes in daily practice. It is at a TRL of 9. Other systems for robotic animal therapy reached the market, such as the catlike NeCoRo (Libin and Cohen-Mansfield 2004) or the doglike AIBO (Banks, Willoughby, and Banks 2008; Tamura et al. 2004) but are no longer commercially available. Many other robots still exist in maturity levels, such as a research prototype (TRL 2–4).

PARO is a good example of a SAR as it provides assistance to human users, but it gives that assistance through social interaction rather than physical interaction. Therefore, PARO can be seen at the upper right corner of the framework in Figure 9.1, supporting the users rather than the professionals in an SAR manner.

ACCOMPANY

The European ACCOMPANY (Acceptable robotiCs COMPanions for AgeiNg Years) Project (http://accompanyproject.eu/) was a 3-year robotic project that aimed to prolong independent living of elderly people by means of a service robot developed by a multidisciplinary consortium.*
The project made use of an existing service robot, the Care-O-bot® (http://www.care-o-bot.de/de/care-o-bot-3.html) (Figure 9.3), with the aim to further develop its functionalities to assist older people to carry out relatively difficult daily tasks on their own again. This robot has an omnidirectional platform with three laser scanners for navigation. A sensor head includes a stereo rig and a three-dimensional (3-D) time-of-flight camera. The sensor head is mounted on an axis that allows it to move back

---

* The consortium consisted of the University of Hertfordshire, United Kingdom; Hogeschool Zuyd, the Netherlands; Fraunhofer, Germany; University of Amsterdam, the Netherlands; University of Sienna, Italy; Maintien en Autonomie à Domicile des Personnes Agées, France; University of Birmingham, United Kingdom; University of Twente, the Netherlands; and University of Warwick, United Kingdom.

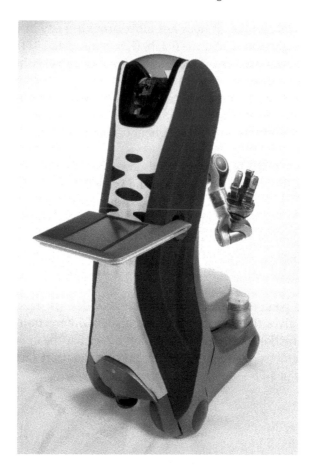

Figure 9.3　Care-O-bot robot of the ACCOMPANY Project. (Reproduced with the permission of the ACCOMPANY Project.)

and forth. The robot torso is on a manipulator with 4 degrees of freedom (DOF), providing more flexibility to position the cameras and enabling the robot to perform body gestures for a more natural interaction with persons. The Care-O-bot also features a 7-DOF robotic manipulator with a dexterous hand with an additional 7 DOF. Interaction with the user is mainly done through a tray for carrying objects. A retractile touch screen is included in the tray. For safety, the robot arm is only used to place and take objects from the tray when no person is detected in the vicinity of the robot.

ACCOMPANY distinguished three types of potential users for its platform: (1) cognitively unimpaired older persons who need some support to remain independent in their own homes, (2) informal caregivers, and (3) professional caregivers. Different aspects were explored, such as empathic and social human–robot interaction; ethical concerns (Bedaf et al. 2016; Draper, Sorell, Bedaf, Gutierrez Ruiz et al. 2014; Draper, Sorell, Bedaf, Syrdal et al. 2014; Sorell and Draper 2014); robot learning and memory visualization (Ho et al. 2013); monitoring of persons and chores at home (Hu, Englebienne, and Kröse 2014; Hu, Lou et al. 2014); and the technological integration of these multiple approaches.

Within the ACCOMPANY Project, the fetch-and-carry task of the Care-O-bot going to the kitchen and getting something to drink was selected as the (initial) scenario task. A total of three subscenarios were carried out that together formed the functionalities of the final robot (Bedaf and Gelderblom 2014). In the first scenario, robot tasks are to remind the user to take his or her medication and to carry a bottle of water to the user. In the second scenario, the robot should be able to seek the user when the doorbell rings, get a parcel from the door, monitor the user to determine whether he or she has been drinking, and fetch and carry a glass of water from the kitchen and place it on the table. Finally, in the third scenario, robot tasks are to play an activity game with the user, recognizing visitors and fetching a vase.

The Care-O-bot robot used in the ACCOMPANY Project can be considered at a TRL of 8. Its utilization as a robotic companion integrated in an intelligent environment, as it was aimed in the ACCOMPANY Project, is still at a TRL of 6–7, having the prototypical system demonstrated in a relevant environment (Duclos and Amirabdollahian 2014).

The aim of the ACCOMPANY Project was to create a robot that would be capable of supporting elderly people in their independent living by focusing not only on how to successfully execute tasks technically but also on the development of acceptable social behavior of the robot while executing these tasks. For example, the robot gives physical feedback to the user to make its intentions clearer (e.g., the robot bows after delivering a parcel or turns its torso when placing the drink on a table). This makes the robot more than just a PAR as it also takes socially acceptable behavior into account. It is therefore placed more toward SAR than PAR on the horizontal line in Figure 9.1. In addition, this robot leans more toward supporting the user than the caregiver and is therefore placed in the upper right quadrant of the framework for robots for care of elderly people.

VictoryaHome

VictoryaHome is a project co-funded by the European Active and Assisted Living (AAL) Program aiming at enabling elderly people to live their lives

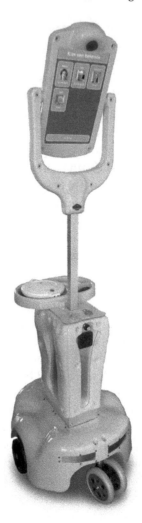

Figure 9.4 VictoryaHome telepresence robot. (Reproduced with the permission of the VictoryaHome Consortium.)

the way they want to (Serrano et al. 2014). With the vision "Be Well, Create Possibilities," a comprehensive support system that monitors the health and safety of older adults and facilitates social contact was devised. The system includes an activity monitor, a fall detector, an automatic pill dispenser, and a mobile telepresence robot. A smartphone app for family and friends providing a general overview of the elderly person's well-being is also included. In addition, professional caregivers can use the system to monitor the user. Technical developments were framed within the following principles: providing the user and caregivers peace of mind, never leaving the user alone, always allowing the user to connect with significant ones, providing safety and security, helping the helpers, sharing feelings and experiences, and making caring for elderly people popular.*

The robot platform used in the VictoryaHome project is called Giraff (see Figure 9.4) and is produced by Giraff Technologies AB (http://www .giraff.org/?lang=en) in Sweden. It allows virtually entering a home from a computer via the Internet and conducting a natural visit without actually being physically present. The platform can move freely in the home, controlled through the caregiver's computer mouse. Videoconferencing with the people in the home is also provided.

The Giraff is a commercially available robotic platform at a TRL of 8–9. Its integration in the VictoryaHome system underwent long-term trials with end users and is at a TRL of 6–7.

VictoryaHome supports both the end user and the caregiver. It is mainly a communication tool, but the mobile platform includes a tray to carry objects (i.e., the pill dispenser), and thus it also provides physical assistance. Therefore, it can be placed in the middle of the axis user-caregiver and more toward SAR than PAR in Figure 9.1.

VGo

Another commercial telepresence system including a teleoperated robot is the VGo (http://www.vgocom.com/) (see Figure 9.5). It provides a means for obtaining health information, improving older adults' social and daily functioning, and giving peace of mind to family members and caregivers who live remotely (Seelye et al. 2012). The VGo robot can be controlled locally through a handheld controller or remotely over the Internet. It has a camera, microphones, speakers, and a video display to establish a video communication connection between different locations. Distance sensors placed on the robot base ensure safety. As with the Giraff, family members, friends, or professional caregivers can access the VGo system to monitor the elderly person's well-being.

Being a relatively new commercially available product, the VGo system is at a TRL of 8–9. In Figure 9.1, it occupies a position to the right of the ACCOMPANY system because no physical assistance is provided.

---

* Input on the VictoryaHome project was received from Dr. J. Artur Serrano, the scientific manager of the VictoryaHome Consortium and currently research scientist at the Norwegian Center for eHealth Research and associate professor of Telemedicine and eHealth Research Group, Faculty of Health Sciences, UiT Arctic University of Norway.

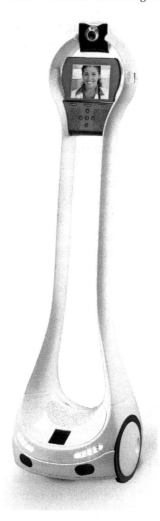

Figure 9.5   VGo telepresence robot. (Reproduced with the permission of Vecna Technologies, Inc.)

My Spoon

The mealtime robot My Spoon, developed by the Japanese company SECOM (http://www.secom.co.jp/english/myspoon/), focuses on people who are unable to eat without the help of others (e.g., due to limited arm/hand function) (see Figure 9.6). It is a robot that provides meal assistance by providing a special plate or bowl that keeps the food and a robot arm with a fork and spoon attached that picks up the food and delivers it to the user. Being unable to independently eat strongly affects one's feelings

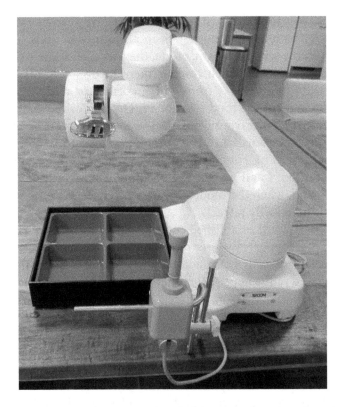

Figure 9.6   My Spoon robot. (Reproduced with permission of Focal Meditech BV.)

of independence and freedom. In addition, it has a negative impact on the nutrition intake, yielding several health problems (e.g., malnutrition) and correspondingly increasing medical-societal costs. Feeding someone is labor intensive and is perceived as embarrassing to some people. It also is aggravating for partners or family members, as they often do not have the time to eat themselves and because meal enjoyment disappears when one is not an equal dinner partner.

My Spoon allows the user to eat with only minimal help from a caregiver, at his or her own speed, and according to his or her own preferences. It creates independence and reduces the amount of care. My Spoon can be operated with a joystick or a button and has three modes: (1) manual mode, (2) semiautomatic mode, and (3) automatic mode (SECOM 2016). Modes differ regarding the freedom/control in scooping the type of food users prefer (from a specific location in one of the four My Spoon compartments). In the manual mode, maximum flexibility and control are obtained by fully controlling the spoon with the joystick. Any food item within the included tray can be eaten in any desired order by moving the joystick in all four directions (up, down, left, right). In the semiautomatic mode, the user operation is simplified. The user chooses from which compartment he or she wants to receive food, but the robot decides from which corner (or middle or border) of the compartment the food is scooped. Only a desired compartment within the included tray and no specific food item can be chosen by using the joystick. Finally, in the automatic mode the My Spoon will automatically select a compartment and grasp a food item by simply pressing a button. In all modes, the spoon will automatically approach the mouth, and, when the mouth comes in contact with the spoon, the fork will automatically retract.

My Spoon is a well-established commercially available robot at a TRL of 9. My Spoon supports the user physically with the eating activity without any social interactions. In addition, My Spoon is user oriented and therefore placed in the upper left corner of the framework in Figure 9.1.

RIBA

RIBA (and its follow-up version ROBEAR) is the product of a collaboration between two Japanese companies: RIKEN and Tokai Rubber Industries Limited (http://rtc.nagoya.riken.jp/RIBA/index-e.html). It is a nursing robot that is able to lift a person from a bed or wheelchair, which is one of the most physically challenging tasks in nursing care (see Figure 9.7).

RIBA features specially created joint positions and link lengths designed for lifting a human. The robot's body is covered with soft materials, and the elbow and waist joints are isolated, making RIBA safe for physical interactions. This softness also contributes to patients' comfort when they are being lifted. A teddy bear shape was deliberately used to put patients at ease and to give a friendly, nonthreatening, appearance. Two cameras and two microphones allow RIBA to follow an operator using visual and audio cues. The nursing robot responds to the operator's voice commands from the basic "hello," "good-bye," and "shake hands," through lifting up and down, to other more intricate moves, such as transferring clients from a bed to a seat. Motion is adjusted and suspended or resumed by touching RIBA's tactile sensors. RIBA's developers claim this is an intuitive control method because the contact position and force direction coincide with those of the desired motion. The robot is on omnidirectional wheels, so it can move in any direction.

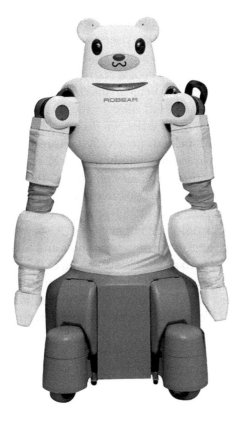

Figure 9.7   ROBEAR nursing robot. (Reproduced with the permission of RIKEN-TRI.)

The RIBA prototype was tested and validated in a laboratory environment; thus, it is at a TRL of 4–5. Its main function is to lift a person, supporting or even taking over caregiver's tasks, which clearly places it in the lower left corner of the framework matrix in Figure 9.1.

Critical Review of the Available Utilization Protocols

Socially assistive robots such as PARO have mainly been used with elderly people with dementia. The underlying idea is to achieve the benefits of animal therapy using a robotic system. However, outcomes of animal therapy with patients with dementia or other pathologies are still under debate, and no established protocols are available (Filan and Llewellyn-Jones 2006;

Nordgren and Engström 2014; O'Haire 2013; O'Haire, Guérin, and Kirkham 2015; Williams and Jenkins 2008). Users are expected to interact with the robotic pets as they would with a real pet. Most studies that evaluated the effect of these SARs on elderly people restricted the use of the robotic systems to specific hours per day (Bemelmans et al. 2012; Mordoch et al. 2013).

Service robots like the Giraff used in the VictoryaHome project, the Care-O-bot used in the ACCOMPANY Project, or the VGo are meant to be used 24/7 in homes for elderly people. Systems include a number of software licenses, such that various family members, friends, and caregivers can access the system through their computers. The system can be connected to a care facility such that possible alarms are directly sent to caregivers, who can then use the robot's telepresence feature to better assess the situation. Long-term studies are not available. Also, it is still necessary to show the economic value of telepresence robots and to develop the appropriate business models. An economic evaluation of the ACCOMPANY system was provided by Duclos and Amirabdollahian (2014).

Envisioned clients for ARs to support caregivers like ROBEAR are care facilities that would like to alleviate personnel from strenuous tasks, such as lifting patients from a mattress at floor level into a wheelchair. However, these robots are still not commercially available, and the concept needs to be validated in real environments (e.g., will ROBEAR be more effective than a mobile hoist?).

Review of User Studies, Outcomes, and Clinical Evidence

Most of the user studies about robots for older people have included the robot PARO (Jøranson et al. 2016). The current applications of the other robots presented in this chapter are not abundant. To the best of our knowledge, there is one study trialing the VGo robot with end users (Seelye et al. 2012) and some user studies with the Care-O-bot robot (Bedaf et al. 2016; Marti and Iacono 2015). Multicountry VictoryaHome user trials are currently being executed (Serrano et al. 2014). No studies were found that implemented the robots RIBA or My Spoon with older adults specifically.

The majority of the studies using PARO have been conducted with older adults with dementia residing in nursing homes or community dwellings. Regarding outcomes, PARO was found to reduce patients' and caregivers' stress. It stimulated the interaction and socialization between patients and caregivers and has been shown to have a positive psychological effect on patients. When older people interacted with PARO, they showed an improvement in their mood (Bemelmans et al. 2015; Shibata,

Kawaguchi, and Wada 2012; Wada et al. 2005; Yu et al. 2015); relaxation (decreasing stress levels) (Jøranson et al. 2015; Wada and Shibata 2007); laughing, positive expressions (Takayanagi, Kirita, and Shibata 2014); and social interactions not only with each other (Chang, Sabanovic, and Huber 2013; Giusti and Marti 2006; Klein and Cook 2012; Robinson et al. 2013; Robinson, Broadbent, and MacDonald 2016; Shibata, Kawaguchi, and Wada 2012, Wada and Shibata 2007) but also with their caregivers (Shibata, Kawaguchi, and Wada 2012). Interacting with PARO encouraged communication and increased elderly people's communicative utterances (Wada et al. 2005) and frequency of talking (Giusti and Marti 2006). The implementation of PARO in daily intramural psychogeriatric care practice with elderly people with dementia increased individually defined therapeutic goals for each participant regarding psychological and psychosocial functioning (Bemelmans et al. 2015). Interventions using PARO have also shown a reduction of symptoms of depression (Wada et al. 2005; Yu et al. 2015) and a tendency to decrease caregivers' burden (Yu et al. 2015).

Some studies have reported the type of reactions toward PARO while older adults interacted with the robot. Using a satisfaction questionnaire, Shibata, Kawaguchi, and Wada (2012) examined people living with PARO. They received 85 responses from persons in all age groups (68% above 60 years old) who owned the PARO robot from 2 to 519 days (average 53.49 days). Most of the participants were female (72%). Researchers investigated the PARO features that were most important for males and females: "Eye blink," "Body shape," "Face," and "Cry" were the most important characteristics for males, while "Tactile texture," "Blink," "Face," and "Cry" were the most important characteristics for females. Both males and females expressed "Healing effect is expected" as the main reason for acquiring PARO. The majority of the participants were satisfied (47%) or very satisfied (34%) with the robot. Jøranson and colleagues (2016) observed behaviors in older adults at different stages of dementia interacting with PARO during 12 weeks. Results revealed that the behavior of "Observing Paro" was more often shown by participants with mild-to-moderate dementia, and "Observing other things" was most commonly shown by elders with severe dementia. Moreover, the behavior "Smile/laughter toward other participants" increased, while "Conversations with PARO on the lap" decreased as the intervention progressed. Yu and colleagues (2015) found that during six 30-minute sessions of occupational therapy using PARO, most of the time older adults with dementia showed neutral expressions, while less time was spent smiling and laughing.

Despite the described positive outcomes, caution is needed before concluding that PARO is in fact a suitable non-pharmacological treatment for neuropsychiatric symptoms of elders with dementia (Bemelmans et al. 2012; Broekens, Heerink, and Rosendal 2009; Mordoch et al. 2013). All studies involved small sample sets and short durations. Only recently are studies using randomization and control groups becoming available (e.g., Jøranson et al. 2015). Several papers on PARO user studies reported partial results from the same study. Often, study methodologies are not clearly described, thus preventing replication. Further research (i.e., independent randomized clinical trials) is still needed to establish the efficacy of SARs such as PARO in the treatment of elderly people.

The robot VGo was placed in the homes of eight older adults who lived alone in their own homes and had no cognitive impairment (Seelye et al. 2012). Results from first user trials indicated that older adults appreciated the potential of telepresence robotic technology of the VGo to support physical health and well-being, social connectedness, and the ability to live independently at home. Friends and adult children of the participants who were able to move the robot remotely appreciated this feature, especially during videoconferencing. However, one participant, who subsequently progressed to a diagnosis of mild cognitive impairment, responded negatively to the robot. The participant became confused by VGo's purpose, requesting the robot to be taken away from her home (Seelye et al. 2012).

Marti and Iacono (2015) designed a graphic user interface for older adults to interact with the robot Care-O-bot. The interface was composed of icons that represented the possible actions that the robot may perform for the person at home. The interface also had a feature that represented the feelings of the robot (e.g., anger, surprise, sadness) by a dynamic mask. The aim of the interface was to facilitate the interaction between the older adult and the robot. The interface was tested with 72 older adults who understood how the interface worked and expressed that the dynamic mask helped them to interact with the robot. Some participants reported that they identified with the robot's feelings displayed in the dynamic mask, which helped them to feel empathy with the robot.

Professionals' attitudes about robotic telepresence technology have been investigated (Boman 2013; Kristoffersson et al. 2011). It is worth noting that there was a large variance in acceptance of the robot between different health professionals (nursing and health subject teachers; nursing, occupational therapy, and audiology students) (Kristoffersson et al. 2011), and that caregivers reported the difficulties of communicating and simultaneously controlling the robot, as well as the possibility of patients being put into a defensive role because the robot is being remotely operated by the caregiver (Boman 2013).

Discussion and Reflection

In this chapter, just a few examples of robots for care of elderly people have been discussed. Looking at the enormous research effort in this area (Bedaf, Gelderblom, and De Witte 2015; Bemelmans et al. 2012; Feil-Seifer and Matarić 2005; Gelderblom et al. 2010; Kachouie et al. 2014; Lehmann et al. 2013; Rabbitt, Kazdin, and Scassellati 2015; Serrano et al. 2014), it is realistic to expect that many more examples will become available within the next few years.

The framework presented may help to structure this field and to enable a sound discussion of the aims of certain robot systems. It is also likely that combinations of assistive robotic platforms and telecare applications such as in the VictoryaHome project will enter the market. These systems will play an important role in care of elderly people in the future. To be effective, however, it is essential that robot systems have functionality that is really supporting the "solution" for these problems. Focused research is needed to obtain this knowledge and to develop the necessary robot functionalities.

The idea of robots playing a role in care raises much discussion among health care professionals and also in the general public. Often, ethical issues are raised (see Chapter 10) and sometimes also the fear of robots taking over the work of health care professionals. The ethical issues are related to dependence on technology in general and to the nonhuman and "cold" character of robots, which is considered to be in contrast with the fundamentals of care (of elderly people). Examples of the PARO and VictoryaHome, however, showed that robot technology is not necessarily inhumane and cold. On the contrary, these examples showed that robots can really add warmth to care, even if it is technical. It is important for the future development of robotics in care of elderly people that these discussions about ethical issues are given sufficient attention. Otherwise, we might be confronted with robots that do not add value to care of elderly people and miss the potential added value of robotics.

STUDY QUESTIONS

1. What are main activities that threaten people's ability to live independently once the activities become problematic?
2. What are PARs?
3. What are SARs?
4. Describe the two dimensions that are used in the framework to categorize different robots for care of elderly people.
5. Give an example of a PAR and explain why it is a PAR.

6. Give an example of an SAR and explain why it is an SAR.
7. What are strong points of using robots in the care of elderly people?
8. What are possible weak points or concerns of using robots in the care of elderly people?
9. In what way(s) can you envision that the work of care professionals will change when robots are used in care practices?
10. What conditions have to be met to successfully integrate robots into care processes?

References

Banks, M.R., L.M. Willoughby, and W.A. Banks. 2008. "Animal-assisted therapy and loneliness in nursing homes: Use of robotic versus living dogs." *Journal of the American Medical Directors Association* 9 (3):173–177.

Bedaf, S., H. Draper, G.J. Gelderblom, T. Sorell, and L. de Witte. 2016. "Can a service robot which supports independent living of older people disobey a command? The views of older people, informal carers and professional caregivers on the acceptability of robots." *International Journal of Social Robotics* 8 (3):409–420.

Bedaf, S., and G.J. Gelderblom. 2014. "ACCOMPANY Project Deliverable 1.5 final report on scenarios and system functionality of the ACCOMPANY system." http://www.rehabilitationrobotics.net/cms2/sites/default/files/ACCOMPANY %20D1.5_report_scenarios_system%20fuct.pdf.

Bedaf, S., G.J. Gelderblom, and L. De Witte. 2015. "Overview and categorization of robots supporting independent living of elderly people: What activities do they support and how far have they developed?" *Assistive Technology* 27 (2):88–100.

Bedaf, S., G.J. Gelderblom, D.S. Syrdal, H. Lehmann, H. Michel, D. Hewson, F. Amirabdollahian, K. Dautenhahn, and L. de Witte. 2014. "Which activities threaten independent living of elderly when becoming problematic: Inspiration for meaningful service robot functionality." *Disability and Rehabilitation: Assistive Technology* 9 (6):445–452.

Bekey, G., R. Ambrose, V. Kumar, A. Sanderson, B. Wilcox, and Y. Zheng. 2006. *WTEC Panel Report on International Assessment of Research and Development in Robotics (Final Report)*. Lancaster, PA: World Technology Evaluation Center.

Bemelmans, R., G.J. Gelderblom, P. Jonker, and L. de Witte. 2012. "Socially assistive robots in elderly care: A systematic review into effects and effectiveness." *Journal of the American Medical Directors Association* 13 (2):114–120.e1.

Bemelmans, R., G.J. Gelderblom, P. Jonker, and L. de Witte. 2015. "Effectiveness of robot Paro in intramural psychogeriatric care: A multicenter quasi-experimental study." *Journal of the American Medical Directors Association* 16 (11):946–950.

Boman, I.L. 2013. Health Professionals' Perceptions of the Robot "Giraff" in Brain Injury Rehabilitation. Assistive Technology: From Research to Practice. AAATE 33, 115.

Broekens, J., M. Heerink, and H. Rosendal. 2009. "Assistive social robots in elderly care: A review." *Gerontechnology* 8 (2):94–103.

Butter, M., A. Rensma, J. van Boxsel, S. Kalisingh, M. Schoone, M. Leis, G.J. Gelderblom et al. 2008. *Robotics for Healthcare: Final Report*. Brussels: European Commission, DG Information Society.

Cameron, C., and P. Moss. 2007. *Care Work in Europe: Current Understandings and Future Directions*. New York: Routledge.

Chang, W.-L., S. Sabanovic, and L. Huber. 2013. "Situated analysis of interactions between cognitively impaired older adults and the therapeutic robot PARO." *Lecture Notes in Computer Science* no. 8239:371–380. British Library Document Supply Centre Inside Serials and Conference Proceedings, EBSCOhost.

Draper, H., T. Sorell, S. Bedaf, C. Gutierrez Ruiz, Hagen Lehmann, Michael Hervé, Gert Jan Gelderblom, Kerstin Dautenhahn, and Farshid Amirabdollahian. 2014. "What asking potential users about ethical values adds to our understanding of an ethical framework for social robots for older people." Paper presented at AISB50—50th Annual Convention of the AISB, April 1–4, London.

Draper, H., T. Sorell, S. Bedaf, D.S. Syrdal, C. Gutierrez-Ruiz, A. Duclos, and F. Amirabdollahian. 2014. "Ethical dimensions of human–robot interactions in the care of older people: Insights from 21 focus groups convened in the UK, France and the Netherlands." *Proceedings of Social Robotics: 6th International Conference, ICSR 2014, Sydney, NSW, Australia*: 135.

Duclos, A., and F. Amirabdollahian. 2014. "ACCOMPANY Project Deliverable 7.3 economic evaluation." http://rehabilitationrobotics.net/cms2/sites/default/files/ACCOMPANY%20D7.3_Economic%20Model.pdf.

Eurostat. 2016. Population data. http://ec.europa.eu/eurostat/web/population-demography-migration-projections/population-data.

Feil-Seifer, D., and M.J. Matarić. 2005. "Defining Socially Assistive Robotics." *Proceedings of the 2005 IEEE 9th International Conference on Rehabilitation Robotics* 2005: 465–468.

Filan, S.L., and R.H. Llewellyn-Jones. 2006. "Animal-assisted therapy for dementia: A review of the literature." *International Psychogeriatrics* 18 (4):597–611.

Fong, T., I. Nourbakhsh, and K. Dautenhahn. 2003. "A survey of socially interactive robots: Concepts, design, and applications." *Robotics and Autonomous Systems* 42 (3–4):143–166.

Gelderblom, G.J., R. Bemelmans, N. Spierts, P. Jonker, and L. de Witte. 2010. "Development of PARO interventions for dementia patients in Dutch psychogeriatric care." In *Social Robotics SE-26*, edited by ShuzhiSam Ge, Haizhou Li, John-John Cabibihan, and YeowKee Tan, 6414:253–258. Lecture Notes in Computer Science. Berlin: Springer.

Giusti, L., and P. Marti. 2006. "Interpretative dynamics in human robot interaction." *Proceedings in the 15th IEEE International Symposium on Robot and Human Interactive Communication*, ROMAN. Hatfield, 111–116.

Ho, W.C., K. Dautenhahn, N. Burke, J. Saunders, and J. Saez-Pons. 2013. "Episodic memory visualization in robot companions providing a memory prosthesis for elderly users." In *Assistive Technology: From Research to Practice: AAATE 2013*, edited by P. Encarnação, 120. Amsterdam: IOS Press.

Hu, N., G. Englebienne, and B. Kröse. 2014. "A two-layered approach to recognize high-level human activities." *RO-MAN the 23rd IEEE International Symposium on Robot and Human Interactive Communication*, August 25–29, 243.

Hu, N., Z. Lou, G. Englebienne, and B. Kröse. 2014. "Learning to recognize human activities from soft labeled data." *Proceedings of Robotics: Science and Systems (RSS)*, July, Berkeley, CA.

Jøranson, N., I. Pedersen, A.M. Rokstad, and C. Ihlebæk. 2015. "Effects on symptoms of agitation and depression in persons with dementia participating in robot-assisted activity: A cluster-randomized controlled trial." *Journal of the American Medical Directors Association* 16 (10):867–873.

Jøranson, N., I. Pedersen, A.M.M. Rokstad, G. Aamodt, C. Olsen, and C. Ihlebæk. 2016. "Group activity with Paro in nursing homes: Systematic investigation of behaviors in participants." *International Psychogeriatrics* 28 (8):1345–1354.

Kachouie, R., S. Sedighadeli, R. Khosla, and M.-T. Chu. 2014. "Socially assistive robots in elderly care: A mixed-method systematic literature review." *International Journal of Human-Computer Interaction* 30 (5):369–393.

Klein, B., and G. Cook. 2012. "Emotional robotics in elder care—A comparison of findings in the UK and Germany." In *Social Robotics,* edited by S. Ge, O. Khatib, J.-J. Cabibihan, R. Simmons, and M.-A. Williams, 108–117. Berlin: Springer.

Kristoffersson, A., S. Coradeschi, A. Loutfi, and K. Severinson-Eklundh. 2011. An Exploratory Study of Health Professionals' attitudes about robotic telepresence technology. *Journal of Technology in Human Services* 29 (4):263–283.

Lehmann, H., D. Syrdal, K. Dautenhahn, G.J. Gelderblom, and S. Bedaf. 2013. "What should a robot do for you?—Evaluating the needs of the elderly in the UK." *Proceedings of ACHI 2013: The Sixth International Conference on Advances in Computer-Human Interactions*, March, 83–88.

Libin, A., and J. Cohen-Mansfield. 2004. "Therapeutic robocat for nursing home residents with dementia: Preliminary inquiry." *American Journal of Alzheimers Disease and Other Dementias* 19 (2):111–116.

Marti, P., and I. Iacono. 2015. "Social and empathic behaviours: Novel interfaces and interaction modalities." *24th IEEE International Symposium on Robot and Human Interactive Communication*. Kobe, Japan: IEEE, 217–222.

Miller, E.A., and W.G. Weissert. 2000. "Predicting elderly people's risk for nursing home placement, hospitalization, functional impairment, and mortality: A synthesis." *Medical Care Research and Review* 57 (3):259–297.

Mordoch, E., A. Osterreicher, L. Guse, K. Roger, and G. Thompson. 2013. "Use of social commitment robots in the care of elderly people with dementia: A literature review." *Maturitas* 74 (1):14–20.

Nordgren, L., and G. Engström. 2014. "Effects of dog-assisted intervention on behavioural and psychological symptoms of dementia." *Nursing Older People* 26 (3):31–38.

O'Haire, M.E. 2013. "Animal-assisted intervention for autism spectrum disorder: A systematic literature review." *Journal of Autism and Developmental Disorders* 43 (7):1606–1622.

O'Haire, M.E., N.A. Guérin, and A.C. Kirkham. 2015. "Animal-assisted intervention for trauma: A systematic literature review." *Frontiers in Psychology* 6:1121.

PARO Robots. 2014. PARO therapeutic robot. http://www.parorobots.com/.

Rabbitt, S.M., A.E. Kazdin, and B. Scassellati. 2015. "Integrating socially assistive robotics into mental healthcare interventions: Applications and recommendations for expanded use." *Clinical Psychology Review* 35:35–46.

Robinson, H., E. Broadbent, and B. MacDonald. 2016. "Group sessions with Paro in a nursing home: Structure, observations and interviews." *Australasian Journal on Ageing* 35 (2):106–112.

Robinson, H., B. Macdonald, N. Kerse, and E. Broadbent. 2013. "The psychosocial effects of a companion robot: A randomized controlled trial." *Journal of the American Medical Directors Association* 14 (9):661–667.

SECOM. 2016. Meal-assistance robot. http://www.secom.co.jp/english/myspoon/.

Seelye, A.M., K.V. Wild, N. Larimer, S. Maxwell, P. Kearns, and J.A. Kaye. 2012. "Reactions to a remote-controlled video-communication robot in seniors' homes: A pilot study of feasibility and acceptance." *Telemedicine and E-Health* 18 (10):755–759.

Serrano, J.A., H. van den Heuvel, O. Bjorkman, S. von Rum, and I. Bierhoff. 2014. "One year of VictoryaHome." *Proceedings of the AAL Forum 2014*, September 9–12, Bucharest, Romania.

Shibata, T., Y. Kawaguchi, and K. Wada. 2012. "Investigation on people living with seal robot at home: Analysis of owners' gender differences and pet ownership experience." *International Journal of Social Robotics* 4 (1):53–63.

Sorell, T., and H. Draper. 2014. "Robot carers, ethics, and older people." *Ethics and Information Technology* 16 (3):183–195.

Takayanagi, K., T. Kirita, and T. Shibata. 2014. "Comparison of verbal and emotional responses of elderly people with mild/moderate dementia and those with severe dementia in responses to seal robot, PARO." *Frontiers in Aging Neuroscience*, 6 (257). Published online September 26, 2014.

Tamura, T., S. Yonemitsu, A. Itoh, D. Oikawa, A. Kawakami, Y. Higashi, T. Fujimooto, and K. Nakajima. 2004. "Is an entertainment robot useful in the care of elderly people with severe dementia?" *Journals of Gerontology. Series A, Biological Sciences and Medical Sciences* 59 (1):M83–M85.

Vlaskamp, F., T. Soede, and G.J. Gelderblom. 2011. *History of Assistive Technology: 5000 Years of Technology Development for Human Needs.* Heerlen, the Netherlands: Zuyd University of Applied Sciences.

Wada, K., and T. Shibata. 2007. "Living with seal robots—Its sociopsychological and physiological influences on the elderly at a care house." *IEEE Transactions on Robotics* 5:972.

Wada, K., T. Shibata, T. Saito, K. Sakamoto, and K. Tanie. 2005. "Psychological and social effects of one year robot assisted activity on elderly people at a health service facility for the aged." *Proceedings of the 2005 IEEE International Conference on Robotics and Automation* (April):2796–2801.

Williams, E., and Jenkins, R. 2008. "Dog visitation therapy in dementia care: A literature review." *Nursing Older People* 20 (8):31–35.

World Health Organization. 2001. *International Classification of Functioning, Disability and Health (ICF)*. Geneva: World Health Organization.

Yu, R., E. Hui, J. Lee, D. Poon, A. Ng, K. Sit, K. Ip et al. 2015. "Use of a therapeutic, socially assistive pet robot (PARO) in improving mood and stimulating social interaction and communication for people with dementia: Study protocol for a randomized controlled trial." *JMIR Research Protocols* 4 (2):e45.

10

Ethical and Social Implications of the Use of Robots in Rehabilitation Practice

Liliana Alvarez and Albert M. Cook

Contents

Learning Objectives

After completing this chapter, readers will be able to

1. Analyze the impact of introducing robots in rehabilitation practice from an ethical perspective.
2. Characterize the major ethical tensions that arise when introducing robots in rehabilitation practice and research.
3. Integrate ethical considerations in the clinical reasoning and clinical decision-making process when introducing robots in rehabilitation practice.
4. Compare and contrast the benefits and limitations of using robots in rehabilitation practice and research from an ethical standpoint.

Introduction

As robotic systems have moved from the lab to the home, clinic, and greater community, individual users will come to increasingly depend on them. This dependence has made the importance of safe and efficacious operation more evident. Because of their increasing role as social companions and helpmates, robots have also been perceived as having a special relationship with the user. The anthropomorphic nature of many of these robots can lead to interpretations and impressions that resemble human-human relationships. When such relationships develop, ethical concerns can arise.

As robots become more and more autonomous and employ decision-making capabilities through artificial intelligence (AI), humans may also experience loss of autonomy and independence. When the AI includes clinical decision making, there are also ethical dilemmas associated with best practices, as human clinicians and AI algorithms may not interpret, enact, and adapt those practices in the same way.

As robots replace human caregivers, there are additional ethical issues that become important. The use of robots as a means of keeping people in their own homes can also raise issues related to autonomy and safety. Social robots have a goal of establishing companionship and a close relationship when interacting with certain populations, such as children with autism or adults with dementia. Overall, such applications have ethical implications that must be considered. This chapter focuses on these ethical questions and the ways in which they are being framed and discussed in the literature and in practice.

Principles

The Ethical Context

Once thought to be the object of advanced scientific endeavors, robots have steadily made their way into the forefront of technological applications. In nations across the world, robots are now regarded as not only a feasible alternative or assistive device for humans, but also as items that are increasingly present in different spheres of human life. In spite of the varied representations of robots that are spread across media outlets, individuals seem to have an overall positive perception of the development and use of robots. For example, in a survey conducted across European nations, most European Union citizens expressed positive views toward robots, with percentages ranging from 54% in Greece to 88% in Denmark and Sweden (European Commission 2012).

In spite of the overall positive perception of the public toward robots, people feel less optimistic about them when it comes to health care, specifically the care of the elderly, those with chronic health care needs, children, and those with disabilities. In fact, the European Commission (2012) found that European respondents highly supported the use of robots in situations that would be too dangerous or too taxing for humans (e.g., manufacturing, military and security, and space exploration). However, "there is widespread agreement that robots should be banned in the care of children, the elderly or the disabled (60%) with large minorities also wanting a ban when it comes to other 'human' areas such as education (34%), healthcare (27%) and leisure (20%)" (p. 4). Similarly, in a national U.S. survey, the Pew Research Center (2014) found that 65% of Americans "think it would be a change for the worse if lifelike robots become the primary caregivers for the elderly and people in poor health" (p. 3). Although the acceptance of technology is believed to be a largely age-dependent phenomenon, Americans across all age groups agreed on the negative implications of using robots in such areas (Pew Research Center 2014).

Although these large data sets did not explore the reasons behind the mistrust toward robots in health, such negative representations seem to spread to other concrete spheres of application, such as robotic-assisted surgery (RS). In a study conducted by Boys and colleagues (2016), 72% of respondents thought RS was safer, faster, more effective, and less painful than conventional surgery. Yet, 55% of respondents would prefer to have conventional surgery instead of RS. The reasons for mistrust toward robots in health care environments may be influenced by several factors.

Perhaps two prominent and interrelated ones are how much people know about robots and their characteristics and the ethical tensions that arise when allowing robots into situations of particular importance and sensitivity for humans, such as health care practices. An example of these tensions is seen more clearly in situations of "algorithm aversion."

Algorithm aversion refers to the phenomenon by which humans prefer and choose a human over an algorithm, even when the algorithm is shown to consistently outperform the human's decision making (Dietvorst, Simmons, and Massey 2014). Several factors can give rise to this phenomenon, such as the ethicality of relying on algorithms to make important decisions or the perceived inability of algorithms to learn from experience (Dawes 1979). Also, significant to the implications of such aversion in the field of robotics in health care is the fact that tolerable human errors become intolerable when made by machines (Dietvorst, Simmons, and Massey 2014). Such errors seem to erode the trust of the public in robots and thus could potentially undermine the uptake of robotic solutions in the field of rehabilitation, such as the ones described in this book. However, as each of the chapters of this book has articulated, the benefits of robotics when applied to rehabilitation are numerous. Such important advantages for human health, and the fact that researchers and developers are actively engaged in considering and negotiating the ethical implications of robotics, are proof of the promising advances that are currently possible and those that will be possible within the next generations.

In the forefront, this section is concerned with the implications and potential for a code of values and norms that can guide the practical decision making of professionals in this field (i.e., professional ethics; Airaksinen 2003). In the background, this section is committed to the imperative reflection on "the constructed norms of internal consistency regarding what is right and what is wrong" or the *ethics* of robotics in health care (Martin, Bengtsson, and Dröes 2010, 65). Although we acknowledge that there may be several approaches to an ethical analysis of a field like this one, this section considers a principles-based approach. We believe this approach particularly lends itself for the purpose of illuminating the current ethical considerations of this emerging and expanding field in a way that articulates both the current applications and the potential of these technologies. When considering the ethics of using robots in rehabilitation practice, at least three dimensions must be considered: the ethics of the person who develops the technology, the ethics of the rehabilitation professional when implementing robots in practice, and the ethical systems built into robots (Aasaro 2006). The following sections consider all three of these, sometimes focusing on one more than the others depending on the principle and its practical considerations in this field.

Autonomy

The principle of autonomy upholds the belief that every person has a right to self-determination and to be free from interference, risks to privacy, or unnecessary constraints. Such a principle has important implications for robotics in rehabilitation. At the very least, adhering to this principle requires that users of robotics-based services in rehabilitation be fully informed and apprised of the capabilities and limitations of the robot. The latter is necessary for the person to make a fully informed decision (and to provide **informed consent**, when applicable).

Providing adequate information about the robot and its role in the care plan and process is fundamental to increase the public trust in robotic applications, as well as fully ensure the person's autonomy is respected. Such information includes, but is not limited to, the capabilities of the robot, proposed role in care, benefits and limitations, length of intervention, alternative options, and safety and privacy concerns. Although adequate information is necessary, such information does not guarantee that ethical tensions will be avoided. Feil-Seifer and Matarić (2011) offered an example that illustrates the possible tensions regarding autonomy, especially applied to socially assistive robots (SARs). In their example, a companion robot is used in a nursing home that does not allow pets. The residents are told that the robot is "just like a pet." Although such information can be true in principle, the residents soon discover that the robot has a limited repertoire of behaviors, which causes the residents to feel lonely and disappointed. Even when adequate information is offered, the interactions of the human and the device can become complex, and altered expectations can emerge. For example, although users are fully informed that the Roomba® serves purposes related to vacuuming, Sung et al. (2007) found that users bond to them and demand that they be fixed and returned when broken, as opposed to fully replaced with a new one. Although this example does not relate directly to the rehabilitation field, the extrapolations to possible tensions in the field are evident. Thus, health care professionals must be aware of the possible autonomy implications of introducing robots and be ready to partner with their clients and developers to negotiate them in the best interest of the client.

Privacy

In addition to issues related to information and self-determination, potential threats to a client's privacy must be discussed and fully addressed. Although some of the robotic systems discussed in this book do not collect personal health information (e.g., Lego® robots for children with physical disabilities), the functions and purpose of certain robotic systems require the comprehensive gathering of personal health and other data. Such is the case for mobile robots intended to help older adults age in place. Alaiad, Zhou, and Koru (2014) found privacy to be one of the determinants of adoption of home health care robots. To ensure the older adult's safety, robots in this context are expected to collect data and to report to a professional or selected contact family member, in some circumstances even to emergency respondents. Although such functionalities are clearly beneficial when it comes to monitoring the health and safety of the person, while enabling independence, being monitored can create feelings of discomfort and has been shown to change the behaviors of older adults. When comparing the effect of a monitoring camera, a stationary robot, and a mobile robot for older adults, Caine, Šabanović, and Carter (2012) found that older adults engaged in privacy-enhancing behaviors (PEBs) (i.e., behaviors that alleviate their privacy concerns), such as censoring speech during phone calls, hiding from the device, and so on. Although this study provided empirical evidence of such concerns, the potential of robots is promising in this regard as Caine and colleagues found that participants were more likely to engage in PEBs when monitored with a camera than with a robot.

In summary, the need to protect the client's autonomy requires a concerted effort between researchers, clinicians, and developers and challenges all parties with seeking the input of clients. Considering privacy-driven design can provide viable options for the development, deployment, and evaluation of robots in rehabilitation.

Paternalism

In addition to the implications for informed consent articulated previously, robotic systems are vulnerable to other well-established risks to informed consent, much as other assistive technologies (ATs; see Cook and Polgar 2015). Such risks include the use of robotic systems with people who may not be able to provide informed consent via conventional methods. Of particular importance for the use of robots in rehabilitation is the risk of paternalism. Paternalism is defined as "the interference of a state or individual in relation to another person, either against their will or when the interference is justified by a claim of better protection for the individual" (Martin, Bengtsson, and Dröes 2010, 71). Paternalism occurs when safety is privileged over freedom of choice and when the assumption that a person needs to be protected from himself or herself is enacted. For example, robotic systems can enhance the safety of people with dementia, but their use may be imposed on the person. Although there are certainly no easy answers regarding what the best path forward is in these circumstances, this section is meant to articulate the complexity and the ethical tension and invite clinicians and developers alike to reflect on them.

Fidelity

Based on loyalty to the client, *fidelity* refers to notions of faithfulness, trustworthiness, and honesty in care (Kitchener 2000). As articulated by Purtilo (2005), fidelity in the context of health care (which includes rehabilitation) implies treating the client with respect; competency of the health care professional; adhering to the professional code of ethics; following regulations, protocols, and procedures; and honoring agreements made with the client. Such implications charge the rehabilitation professional with the responsibility of acting transparently, regardless of the methods for assessment and intervention, but warrant specific considerations pertaining to robotics in rehabilitation. As a fundamental aspect of fidelity, rehabilitation professionals must be fully competent in operating the robotic system and providing the necessary information about it and have adequate information to provide at least some basic troubleshooting options when needed. Thus, developers must ensure that training is provided and rehabilitation professionals feel comfortable with the technology and its applications.

As with any other technologies, both therapists and developers must be alert to potential conflicts of interest and avoid situations that could threaten the ethical fidelity of the procedure. For example, a therapist who is paid by the developer to provide training to other therapists interested in purchasing the robotic system must fully disclose his or her role and ensure that comprehensive and accurate information about the benefits, limitations, and risks is provided. Of particular importance in this emerging field, and given the rapid changes in robotic technology, clinicians, developers, and researchers must inform the clients of the *unknowns*. For example, researchers or clinicians may not know the effects of using certain robots on the emotional bonding of participants throughout the treatment or study as this may remain unexplored. However, full disclosure of this fact must be provided when obtaining informed consent.

Fundamental to the principle of fidelity within the field of robotics, especially when it comes to human–robot interactions (HRIs), is the Wizard-of-Oz (WoZ) technique. The WoZ technique is a widely used robot evaluation technique, designed to acquire input and feedback from potential robot users before a fully functioning robot prototype is completed (Dautenhahn 2014). Used by both developers and researchers, in the WoZ technique, a human remotely controls the robot prototype version, unknown to the participants or users. Although the technique enables the researcher, developer, or even the practitioner to acquire important information pertaining to the reactions and characteristics of the HRI, such a technique raises concerns due to its inherent social deception. For example, participants may experience discomfort after they learn that the robot was being operated by a human. Potential feelings of embarrassment can negatively affect the interaction and reduce the person's intention and willingness to use the robot (Fraser and Gilbert 1991). Some client populations may also be more at risk for *Turing deceptions* resulting from WoZ techniques. Box 10.1 provides a description of Turing deceptions (Turing 1950). A Turing deception is a deception that occurs when a person is unable to determine whether he or she is interacting with a machine or a person (Miller 2010; Riek and Watson 2010). The WoZ technique can easily result in such deceptions, which may be harmful for clients, such as those with dementia or with mental health concerns (Luxton, Anderson, and Anderson 2016).

In 2010, the United Kingdom's Engineering and Physical Sciences Research Council (EPSRC) developed five ethical rules for robotics, a living document that challenges practitioners to think about the ethical standards for design, development, research, and implementation of robots in all dimensions of human life (see Box 10.2). Rule 4 specifically addresses

---

BOX 10.1   TURING DECEPTIONS

In his article "Computing Machinery and Intelligence," Alan Turing (1950) proposed the Turing Test, aimed at determining whether a machine can think. First, Turing proposed what is known as the imitation game. In this game, an interrogator is given the task, through written questions to which he receives written answers, of determining which of the two respondents to his questions is the man and which is the woman. Turing then poses the question of whether one could expect an interrogator to accurately identify the respondents when these are changed to a man and a machine (the latter of which would have adequate speed and programming to respond). Would the interrogator be able to tell them apart? Or, would he or she be deceived by the machine (thus engendering the term *Turing deception*)?

BOX 10.2   ENGINEERING AND PHYSICAL SCIENCES RESEARCH COUNCIL'S FIVE ETHICAL RULES FOR ROBOTICS*

1. Robots should not be designed as weapons, except for national security reasons.
2. Robots should be designed and operated to comply with existing law, including privacy.
3. Robots are products: As with other products, they should be designed to be safe and secure.
4. Robots are manufactured artifacts: The illusion of emotions and intent should not be used to exploit vulnerable users.
5. It should be possible to find out who is responsible for any robot.

---

* Adapted from Engineering and Physical Sciences Research Council, 2010. *Principles of Robotics: Regulating Robots in the Real World*. Retrieved from https://www.epsrc.ac.uk /research/ourportfolio/themes/engineering/activities/principlesofrobotics.

the concerns raised by WoZ techniques, and it states that "robots are manufactured artefacts: the illusion of emotions and intent should not be used to exploit vulnerable users" (EPSRC 2010). Thus, all users must be aware of whether the robot is being remotely operated by a human or if the interaction taking place involves only the robot under its specific programming conditions.

Beneficence and Nonmaleficence

Overall, the principles of beneficence and nonmaleficence govern the behavior of health care professionals by ensuring that the benefits of any treatment, procedure, or intervention outweigh the risks. These principles imply that the professional will strive to do good and abstain from any action that may harm the client. In the context of rehabilitation robotics, such principles can (and should) be considered from the perspective of a professional choosing to use a robot as part of the intervention with a client. In such circumstances, these principles must be enacted in line with the considerations for all types of ATs (see Cook and Polgar 2015). However, an angle specific to rehabilitation robotics is that of the actions and processes that the robot performs. When analyzing the practical applications of beneficence and nonmaleficence in this area, the robot's programming must ensure that the interaction with the human always seeks the well-being of the client. Also, the robot must not perform any action that can harm the person. Although such considerations seem obvious, they are at the forefront of what has concerned researchers, developers, and the general public since the materialization of robotics.

In a famous science fiction novel of 1942, *Runaround*, Russian American writer Isaac Asimov articulated the "Three Laws of Robotics," listed in Box 10.3 (Asimov 1950, 26). Although Asimov used such rules to expand on the richness of his fictional work, the rules gained wide adoption and are considered a paramount aspect in the field of robotics and machine ethics (Anderson 2008). Asimov's Laws adhere specifically to the principle of nonmaleficence. However, such distinctions are not always straightforward when it comes to rehabilitation and health care. For example, when a robot is programmed to remind a person to take his or her medication, the most appropriate action if the person refuses can be difficult to discern. Allowing a person to miss a dose might be harmful for the person, but insisting or forcing the action violates the person's autonomy (Deng 2015). Programming the robot to negotiate such circumstances can be challenging. An answer to this and other similar ethical tensions in robotics has been partially addressed by exploring machine learning and the ways in which robots can learn.

Anderson and Anderson (2007) conducted a study in which the commercially available NAO™ robot was programmed to remind people of their medications. To help NAO negotiate these issues, the authors provided multiple examples of cases in which bioethicists had resolved conflicts involving a person's autonomy, beneficence, and nonmaleficence. With the use of learning algorithms, they identified patterns that could guide NAO in new situations. Although such approaches are promising, concerns remained regarding the fact that a learning algorithm provides flexibility to the robot and the pattern that will be identified and used by the robot would remain unknown to the programmer or clinician. What then prevents a robot from drawing a certain conclusion that may not be in the best interest of clients? These and other considerations remain the focus of important debates in the field of robotics (Deng 2015), all of which

---

BOX 10.3   ASIMOV'S THREE LAWS OF ROBOTICS

1. A robot may not injure a human being or, through inaction, allow a human being to come to harm.
2. A robot must obey orders given it by human beings except where such orders would conflict with the First Law.
3. A robot must protect its own existence as long as such protection does not conflict with the First or Second Law.

have profound effects on rehabilitation practice. Meanwhile, rehabilitation professionals are faced with the need to utilize the great technology advancements provided by robots, which, in accordance with beneficence, have been shown to provide great benefits to different client populations. To do so, it is imperative that professionals remain open and up to date with the developments of both the technology and the research, and above all, that they continue to infuse transparency and client centeredness in their evidence-based practice to uphold clients' autonomy.

Stigma

Stigma is a sign of social unacceptability derived from shame or disgrace that is associated with something specific that is considered to be socially unacceptable (Perry, Beyer, and Holm 2009). Although ATs enable and facilitate participation for people with disabilities, AT users can experience stigma as a negative outcome (Zwijsen, Niemeijer, and Hertogh 2011). In such circumstances, AT users are perceived as weak or less able, attributes that in modern societies are assigned greater value than others. As a result, using the AT increases the visibility of conditions that others choose to discriminate and stigmatize. Although the dynamics of stigmatization associated with AT use has not been explored in regard to robots, it is possible that such behaviors of discrimination may extend to those who use robots as part of their rehabilitation processes. In addition, stigmatizing views may arise from users themselves as they interact with these novel technologies. For example, in a study conducted with 57 adults over the age of 40 who had their blood pressure taken by a medical student and a robot, Broadbent and colleagues (2010) found that participants had concerns regarding reliability, safety, and loss of personal care when the measurement was made by the robot. The readings of blood pressure did not differ between robot and medical student.

Efforts in individualizing and customizing AT have been shown to reduce stigma for people with disabilities (Sanford 2012) and hold promise for rehabilitation robotics. For example, attention to characteristics such as ethnicity and race of anthropomorphic robots may decrease stigma (see the section on robot morphology and behavior).

Justice

In the context of principle-based ethics, *justice* refers to "the moral obligation to act on the basis of fair adjudication between competing claims"

(Gillon 1994, 3). As proposed by Gillon, fair adjudication in health care settings implies **distributive justice** (i.e., fairly distribute scarce resources); rights-based justice (i.e., the respect for people's rights); and legal justice (i.e., respecting laws that are morally acceptable). Such an approach to justice overcomes the common pitfall of equating justice with equality, which ignores the fact that people can still be treated unjustly even when treated equally (McKeon 1941). In the context of health care, justice is the source of heated political debates, and when applied to rehabilitation robotics, it raises important concerns.

Given the high cost of robotic technologies and the recent emergence of several of its applications in the field of rehabilitation, it is reasonable to expect that access to several of the devices discussed in this book is limited to developed countries (and health care systems that can afford such innovations). Even within such systems, it is reasonable to expect that some users may be able to benefit from the implementation of these technologies, while others may have to wait, sometimes for a certain period of time (if the robot is in the process of development and access was given only to research participants) or perhaps indefinitely (if social insurance systems do not cover such interventions as part of the standard of care). The dynamics created by this distribution of resources challenges practitioners and developers to design low-cost options that can ensure broader access (e.g., the Compact Rehabilitation Robot [CR2]; Khor et al. 2014). Lego robots (described in Chapter 7) for children with disabilities represent an alternative to more expensive robots, and while still unaffordable in some regions and for some populations, they provide one possible avenue in thinking broadly about justice in the context of rehabilitation robotics.

Ethical Implications for the Use of Robots

Derived from the ethical tensions that uniquely result from the transition of robots into more human environments and the increasing interaction of humans with robotic systems, Riek and Howard (2014) proposed a code of ethics for the HRI profession (p. 6). The principles of this code of ethics (outlined in Box 10.4) provide an opportunity for rehabilitation professionals to reflect on the many ethical considerations of incorporating robots in their practice. In fact, Riek and Howard's code is meant to broaden the scope of robot ethics beyond the research and product development arena and to involve practitioners. Thus, readers are encouraged to carefully review the proposed code and consider that the ethical tensions it reflects will expand as robot autonomy increases.

BOX 10.4   RIEK AND HOWARD'S CODE OF ETHICS FOR THE HUMAN–ROBOT INTERACTION (HRI) PROFESSION

PRINCIPLES OF HRI PROFESSION CODE (AS PROPOSED BY RIEK AND HOWARD 2014)

Human Dignity Considerations

(a) The emotional needs of humans are always to be respected.

(b) The human's right to privacy shall always be respected to the greatest extent consistent with reasonable design objectives.

(c) Human frailty is always to be respected, both physical and psychological.

Design Considerations

(d) Maximal, reasonable transparency in the programming of robotic systems is required.

(e) Predictability in robotic behavior is desirable.

(f) Trustworthy system design principles are required across all aspects of a robot's operation, for both hardware and software design, and for any data processing on or off the platform.

(g) Real-time status indicators should be provided to users to the greatest extent consistent with reasonable design objectives.

(h) Obvious opt-out mechanisms (kill switches) are required to the greatest extent consistent with reasonable design objectives.

Legal Considerations

(i) All relevant laws and regulations concerning individuals' rights and protections (e.g., FDA [Food and Drug Administration], HIPAA [Health Insurance Portability and Affordability Act], and FTC [Federal Trade Commission]) are to be respected.

(j) A robot's decision path must be re-constructible for the purposes of litigation and dispute resolution.

(k) Human informed consent to HRI is to be facilitated to the greatest extent possible consistent with reasonable design objectives.

Social Considerations

(l) Wizard-of-Oz should be employed as judiciously and carefully as possible and should aim to avoid Turing deceptions.

(m) The tendency for humans to form attachments to and anthropomorphize robots should be carefully considered during design.

(n) Humanoid morphology and functionality is permitted only to the extent necessary for the achievement of reasonable design objectives.

(o) Avoid racist, sexist, and ableist morphologies and behaviors in robot design.

But, such ethical tensions are not meant to scare or shy practitioners away from considering the use and application of robots in their rehabilitation practice. Instead, we argue that the entirety of this chapter is meant to promote continued critical reflection on the implications of the use of robots given the evidence-based benefits that are thoroughly outlined in each chapter of this book.

The following sections describe the ethical implications of using robots in several settings of rehabilitation practice; the attempt is to illustrate the unique considerations that pertain to each. Although the following list is not exclusive, it is meant to frame the discussions and reflections around the most salient settings of rehabilitation robotics practice.

As is described in previous chapters, advances in assistive robotics that have the potential for assisting persons with disabilities are commonly divided into two broad categories: physically assistive robots (PARs) or Socially Assistive Robots (SARs). PARs are designed to provide assistance with manipulation of objects or mobility of the person. Feil-Seifer and Matarić (2005) defined SARs as robotic devices whose goal is "to create close and effective interaction with a human user for the purpose of giving assistance and achieving measurable progress in convalescence, rehabilitation, and rehabilitation, and learning" (Feil-Seifer and Matarić 2005, 465).

Physically Assistive Robots

As described in the other chapters of this book, robots that provide physical assistance place the human operator at the center of the process. The goal is to enhance the ability to manipulate objects and to function independently. This relationship between robot and person raises ethical questions.

Robots can operate at different levels of autonomy with respect to the control exerted by the user. At one extreme, the robot can accept high-level commands that define a task to be completed (e.g., take a glass from the shelf, fill it with water, and bring it to the user). The robot will perform whatever subtasks are necessary and make necessary decisions (e.g., determine if the glass is full) without requesting any human intervention. This is referred to as being *fully autonomous*. Alternatively, the user can have direct control over the robot movements at each step in the task. This is referred to as *teleoperation*.

Between these two extremes of autonomy (autonomous and teleoperated robot), several levels of autonomy can be defined (see Chapter 2)

(Parasuraman, Sheridan, and Wickens 2000). Assistive robots are often employed at a midrange of autonomy, in which the user merely needs to hit or press and hold a switch to replay a prestored movement.

Rather than just compensating for lost function, ATs should contribute to growth and independence for persons with disabilities and the elderly. The potential benefits of technologies such as robotics must be balanced with the ethical concerns of autonomy and privacy (Remmers 2010). Fundamental to self-determination is enlisting the help of others as needed. Independence means having the opportunity to make a choice of how and when daily functions such as taking a shower, bathing, dressing and undressing, using the toilet, and eating are carried out as well as completing activities such as shopping, cleaning, preparing meals, or taking care of financial affairs.

Socially Assistive Robots

Supervision

Socially assistive robots have the goal of automating supervision, coaching, motivation, and companionship in one-on-one interactions with individuals (Feil-Seifer and Matarić 2011). They are targeted at persons who experience cognitive impairments as a consequence of aging, stroke, dementia, or autism spectrum disorder, among many other etiologies, opening up a range of ethical concerns. Benefits of an ethical treatment should exceed the risks if the ethical principles of beneficence and nonmaleficence are followed. These robots are not in clinical use, but there have been research studies with potential client groups.

One of the areas of robotic application is the provision of care by devices that include clinical decision making based on sensing and AI. These devices may be developed in the form of "carebots." From an ethical point of view, there are two distinct approaches: replacement of human care by ATs and care assisted by AI technologies but without replacing human care. The latter is far less controversial than the former (Coeckelbergh 2010). In this section, we discuss both the current clinical application and the possible future implications for this type of care because the ethical issues raised are far reaching and could affect future AT application in general.

Companions

If a user becomes emotionally attached to the robot, it can cause a significant ethical dilemma (Feil-Seifer and Matarić 2011). If the robot is removed due to lack of adaptation or failure in the robot software or electronics, then the emotional contact benefit is lost, and there can be a sense of loss by the user, especially if the user cannot understand the causes for the robot's removal. For example, research with SARs has shown that elderly users and users with Alzheimer's disease engage with robots and miss them when they are removed. Because there is a demonstrated emotional attachment, the question, "Is there deception inherent in the personification of a robot by a user or a caregiver?" has been proposed (Feil-Seifer and Matarić 2011, 8). There are a number of factors that relate to the personification of robots. The actual design of the robot may or may not be purposefully manipulated to alter the perceptions of the user toward therapeutic goals (Feil-Seifer and Matarić 2011). The physical appearance, including human-like features, can influence how the robot is perceived. Larger robots are more fearsome and smaller are perceived as more friendly. How the robot is dressed and the type of voice also affect user responses. Feminine voices are more soothing, and the presence of a lab coat could indicate authority. As other features such as gestures, coordinated body movements, and facial expressions are added, the personification is increased.

Different groups have different reactions to SARs (Feil-Seifer and Matarić 2011). While some participants interacting with robots can correctly distinguish between robot activities and the equivalent capabilities in a person or pet, other users form emotional attachments to the SARs, leading to misconceptions about the robots' emotional capabilities. One danger in this type of attachment is emotional loss; for example, one participant thought the robot would miss him when he was not there—something the robot could not do. Another risk is that the user might believe that the robot could assist him as a human would do, for example, telling the robot about symptoms that should be told to a clinician.

This deception has been viewed negatively because our interests are not likely to be served by illusions. In considering the potential ethical impact of SARs, Sparrow and Sparrow (2006), wrote: "What most of us want out of life is to be loved and cared for, and to have friends and companions, not merely to believe that we are loved and cared for, and to believe that we have friends and companions, when in fact these beliefs are false" (p. 155). Their concerns are on several levels. First, they believe that it is unethical to intend to deceive others, even for their own subjective benefit. They also are concerned that people will be deceived when they are given SARs that have human or animal-like features. They consider these deceptions to be unethical, especially when the result of the deception could harm the individual who is being deceived. Others disagree, "since in practice most of the time people are very much aware that a certain AI autonomous system such as a robot is not really human, even if the robot has a human appearance and even if they respond to the robot as if it were human" (Coeckelbergh 2010, 187). This discussion reinforces the patient-centered concept discussed previously.

Sparrow and Sparrow (2006) did acknowledge that robots may have a part to play in roles when they might physically assist an individual but not replace human carers. But, even this more limited role proposed for robots to provide care of sufficient quality to replace human care providers also leads to a concern for the overall reduction in human social interaction for this vulnerable population (Sparrow and Sparrow 2006). Even the PARs that carry out tasks of daily living might deprive a person of human contact. For some individuals in home care, the only human contact they have is with the cleaning staff who comes weekly because all other care can be provided remotely. If a robot cleaning system, currently available (see http://www.irobot.com/ for an example), is used to vacuum their house, then even the weekly appearance of a human cleaning assistant might disappear.

Coeckelbergh (2010) defined care where AT provides functional gain but does not really emotionally relate to the person as "shallow care." In contrast, "deep care" is care that includes feeling for the person that is reciprocal. It is the area of deep care that causes the major ethical controversy. "The problem is not the technologies themselves, not replaceability as such, and not the (potential violation of) the principles of privacy or autonomy alone, but the question of what good care and the good life are for us as humans, for us in this context, and for us as the unique persons that we are" (Coeckelbergh 2010, 190). Coeckelbergh described "good care" as meeting social and emotional needs of patients. Although in certain situations a person might prefer the use of a robot, Coeckelbergh's description leads many to argue that AT alone is not satisfactory for replacing human care (e.g., nursing care for seniors). Thus, the social and emotional needs of the potential user must be carefully considered. Among the potential objections are the following (Coeckelbergh 2010):

1. An AI robot or an AI monitoring system is able to deliver care, but it will never really care about the human.
2. AI technologies cannot provide good care because that requires contact with humans who have social and emotional needs.
3. Even if AI ATs do provide good care, they will violate the fundamental principle of privacy in doing so, which is why they should be banned.
4. AI assistive robots provide "fake" care, and they are likely to "fool" people by making people think they receive real care.

Coeckelbergh (2010) also cautioned us not to "set the standards of care too high when evaluating the introduction of AI assistive technologies in health care, since otherwise we would have to reject many of our existing, low-tech health care practices" (p. 181). It is worth noting that some of the concerns mentioned may have implications for care more broadly, even when in the hands of a human caregiver. For example, privacy may be infringed when care is provided by a formal caregiver. Thus, these cautions invite us to reflect on the implications and assumptions around rehabilitation care and the potential specific applications of robotics within that framework.

As Companions: Ascribing Human Attributes

Robot companions are designed with the goal of supporting individuals (especially older adults or people with disabilities) to live independently by providing companionship, monitoring health, maintaining safety, and assisting with activities of daily living, such as eating, bathing, or dressing (Heerink, Kröse, Evers, and Wielinga 2008). With the major demographic shifts in the world population, by which aging is now at the forefront of health planning and policy, robot companions hold the promise of opportunities. However, practitioners face important considerations regarding the implications of robots as companions.

When interacting with a robot, people ascribe human attributes to the robot, including intelligence, intentionality, and responsibility. As such, interactions with robots are currently modeled after human-human interactions (de Graaf 2015). Although such interactions are not intrinsically harmful, it can result in misrepresentations and false expectations of what robots can and are designed to do for the person. For example, individuals who use a robot as a companion may find their interaction with the robot replacing their relationships with other people, leading to isolation (Sparrow and Sparrow 2006). Although robots can certainly assist in certain tasks that can maintain overall health and safety, rehabilitation practitioners must keep in mind that such interactions cannot meet the emotional needs of older adults or people with disabilities (Sparrow and Sparrow 2006). Strategies must be put in place to ensure that robot companionship and services do not substitute for human social interaction and care.

In Research and Practice: Participant Bonding and Placebo Effects

When introducing a robot in both research and practice settings, participants/clients may develop strong emotional or psychological bonds with the robot, especially given the ways in which the robot enables, facilitates, or assists with their engagement in important activities of daily living. At the end of the project or intervention plan, taking away the robot may have adverse effects on the person that practitioners need to consider.

Certain populations are more vulnerable to such effects, including children, older adults, and people who are in situations of vulnerability (such as those who may be in environments in which, other than the robot, there is a lack of human companionship) (Riek and Howard 2014). For example, a study by Gross and colleagues (2015) investigated the effects of introducing a robot companion for domestic health assistance for older adults. The study found that older adults formed emotional bonds with the robot and were sad after the project concluded and the robots were removed. Evidence of the emotional bonds they created were observed in the fact that most of the participants named the robot, treated it as a social being, praised it for a task well done, and felt sorry when the robot failed to do something appropriately. Similarly, Robins, Dautenhahn, and Dubowski (2005) articulated their concerns resulting from studies of robot use for children with autism spectrum disorder, in which certain isolation behaviors were observed. Specifically, children sought exclusive relationships with the robot, sometimes ignoring their peers or the experimenter. Thus, researchers and practitioners must carefully consider the effects of emotional bonding for the participants/clients and must articulate those when obtaining informed consent.

Another important consideration when evaluating the effects of robot-assisted therapies is that of the placebo effect. A placebo effect is a change in a symptom or condition that occurs as a result of a procedure aimed at pleasing the patient and not at excreting specific effects (Price, Finniss, and Benedetti 2008). When comparing the effects of a robot-based intervention with other modalities (including a therapist-only procedure), the results may be affected by the perceptions of the participant, who may favor one over the other. Such potential risks to successfully evaluating efficacy and effectiveness must be considered when interpreting data, implementing rehabilitation strategies, and monitoring their results.

Among the populations that can benefit from rehabilitation robotics, children are prominent potential users. As described in several of the chapters of this book, practitioners, developers, and researchers are exploring the benefits of robot-assisted therapies or strategies for children with physical (Cook et al. 2012), developmental (Scassellati, Admoni, and Matarić 2012), and cognitive disabilities (Robins et al. 2012). Nevertheless, there are certain ethical concerns that may affect the way parents and therapists respond to the use of robots in pediatric rehabilitation practice. Specifically, the autonomy of the robot raises important concerns, as well as issues regarding trust.

First, robot autonomy has ethical implications in the work with children, which can be considered from two opposite perspectives. On one hand, the more autonomous the robot is, the better it may be able to accommodate the needs of children who require greater or varied support in an activity. For example, a robot that supports children as they play can interact with the child in accordance with the child's needs, and as the needs of the child change, the robot can adapt to them. An autonomous robot is therefore optimally positioned to release control of the activity to the child, as the child further develops the required skills or is better able to perform the therapeutic task. Under this lens, increased robot autonomy is an ideal feature that, from an ethical perspective, enhances children's autonomy while providing the necessary therapeutic support.

On the other hand, increased robot autonomy raises concerns regarding responsibility. If the child-robot interaction is largely dependent on robot autonomy, the therapist may not have full control of such interaction. In this case, the responsibility for the robot's actions and its effects can be questionable (Coeckelbergh et al. 2015). In addition to the inherent ethical tensions resulting from robot autonomy, such tensions also give rise to questions regarding trust. Specifically, potential feelings of mistrust on behalf of parents, who are presented with the option of having a robot "in control" of the therapeutic interaction, are possible (Coeckelbergh et al. 2015).

A potential solution to such conflicting interests is that of supervised autonomous interaction. In a supervised autonomous interaction, such as the one developed by the "Development of Robot-Enhanced therapy for children with AutisM spectrum disorders" (DREAM) project (Thill et al. 2012), the therapist assigns the robot specific goals that the robot then works to autonomously achieve with the child. In this case, the robot operates autonomously for short periods of time while under the instruction and supervision of the therapist (also avoiding full WoZ techniques). Such solutions can represent a possible compromise toward achieving more ethically solid robot-assisted therapy strategies.

Future Issues

Increasing Autonomy of Robotic Systems

As technologies become more sophisticated, robots will be more human-like, with smoother motions, more integrated functions, and anthropomorphic features that mimic humans closely. They will also have sophisticated decision-making capabilities. These features will begin to blur the distinction between care by humans and care by robots. Robot-based care with highly autonomous devices can reduce the autonomy of the person using the robot. The challenge is to balance the person's goals and needs with the capabilities of the robotic systems to ensure that it is the functional independence of the person that is paramount, not just the capability of the robot.

Artificial Intelligence in Decision Making

The fidelity of care is also important as robots' clinical decision-making capabilities increase. The meaning and scope of beneficence may also change, expand, or possibly contract as more autonomous robots play a more prominent role in the provision of rehabilitation assistance. Issues of nonmaleficence will be related not only to safety of the robots but also to the efficacy and safeguards built into the AI algorithms controlling the robots. Decisions made by and executed by an AI-controlled robot will not necessarily conform to standards of clinical practice as promoted by disciplines related to rehabilitants. This disconnect can lead to ethical dilemmas for the clinician and the consumer.

Allocation of Responsibility

Allocation of responsibility is a critical concern for rehabilitation professionals. As practitioners, rehabilitation professionals must abide by the code of ethics of their respective professions and are responsible for ensuring the safety of the procedures they choose to implement. With increased robot autonomy, rehabilitation professionals face ethical dilemmas regarding who is responsible for the procedure and the actions of the robot. The issue of responsibility for the robot extends not only to the therapist but also to developers, researchers, manufacturers, and users (Datteri and Tamburrini 2009). Specifically, as learning algorithms are implemented in more autonomous robots, there is a limited ability to predict the behavior of the robot in a given situation. This has important implications regarding liability insurance, as well as moral responsibility (Datteri and Tamburrini 2009). Although no definitive answer can be provided at the moment, researchers and ethicists continue to consider such implications. When implementing robots in their practice, rehabilitation professionals are encouraged to clarify the capabilities of the robot, the responsibility and coverage of any potential adverse effects.

Robot Morphology and Behavior: Ethical Implications Concerning Race, Ethnicity, and Cultural Diversity

As robotic technologies continue to advance and robots' anthropomorphism increases, it is imperative that developers, researchers, and practitioners consider issues regarding a potential lack of diversity in the characteristics of robots, such as gender, race, and ethnicity. The impact of stereotypes in robot development is of great importance, considering evidence showing that humans respond to robots much as they do with other social entities and ascribe similar stereotypes regardless of robot capacity. For example, Tay et al. (2013) investigated the effects of gender stereotypes in users' acceptance of social robots. When considering a security robot, their study indicated that users preferred a male robot and perceived it as more useful and acceptable. Similarly, Carpenter and colleagues (2009) investigated people's expectations of humanoid robots designed for home use. In the study, preference for the female robot was observed. Also, when interacting with a robot designed to be gender neutral, such as NASA's Robonaut, 99 of 100 people identify it with a male pronoun (Dattaro 2015). As a result, practitioners must carefully consider the implications of gender stereotypes and preferences of users.

In addition to stereotypes regarding gender, the current status of robotic technology development is already exhibiting biases regarding race and ethnicity. In fact, most current anthropomorphic robots have Caucasian or Asian features, and their appearance and behavior seem to be explicitly Eurocentric (Riek and Howard 2014). Although it is possible that such characteristics are a result of the origin of the current developers of the technologies, it is unlikely that the capacity to develop and commercialize robot technologies will spread to developing countries, and as such, design may continue to be racially biased. It is important that, when working with a client, therapists consider the impact of such features on the client-robot interaction and on the extended effects of such stereotype-reinforcing strategies.

STUDY QUESTIONS

1. What is algorithm aversion, and how does it relate to potential issues of mistrust toward robots?
2. How do Asimov's rules of robotics relate to the ethical principles discussed in this chapter?
3. What are WoZ techniques, and how do they relate to the ethical principle of fidelity?
4. Discuss three prominent ethical issues that a rehabilitation practitioner should consider when incorporating robotics in his or her practice.
5. Remmers (2010) stated that the challenge is to balance the potential benefits of **ambient environments**, AI, and technologies like robotics with ethical concerns of autonomy and privacy, but the stakes are higher because of the pervasive nature of the technology. What does this mean in terms of ethical principles?
6. Coeckelbergh (2010) raised four objections to the use of AI-based devices (including robots). What are they? Do you agree or disagree with this analysis? Why?
7. For intelligent technologies, we can view the concept of autonomy from the point of view of either the device or the person. What ethical principles are implicated by the levels of autonomy shown in Table 1.1 in Chapter 1?

References

Aasaro, P. "What should we want from a robot ethic?" *International Review of Information Ethics* 6 (2006): 2–15.

Airaksinen, T. "The philosophy of professional ethics." In *Encyclopedia of Life Support Systems* (EOLSS). Developed under the auspices of UNESCO, EOLSS, Paris, (2003): 1–6.

Alaiad, A., Zhou, L., Koru, G. "An exploratory study of home healthcare robots adoption applying the UTAUT model." *International Journal of Healthcare Information Systems and Informatics* 9(4) (2014): 44–59.

Anderson, M., Anderson, S.L. "Machine ethics: Creating an ethical intelligent agent." *AI Magazine* 28 (2007): 15–26.

Anderson, S.L. "Asimov's 'Three Laws of Robotics' and machine metaethics." *AI & Society* 22(4) (2008): 477–493.

Asimov, I. *I, Robot*. New York: Doubleday, 1950.

Boys, J.A., Alicuben, E.T., DeMeester, M.J., Worrell, S.G., Oh, S.S., Hagen, J.A., DeMeester, S.R. "Public perceptions on robotic surgery, hospitals with robots, and surgeons that use them." *Surgical Endoscopy* 30(4) (2016): 1310–1316.

Broadbent, E., Kuo, I.H., Lee, Y.I., Rabindran, J., Kerse, N., Stafford, R., MacDonald, B.A. "Attitudes and reactions to a healthcare robot." *Telemedicine Journal and e-Health* 16(5) (2010): 608–613.

Caine, K., Šabanović, S., Carter, M. "The effect of monitoring by cameras and robots on the privacy enhancing behaviors of older adults." Proceedings of HRI 2012, Boston, March 2012.

Carpenter, J., Davis, J.M., Erwin-Stewart, N., Lee, T.R., Bransford, J.D., Vye, N. "Gender representation and humanoid robots designed for domestic use." *International Journal of Social Robotics* 1 (2009): 261–265.

Coeckelbergh, M. "Health care, capabilities, and AI assistive technologies." *Ethical Theory and Moral Practice* 13 (2010): 181–190.

Coeckelbergh, M., Pop, C., Simut, R., Peca, A., Pintea, S., David, D., Vanderborght, B. "A survey of expectations about the role of robots in robot-assisted therapy for children with ASD: Ethical acceptability, trust, sociability, appearance, and attachment." *Science and Engineering Ethics* 1(22) (2015): 1–19.

Cook, A., Adams, K., Encarnação, P., Alvarez, L. The role of assisted manipulation in cognitive development. *Developmental Neurorehabilitation* 15 (2012): 136–148.

Cook, A., Polgar, J. *Assistive Technologies: Principles and Practices*. 4th ed. St. Louis, MO: Elsevier, 2015.

Datteri, E., Tamburrini, G. "Ethical considerations on health care robotics." In *Ethics and Robotics*, R. Capurro, M. Nagenborg (eds.). Amsterdam: IOS Press, (2009): 35–48.

Dattaro, L. "Bot looks like a lady." Future Tense: The Citizen's Guide to the Future. *SLATE: USA*. February 4, 2015. http://www.slate.com/articles/technology /future_tense/2015/02/robot_gender_is_it_bad_for_human_women.html.

Dautenhahn, K. "Human–robot interaction." In *The Encyclopedia of Human-Computer Interaction*, 2nd ed., M. Soegaard, R.F. Dam (eds.). Aarthus, Denmark: Interaction Design Foundation, 2014. Retrieved from https:// www.interaction-design.org/literature/book/the-encyclopedia-of-human -computer-interaction-2nd-ed.

Dawes, R.M. "The robust beauty of improper linear models in decision making." *American Psychologist* 34 (1979): 571–582.

De Graaf, M.M.A. "The ethics of human–robot relationships." Presented at the New Friends Conference, Almere, the Netherlands, October 22–25, 2015.

Deng, B. "Machine ethics: The robot's dilemma." *Nature* 523(7558) (2015). http:// www.nature.com/news/machine-ethics-the-robot-s-dilemma-1.17881.

Dietvorst, B.J., Simmons, J.P., Massey, C. "Algorithm aversion: People erroneously avoid algorithms after seeing them err." *Journal of Experimental Psychology: General* 144(1) (2014): 114–126.

Engineering and Physical Science Research Council (EPSRC). *Principles of Robotics: Regulating Robots in the Real World*. Technical Report. Swindon, U.K.: EPSRC, 2010. Retrieved from: https://www.epsrc.ac.uk/research/ourportfolio/themes /engineering/activities/principlesofrobotics/.

European Commission. "Public attitudes towards robots." 2012. http://ec.europa .eu/public_opinion/archives/ebs/ebs_382_en.pdf.

Feil-Seifer, D.J., Matarić, M.J. "Defining socially assistive robotics." Proceedings of the IEEE 9th International Conference on Rehabilitation Robotics, June 28–July 1, Chicago, USA (2005): 465–468.

Feil-Seifer, D.J., Matarić, M.J. "Ethical principles for socially assistive robotics." *IEEE Robotics & Automation Magazine*, Special issue on Roboethics 18(1) (2011): 24–31.

Fraser, N.M., Gilbert, G.N. "Simulating speech systems." *Computer Speech & Language* 5(1) (1991).

Gillon, R. "Medical ethics: Four principles plus attention to scope." *BMJ* 309 (1994): 1–8.

Gross, H.M., Mueller, S., Schroeter, C., Volkhardt, M., Scheidig, A., Debes, K., Ritcher, K. et al. "Robot companion for domestic health assistance: Implementation, test and case study under everyday conditions in private apartments." Proceedings of the IEEE/RSJ International Conference on Intelligent Robots and Systems (IROS), Hamburg, Germany, September 28–October 2, 2015.

Heerink, M., Kröse, B.J.A., Evers, V., Wielinga, B.J. "The influence of social presence on enjoyment and intention to use of a robot and screen agent by elderly users." Proceedings RO-MAN, Munich, Germany, August 1–3, 2008.

Khor, K.X., Rahman, H.A., Fu, S.K., Sim, L.S., Yeong, C.F., Su, E.L.M. "A novel hybrid rehabilitation robot for upper and lower limbs rehabilitation training." *Procedia Computer Science* 42 (2014): 293–300.

Kitchener, K.S. *Foundations of Ethical Practice, Research, and Teaching in Psychology*. Mahwah, NJ: Erlbaum, 2000.

Luxton, D.D., Anderson, S.L., Anderson, M. "Ethical issues and artificial intelligence technologies in behavioral and mental health care." In *Artificial Intelligence in Behavioral and Mental Health Care*, D.D. Luxton (ed.). San Diego: Academic Press, (2016): 255–276.

Martin, S., Bengtsson, J.E., Dröes, R.-M. "Assistive technologies and issues relating to privacy, ethics and security." In *Supporting People with Dementia Using Pervasive Health Technologies*, M.D. Mulvenna, C.D. Nugent (eds.). London: Springer, (2010): 63–76.

McKeon, R. (ed.). "Aristotle politics. Book 3, chapter 9." In *The Basic Works of Aristotle*. New York: Random House, 1941.

Miller, K.W. "It's not nice to fool humans." *IT Professional*, 12(1) (2010): 51.

Parasuraman, R., Sheridan, T., Wickens, C.D. "A model for types and levels of human interaction with automation." *IEEE Transactions on Systems, Man, and Cybernetics—Part A: Systems and Humans* 30(3) (2000): 286–297.

Perry, J., Beyer, S., Holm, S. "Assistive technology, telecare and people with intellectual disabilities: Ethical considerations." *Journal of Medical Ethics*. 35 (2009): 81–86.

Pew Research Center. "U.S. views of technology and the future." April 17, 2014. http://www.pewinternet.org/2014/04/17/us-views-of-technology-and-the-future/.

Price, D.D., Finniss, D.G., Benedetti, F. "A comprehensive review of the placebo effect: Recent advances and current thought." *Annual Review of Psychology* 59 (2008): 565–590.

Purtilo, R. *Ethical Dimensions in the Health Professions*. Philadelphia: Elsevier Saunders, 2005.

Remmers, H. "Environments for ageing, assistive technology and self-determination: Ethical perspectives." *Informatics for Health & Social Care* 35(3–4) (2010): 200–210.

Riek, L., Howard, D. "A code of ethics for the human–robot interaction profession." In: *Proceedings of We Robot*. 2014. http://robots.law.miami.edu/2014/wp-content/uploads/2014/03/a-code-of-ethics-for-the-human-robot-interaction-profession-riek-howard.pdf.

Riek, L.D., Watson, R.N.W. "The age of avatar realism." *IEEE Robotics & Automation* 17(4) (2010): 37–42.

Robins, B., Dautenhahn, K., Dubowski, J. "Robots as isolators or mediators for children with autism? A cautionary tale." Proceedings of the AISB 05 Symposium on Robot Companions: Hard Problems and Open Challenges in Robot-Human Interaction (April 1–4, 2005): 82–88.

Robins, B., Dautenhahn, K., Ferrari, E., Kronreif, G., Prazak-Aram, B., Marti, P., Iacono, I. et al. "Scenarios of robot-assisted play for children with cognitive and physical disabilities." *Interaction Studies* 13:2 (2012): 189–234.

Sanford, J.A. *Universal Design as a Rehabilitation Strategy*. New York: Springer, 2012.

Scassellati, B., Admoni, H., Matarić, M. "Robots for use in autism research." *Annual Review of Biomedical Engineering* 14 (2012): 275–294.

Sparrow, R., Sparrow, L. "In the hands of machines? The future of aged care." *Minds and Machines* 16(2), (2006): 141–161.

Sung, J.Y., Guo, L., Grinter, R.E., Christensen, H.I. "'My Roomba is Rambo': Intimate home appliances." Proceedings of the 9th International Conference, Ubiquitous Computing, Innsbruck, Austria, September 16–19, 2007.

Tay, B.T.C., Park, T., Jung, Y., Tan, Y.K., Yee Wong, A.H. "When stereotypes meet robots: The effect of gender stereotypes on people's acceptance of a security robot." Proceedings of the 10th International Conference on Engineering Psychology and Cognitive Ergonomics: Understanding Human Cognition 8019 (2013): 261–270.

Thill, S., Pop, C.A., Belpaeme, T., Ziemke, T., Vanderborght, B. "Robot-assisted therapy for autism spectrum disorders with (partially) autonomous control: Challenges and outlook." *Paladyn, Journal of Behavioral Robotics* 3(4) (2012): 209–217.

Turing, A. "Computing machinery and intelligence." *Mind* 59(236) (1950): 433–460.

Zwijsen, S.A., Niemeijer, A.R., Hertogh, C. "Ethics of using assistive technology in the care for community-dwelling elderly people: An overview of the literature." *Aging Mental Health* 15(4) (2011): 419–427.

Glossary

activities of daily living (ADL): tasks performed by people in a typical day that allow independent living. Basic activities of daily living (BADL) include feeding, dressing, hygiene, and mobility. Instrumental activities of daily living (IADL) include more advanced skills, such as managing personal finances, using transportation, telephoning, cooking, performing household chores, doing laundry, and shopping.

ambient environment: a network-based connectivity in which every electronic device used on a regular basis both has computing power and is linked to other devices through local networks (e.g., Wi-Fi) or the Internet.

assisted living: long-term care option that combines housing, support services, and health care, as needed, for individuals who require assistance with activities of daily living.

assistive robot (AR): robot that gives aid or support to a human user.

assistive robotic manipulator (ARM): any robotic arm that is not body bound and with a minimum of 6 degrees of freedom and a gripper, which is safe to interact with humans, especially humans with special needs or a disability, and can assist with several activities under the control of the user.

assistive technology (AT): technology designed to be utilized in an assistive technology device or assistive technology service.

assistive technology device: any item, piece of equipment, or product system, whether acquired commercially, modified, or customized, that is used to increase, maintain, or improve functional capabilities of individuals with disabilities.

assistive technology service: any service that directly assists an individual with a disability in the selection, acquisition, or use of an assistive technology device.

augmentative and alternative communication (AAC) device: devices that produce voice output by either recorded speech or electronic speech synthesis. They might have symbols, letters, words, or phrases to choose from to make phrases, and can be accessed by pressing a display or by using an alternative access method.

augmentative manipulation: a system that supplements (augments) the existing manipulation skills of the user and compensates for limitations in manipulation.

autism spectrum disorder (ASD): range of neurodevelopmental conditions characterized by persistent significant impairment in the social-communication domain along with restricted, repetitive patterns of behavior, interests, and activities.

autonomy: an ethical principle that upholds the belief that every person has a right to self-determination and to be free from interference, risks to privacy, or unnecessary constraints.

beneficence: ethical principle that governs the behavior of health care professionals by ensuring that the benefits of any treatment, procedure, or intervention outweigh the risks. Implies that the professional will strive to do good and abstain from any action that may harm the client.

Cartesian control: assistive robotic manipulator control modality in which the user controls the position of the assistive robotic manipulator end-effector in the Cartesian space.

cerebral palsy (CP): neurological disorder caused by a nonprogressive brain injury or malformation that occurs while the child's brain is under development. Cerebral palsy affects body movement, muscle control, muscle coordination, muscle tone, reflex, posture, and balance. It can also affect fine motor skills, gross motor skills, and oral motor functioning.

compliant control: control strategy in which deviations from equilibrium are allowed depending on the applied external forces. This allows robots to comply with the environment, react to the force acting on the end-effecter, or adapt its motion to uncertainties of the environment.

cosmesis: in the context of prosthetic interventions, an artificial limb designed to closely replicate a user's biological limb in appearance (e.g., a limb with materials and finishing carefully chosen to match a user's skin tone, hair patterning, and other skin markings).

degrees of freedom (DOF): number of independent variables that need to be specified to locate all parts of a robot.

distributive justice: principles of distributive justice are normative principles designed to guide the allocation of the benefits and burdens of economic activity.

elder care: fulfillment of the special needs and requirements that are unique to senior citizens. This broad term encompasses such services as assisted living, adult day care, long-term care, nursing homes, hospice care, and home care.

electromyographic (EMG) recording: recording of electrical activity from muscle tissue at the surface of the skin (sEMG) or inside the muscle tissue (iEMG). See also *myoelectric control.*

embodiment: the feeling that a device (e.g., a prosthesis) is a part of or an extension of the body; a feeling of ownership over a device wherein the user believes it to be an integrated part of their body.

end-effector: device that is attached to a manipulator's wrist (e.g., spoon, a cup bearing a forearm, or a gripper).

engagement: in the context of robots, engagement is the process by which a human user establishes, maintains, and ends his or her perceived connection with the robot itself or the task.

exoskeleton: powered robotic orthosis for people with disabilities, designed to move at least two joints in concert.

fidelity: ethical principle that encompasses treating the client with respect; competency of the health care professional; adhering to the professional code of ethics; following regulations, protocols, and procedures; and honoring agreements made with the client.

forward kinematics: computing the position of the assistive robotic manipulator end-effector in the Cartesian space from the assistive robotic manipulator joint positions.

functional play: the type of play where a child uses the objects according to the function designed for them and as they would be used in reality (e.g., a ball is used as a ball).

games with rules: involves structured play and play activities having rules that need to be followed by each player.

Human Activity Assistive Technology (HAAT) model: model of an assistive technology system representing a person with a disability doing an activity using an assistive technology within a context.

human–robot interaction (HRI): multidisciplinary field that focuses on designing, implementing, and evaluating robot systems that interact with humans.

impedance control: compliant control strategy that imposes a desired dynamic to the interaction between the robot end-effector and the object being manipulated, instead of directly controlling the exerted forces or the end-effector position.

independent living: residential living setting for senior adults that may or may not provide hospitality or supportive services. Under this living arrangement, the senior adult leads an independent lifestyle that requires minimal or no extra assistance. Generally referred to as elder housing in the government-subsidized environment, independent living also includes rental-assisted or market rate apartments or cottages where residents usually have complete choice in whether to participate in the community's services or programs.

informed consent: includes two aspects: (1) not subjecting the individual to control by others without the individual's explicit consent and (2) respectful interaction when presenting information, probing for understanding, and attempting to enable autonomous decision making.

International Classification of Functioning, Disability, and Health (ICF): World Health Organization international classification system that reflects a biopsychosocial model of disability, where disability is the expression of the negative aspects of the interaction between the individual's health condition and contextual factors, while functionality denotes the positive or neutral aspects of the interaction between the individual's health condition and that individual's contextual factors.

inverse kinematics: computing the assistive robotic manipulator joint positions from the assistive robotic manipulator end-effector position in the Cartesian space.

joint control: assistive robotic manipulator control modality in which the user directly controls the assistive robotic manipulator joints.

level of autonomy: degree to which a robot is autonomous in performing the different tasks, ranging from teleoperated (the human completely controlling the robot) to fully autonomous (the robot performing the action without any human intervention).

lower limb exoskeleton (LLE): a multijoint orthosis that uses an external power source to move at least two joints on each leg, which is portable, and can be used independent of a treadmill or body-weight support.

manipulation: involves the use of arms, hands, and fingers to manipulate objects in the environment for a variety of reasons, but usually related to performing activities of daily living.

mobility: the ability to move in one's environment with ease and without restriction.

myoelectric control: use of sampled electrical signals generated by muscle tissue in the user's residual limb or adjacent regions to control a robotic prosthesis.

nonmaleficence: do no harm—the professional will abstain from any action that may harm the client.

object play: play in which the child interacts with objects.

osseointegration: direct structural and functional connection between living bone and the surface of an artificial metal implant.

participation: involvement in a life situation.

pattern recognition: in the context of prosthetic interventions, the use of supervised machine learning to map patterns of muscle activity (electromyographic signals) recorded in a user's residual limb or other tissue to different movements of a multiactuator robotic prosthesis, such as, hand open/close, wrist movement, elbow movement. An advanced form of myoelectric control.

personal service robot: service robots for personal use, used for a non-commercial task, usually by laypersons.

physically assistive robot: robot designed to provide assistance with manipulation of objects or mobility of the person.

playfulness: the disposition to play.

population aging: shift in distribution of a country's population toward older ages.

pretend play or symbolic play: a cognitive play skill of representing knowledge, experience, and objects symbolically. In pretend play, the child uses an object as if it was a different object (e.g., using a block as if it was a car).

professional service robot: service robots for professional use, used for a commercial task, usually operated by a properly trained operator.

rehabilitation: the process aimed at enabling people with disabilities to reach and maintain their optimal physical, sensory, intellectual, psychological, and social functional levels.

robot: actuated mechanism programmable in two or more axes with a degree of autonomy, moving within its environment, to perform intended tasks.

robot autonomy: robot ability to perform intended tasks based on current state and sensing, without human intervention.

robotic assistive technologies: robots used to increase, maintain, or improve functional capabilities of individuals with disabilities.

robotic prosthesis: robotic device that is attached to a user's body throughout daily life to replace the functions of the user's missing limb.

robotics: the science or study of the technology associated with the design, fabrication, theory, and application of robots.

scanning: in scanning, the user waits for selections to be presented to him or her. Scanning can be with one switch or more switches. In one-switch row-column scanning, the switch initiates the scanning, and highlighting will automatically move from one row to another, the switch is pressed to indicate the desired row, and then the highlighting moves across the row. Subsequently, the switch is used to select the desired cell when highlighted. In two-switch row-column scanning, one switch is used to initiate the scanning and to step from one row to another (the "move" switch), and the other switch is used to indicate the desired row (the "select" switch). Subsequently, the move switch is used to step along the columns and the select switch to choose the desired cell.

security: the state of being protected or safe from harm.

service robot: robot that performs useful tasks for humans or equipment, excluding industrial automation applications.

smart wheelchair: powered wheelchair with a range of functions aimed at increasing safe and effective navigation, including, for example, collision avoidance, autonomous navigation to locations, wall following, and virtual path following.

socially assistive robot (SAR): robot that provides assistance to human users through social interaction.

socially interactive robot (SIR): robot for which social interaction plays a key role.

socket: the part of the prosthesis that affixes to the body of a user with an amputation.

stigma: a sign of social unacceptability derived from shame or disgrace that is associated with something specific considered to be socially unacceptable.

surveillance: in the context of AT, refers to monitoring an individual's actions; may occur in a living facility or in the broader community.

targeted reinnervation (TR): surgical procedure that redirects the amputated nerve endings that are used to innervate a missing limb (e.g., hand and wrist muscles) to new muscle sites, thereby providing physiologically natural motor command signals for myoelectric control (targeted muscle reinnervation, TMR); also used with sensory nerves to enable physiologically natural sensory feedback from the robotic prosthesis to reinnervated sites on the skin (targeted sensory reinnervation, TSR).

technology readiness scale: scale, usually with nine levels, used to describe the level of maturity of a technology.

tool: an item that expands the functional range of a human, allowing an individual to manipulate some aspect of the environment.

tool use: a landmark cognitive skill that involves understanding the properties of objects and how they relate to each other as a means to achieve a goal.

upper limb exoskeleton (ULE): a wearable, portable, and autonomously operated multijoint orthosis that uses an external power source to move at least two joints on the upper limb for use in daily life scenarios.

user compliance: extent to which people interact with a robot in the expected manner.

The following sources were consulted during the preparation of this Glossary:

American Heritage Dictionary of the English Language. 5th Edition. S.v. "robotics." Accessed July 13, 2016. http://www.thefreedictionary.com/robotics.

American Psychiatric Association. 2013. *Diagnostic and Statistical Manual of Mental Disorders* (DSM-5). Washington, DC: American Psychiatric Association.

American Speech-Language-Hearing Association (ASHA). "Augmentative and alternative communication (AAC)." Accessed July 13, 2016. http://www.asha.org/public/speech/disorders/AAC/.

Argentum. "Assisted living." Accessed July 13, 2016. http://www.alfa.org/alfa/Assisted_Living_Information.asp.

Argentum. "Senior living glossary of terms." Accessed July 13, 2016. http://www.alfa.org/alfa/Glossary_of_Terms.asp.

Barton, E. 2010. "Development of a taxonomy of pretend play for children with disabilities." *Infants and Young* 23(4): 247–261.

Buttelmann, D., Carpenter, M., Call, J., Tomasello, M. 2008. "Rational tool use and tool choice in human infants and great apes." *Child Development,* 79: 609–626.

Castellano, G., Leite, I., Pereira, A., Martinho, C., Paiva, A., and McOwan, P. W. 2012. Detecting engagement in HRI: An exploration of social and task-based context. ASE/IEEE International Conference on Social Computing and ASE/IEEE International Conference on Privacy, Security, Risk and Trust, 421–428.

Farlex Partner Medical Dictionary. S.v. "activities of daily living." Retrieved July 13, 2016. http://medical-dictionary.thefreedictionary.com/activities+of+daily+living.

Feil-Seifer, D., Matarić, M. 2005. "Defining socially assistive robotics." In *Proceedings of the 2005 IEEE 9th International Conference on Rehabilitation Robotics.* Chicago: IEEE, 465–468.

Fong, T., Nourbakhsh, I., Dautenhahn, K. 2003. "A survey of socially interactive robots." *Robotics and Autonomous Systems* 42(3): 143–166.

Goodrich, M.A., Schultz, A.C. 2007. "Human–robot interaction: A survey." *Foundations and Trends in Human-Computer Interaction* 1(3): 203–275.

Gowen, J.W., Jonhson-Martin, N., Davis Goldman, B., Hussey, B. 1992. "Object play and exploration in children with and without disabilities: A longitudinal study." *American Journal of Mental Retardation* 97: 21–38.

Greif, M.L., Needham, A. 2011. "The development of human tool use early in life." In T. McCormack, C. Hoerl, S. Butterfill (eds.), *Tool Use and Causal Cognition*. Oxford, U.K. Oxford University Press, 51–68.

International Organization for Standardization (ISO). *ISO 13482 International Standard: Robots and Robotic Devices—Safety Requirements for Personal Care Robots*. Geneva: ISO, 2014.

Lamont, J., Favor, C. "Distributive justice." *Stanford Encyclopedia of Philosophy.* Accessed July 13, 2016. http://plato.stanford.edu/entries/justice-distributive/.

Louie, D.R., Eng, J.J., Lam, T., Spinal Cord Injury Research Evidence (SCIRE) Research Team. 2015. "Gait speed using powered robotic exoskeletons after spinal cord injury: A systematic review and correlational study." *Journal of Neuroengineering and Rehabilitation* 12: 82-015-0074-9.

Miller-Keane Encyclopedia and Dictionary of Medicine, Nursing, and Allied Health. 7th Edition. S.v. "mobility." Accessed July 13, 2016. http://medical-diction ary.thefreedictionary.com/mobility.

Perry, J., Beyer, S., Holm, S. 2009. "Assistive technology, telecare and people with intellectual disabilities: Ethical considerations." *Journal of Medical Ethics* 35: 81–86.

Piaget, J. *Play, Dreams and Imitation*. New York: Norton, 1951.

Public Law 108–364. "Assistive Technology Act of 1998, as amended." 2004.

Purtilo, R. 2005. *Ethical Dimensions in the Health Professions*. Philadelphia: Elsevier Saunders.

Skard, G., Bundy, A. 2008. "Test of playfulness." In L.D. Parham, L.S. Fazio (eds.), *Play in Occupational Therapy for Children*. St. Louis, MO: Mosby Elsevier, 71–93.

Stagnitti, K., Unsworth, C. 2004. "The test–retest reliability of the Child-Initiated Pretend Play Assessment." *American Journal of Occupational Therapy* 58: 93–99.

Stern, K. "Definition of cerebral palsy—What is CP?" Accessed July 13, 2016. http://www.cerebralpalsy.org/about-cerebral-palsy/definition.

Wikipedia. "Elderly care." Accessed July 13, 2016. https://en.wikipedia.org/wiki /Elderly_care.

World Health Organization. "Health topics: Rehabilitation." Accessed July 13, 2016. http://www.who.int/topics/rehabilitation/en/.

World Health Organization. "Media Centre—Ageing and health. Fact Sheet no. 404." Accessed July 13, 2016. http://www.who.int/mediacentre/factsheets /fs404/en/.

World Health Organization. "Towards a common language for functioning, disability and health." Accessed July 13, 2016. http://www.who.int/classifications/icf /icfbeginnersguide.pdf?ua=1.

Index

Page numbers followed by f, t, and b indicate figures, tables, and boxes, respectively.

367